Advanced Fitness Assessment and Exercise Prescription

Fourth Edition

Vivian H. Heyward, PhD
University of New Mexico

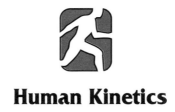

Human Kinetics

Library of Congress Cataloging-in-Publication Data

Heyward, Vivian H.
  Advanced fitness assessment and exercise prescription / Vivian H. Heyward.--4th ed.
    p. cm.
  Rev. ed. of Advanced fitness assessment & exercise prescription. 3rd ed. c1998.
  Includes bibliographical references and index.
  ISBN 0-7360-4016-1
    1. Physical fitness--Testing. 2. Exercise tests. 3. Health. I. Heyward, Vivian H.
  Advanced fitness assessment & exercise prescription. II. Title.

  GV436 .H48 2002
  613.7--dc21

                        2002017210

ISBN: 0-7360-4016-1

Acquisitions Editor: Michael S. Bahrke, PhD; **Developmental Editor:** Elaine H. Mustain; **Assistant Editor:** Maggie Schwarzentraub; **Copyeditor:** Joyce Sexton; **Proofreader:** Red Inc.; **Indexer:** Craig Brown; **Permission Manager:** Dalene Reeder; **Graphic Designer:** Fred Starbird; **Graphic Artist:** Denise Lowry; **Photo Manager:** Leslie A. Woodrum; **Cover Designer:** Keith Blomberg; **Photographer (interior):** Swede Scholer, figure 6.3a, Linda K. Gilkey, all other photos; **Art Manager:** Carl D. Johnson; **Illustrators:** Keith Blomberg, Craig Ronto, and Kristin Darling; **Printer:** Sheridan Books Inc.

Printed in the United States of America   10 9 8 7 6 5 4

Human Kinetics
Web site: www.HumanKinetics.com

United States: Human Kinetics, P.O. Box 5076, Champaign, IL 61825-5076
800-747-4457
e-mail: humank@hkusa.com

Canada: Human Kinetics, 475 Devonshire Road, Unit 100, Windsor, ON N8Y 2L5
800-465-7301 (in Canada only)
e-mail: orders@hkcanada.com

Europe: Human Kinetics, 107 Bradford Road, Stanningley
Leeds LS28 6AT, United Kingdom
+44 (0) 113 255 5665
e-mail: hk@hkeurope.com

Australia: Human Kinetics, 57A Price Avenue, Lower Mitcham, South Australia 5062
08 8277 1555
e-mail: liaw@hkaustralia.com

New Zealand: Human Kinetics, Division of Sports Distributors NZ Ltd.
P.O. Box 300 226 Albany, North Shore City, Auckland
0064 9 448 1207
e-mail: blairc@hknewz.com

*In memory of Mom—for her gentle encouragement
and unwavering confidence in me.*

Contents

Preface   xi
Acknowledgments   xiii

Chapter 9   Designing Weight Management and Body Composition Programs   **197**

Chapter 10   Assessing Flexibility and Designing Stretching Programs   **227**

Chapter 11   Assessing and Managing Stress   **251**

Appendix F   Flexibility Exercises, Low Back Care Exercises, and Stress Assessment   **335**

Preface

Expanding public awareness of the importance of physical activity for optimal health and longevity has led to an increased need for highly qualified exercise scientists to provide leadership for health promotion and physical fitness programs in the public and private sectors. Universities have responded to this need by offering graduate degree programs in exercise science.

The fourth edition of *Advanced Fitness Assessment and Exercise Prescription* is written for exercise science students enrolled in advanced professional courses that deal with physical fitness appraisal and exercise prescription. Previous editions of this text have been adopted for course use by numerous universities and colleges and have been translated into Greek, Italian, Korean, Portuguese, and Spanish.

A primary focus of this book is to provide exercise scientists with the knowledge and skills needed to assess physical fitness status of apparently healthy individuals rather than individuals who have suspected or documented cardiovascular disease. Since this text is not clinically oriented, it contains limited information regarding the etiology and pathophysiology of chronic diseases, screening tests for cardiopulmonary disorders, and the reading and interpretation of electrocardiograms. Exercise scientists working with clinical populations are encouraged to consult clinically oriented books that provide detailed information on exercise testing and exercise prescriptions for these populations.

Advanced Fitness Assessment and Exercise Prescription provides a well-balanced approach to the assessment of physical fitness, addressing five components of physical fitness:

- Cardiorespiratory endurance
- Muscular fitness
- Body weight and composition
- Flexibility
- Neuromuscular relaxation

This text is unique in its scope and in the depth of its content, organization, and approach to the subject matter. Introductory texts typically focus on field testing to evaluate physical fitness. Although this text includes some field tests, it emphasizes laboratory techniques for the assessment of physical fitness components. The scope and depth of information presented make this text an important resource for practitioners—especially those employed in health and fitness settings. The text is organized such that for each physical fitness component, a chapter on assessment is followed by a chapter on exercise prescription. At the end of each chapter, you will find sources for purchasing equipment and supplies related to fitness assessment, as well as an extensive list of references. This text uses a multidisciplinary approach that synthesizes concepts, principles, and theories based on research in exercise physiology, kinesiology, measurement, psychology, and nutrition. The net result is a direct and clear-cut approach to physical fitness assessment and exercise prescription.

Although the scope and organization of the fourth edition of this text are not substantially different from the previous edition, new pedagogical tools are included. In addition to *Key Questions* at the beginning of each chapter, you will find *Key Points, Review Questions,* and a list of *Key Terms* at the end of each chapter. Each of the key terms is defined in the *Glossary of Terms* in the back of the book. The glossary also includes definitions of medical terms used in the text. These pedagogical tools were added to help you identify the key terms and concepts and to test your knowledge and understanding of the material in each chapter.

Throughout the text, the latest information from the sixth edition of *ACSM's Guidelines for Exercise Testing and Prescription* (2000) is incorporated. Updated addresses, phone numbers, and Web sites are included for equipment manufacturers and suppliers, as well as Web sites for professional organizations. The following list highlights some of the changes for each chapter.

Chapter 1

- Recent global and U.S. statistics on the prevalence of various types of chronic diseases
- New research substantiating the link between physical activity and disease risk
- Information about the dose-response relationship between physical activity and health benefits

Chapter 2

- Modified criteria for evaluating risk factors for coronary heart disease
- New terminology for classifying blood pressure and lipoproteins
- ACSM's risk stratification criteria
- ACSM's guidelines for medical examination and exercise testing
- CSEP's physical activity readiness medical examination questionnaire (PARmed-X)
- CSEP's Fantastic Lifestyle assessment form

Chapter 3

- Psychological theories related to lifestyle behavior change
- Application of these theories to exercise program adherence

Chapter 4

- Latest 2000 ACSM guidelines for exercise testing
- Revised ACSM equations for metabolic calculations

Chapter 5

- The concept of $\dot{V}O_2$ reserve as a method for prescribing intensity of aerobic exercise
- Elliptical training and Treading™ as alternative modes of aerobic exercise

Chapter 6

- Updated strength and muscle endurance norms for adult women
- Revised ACSM protocols and norms for push-up and partial curl-up tests

Chapter 7

- ACSM's latest guidelines for designing resistance training programs for older adults
- Guidelines for developing periodized resistance training programs
- Information about creatine supplementation and strength gains

Chapter 8

- Air displacement plethysmography as a possible reference method for body composition assessment
- New body fat standards for adults, children, and physically active individuals
- Validity of upper-body and lower-body bioimpedance analyzers marketed for home use

Chapter 9

- Latest recommendations for vitamin and mineral intakes, including RDAs, adequate intakes, and tolerable upper limits for some nutrients
- Use of resistance training exercise in weight management programs

Chapter 10

- Sit-and-reach tests suitable for assessing the flexibility of middle-aged and older adults
- New approach (i.e., lumbar stabilization) and exercises for low back care exercise programs

Chapter 11

- Updated information about the effectiveness of exercise in reducing psychological stress and regulating mood behaviors
- Use of tai chi in stress management programs

Appendixes

- Revised MET values for conditioning exercises, sports, and recreational activities
- An extensive list of dynamic resistance training exercises with variations for specific muscle groups
- Additional exercises for low back care programs

These updates and additions are intended to provide a more comprehensive and advanced approach to physical fitness appraisal and exercise prescription. I hope you will use the information in this book to improve your knowledge, skill, and professional competence as an exercise scientist.

Acknowledgments

In the evolution of this text, many people have made unique and important contributions. In addition to all of the individuals acknowledged in previous editions of this book, I would like to recognize and thank the following individuals for their contributions to the fourth edition: Virginia Wilmerding and Toryanno Gordon, for serving as models for photographs; Linda Gilkey, for taking the photographs; Cristine Mermier, for assisting with equipment setup for photographs and computer graphics; Len Kravitz, Donna Lockner, and Virginia Wilmerding, for sharing their ideas and expertise; and Elaine Mustain and Maggie Schwarzentraub, for carefully and meticulously editing this book.

I am indebted to each of you and truly appreciate your effort, cooperation, and support.

chapter 1

Physical Activity, Health, and Chronic Disease

KEY QUESTIONS

- Are adults in the United States getting enough physical activity?
- What diseases are associated with a sedentary lifestyle, and what are the major risk factors for these diseases?
- What are the benefits of regular physical activity in terms of disease prevention, and how does physical activity improve health?

- How much physical activity is needed for improved health benefits?
- What kinds of physical activities are suitable for typical people, and how often should they exercise?

Although physical activity plays an important role in the prevention of chronic diseases, an alarming percentage of adults in the United States report no physical activity during leisure time. One of the national health objectives for the year 2010 is to increase to 30% the proportion of people aged 18 years and older who regularly (preferably daily) engage in moderate physical activity at least 30 min per day (U.S. Department of Health and Human Services 2000). According to recent data from major national health surveys, we are far from reaching this objective. At present, only 15% of U.S. adults get the recommended amount of physical activity (U.S. Department of Health and Human Services 2000). Approximately 23% to 29% of the American population report no physical activity during leisure time (Crespo, Ainsworth, Keteyian, Heath, and Smit 1999; Pratt, Macera, and Blanton 1999), and over 60% of all American adults do not get the amount of physical activity recommended for health benefits (Pratt et al. 1999; U.S. Department of Health and Human Services 2000). Also, women report less leisure-time physical activity than men, and the leisure-time physical activity of older adults is less than that of younger adults (Crespo et al. 1999). Thus, as an exercise specialist, you have the challenging role of educating and motivating your clients to incorporate physical activity and regular exercise as an integral part of their lifestyles.

This chapter deals with physical activity trends, risk factors associated with chronic diseases, the role of regular physical activity in disease prevention and health, and physical activity recommendations for improved health. For definitions of terminology used in this chapter, see "Glossary of Terms," page 349.

PHYSICAL ACTIVITY, HEALTH, AND DISEASE: AN OVERVIEW

Our increased reliance on technology has substantially lessened work-related physical activity, as well as the energy expenditure required for activities of daily living like cleaning the house, washing clothes and dishes, mowing the lawn, and traveling to work. What would have once required an hour of physical work now can be accomplished in just a few seconds by pushing a button or setting a dial. As a result, more time is available to pursue leisure activities. The unfortunate fact, however, is that many individuals do not engage in physical activity during their leisure time.

Although the human body is designed for movement and strenuous physical activity, exercise is not a part of the average lifestyle. One cannot expect the human body to function optimally and to remain healthy for extended periods if the body is abused or is not used as intended. Physical inactivity has led to a rise in chronic diseases. Individuals who do not exercise regularly are at greater risk than others of developing chronic diseases such as coronary heart disease, hypertension, hypercholesterolemia, cancer, obesity, and musculoskeletal disorders (see figure 1.1).

For years, exercise scientists and health/fitness professionals have maintained that regular physical activity is the best defense against the development of many diseases, disorders, and illnesses. The importance of regular physical activity in preventing disease and premature death and in maintaining a high quality of life received recognition as a national health objective in the first U.S. Surgeon General's report on physical activity and health (U.S. Department of Health and Human Services 1996). This report identifies physical inactivity as a serious nationwide health problem, provides clear-cut scientific evidence linking physical activity to numerous health benefits, presents demographic data describing physical activity patterns and trends in the U.S. population, and makes physical activity recommendations for improved health (see page 3).

The need for a national initiative to address physical inactivity in Canada was also evident at this time. In 1998, Health Canada and the Canadian Society for Exercise Physiology (CSEP) released *Canada's Physical Activity Guide to Healthy Active Living* (Health Canada and CSEP 1998). They recommended that people accumulate 60 min of light-effort physical activity every day such as walking or gardening, or 20-30 min of vigorous-effort activities such as jogging or aerobics. This recommendation follows the current literature that supports increasing the volume of low-intensity physical activity for improved health benefits (Bouchard 2001).

People can realize modest health benefits by exercising enough to burn as few as 150 kilocalo-

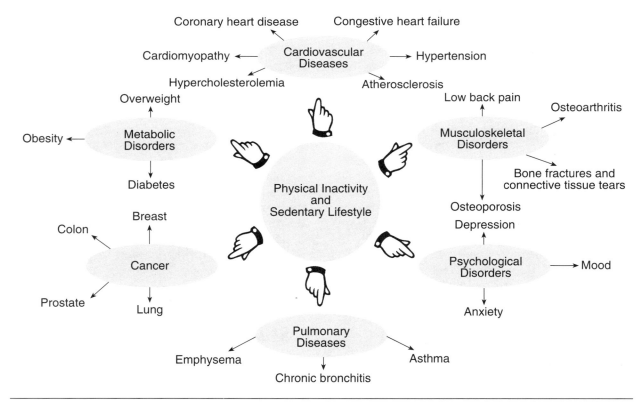

Figure 1.1 Role of physical activity and exercise in disease prevention and rehabilitation.

Health Benefits of Physical Activity

Reduced Risk of

- dying prematurely,
- dying prematurely from heart disease,
- developing diabetes,
- developing high blood pressure, and
- developing colon cancer.

Reduction of

- blood pressure in people who already have high blood pressure, and
- feelings of depression and anxiety.

Help in

- controlling body weight;
- building and maintaining healthy bones, muscles, and joints;
- developing strength and agility in older adults, so they are better able to move about without falling; and
- creating a sense of psychological well-being.

Data from U.S. Department of Health and Human Services, 1996, *Physical Activity and Health: A Report of the Surgeon General–At a Glance* (Washington, DC: Author).

ries (kcal) a day, or 1000 kcal a week. This amount of physical activity decreases the risk of coronary heart disease by 50% and the risk of hypertension, diabetes, and colon cancer by 30% (U.S. Department of Health and Human Services 1996). The Centers for Disease Control and the American College of Sports Medicine (ACSM) have endorsed the following statement regarding physical activity (Pate et al. 1995):

Every U.S. adult should accumulate 30 min or more of moderate-intensity physical activity on most, preferably all, days of the week.

Participation in moderate-intensity physical activity on a daily basis produces significant health benefits, even if fitness levels do not increase. Improvements in health benefits depend on the volume (i.e., combination of frequency, intensity, and duration) of physical activity. This is known as the **dose-response relationship** (Bouchard 2001; Canadian Society of Exercise Physiology 1998; Kesaniemi et al. 2001). Figure 1.2 illustrates the general dose-response relationship between the volume of physical activity participation and selected health benefits that do not require a minimal threshold intensity for improvement like muscular strength and aerobic fitness. The volume of

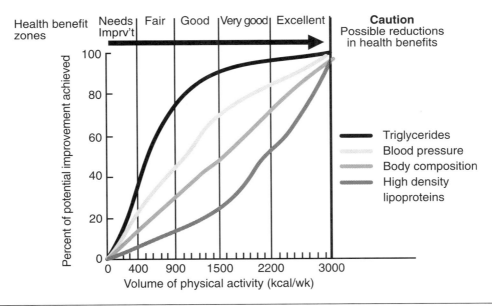

Figure 1.2 Dose-response relationship and health benefit zones for health benefits and volume of physical activity participation.
"Source: *The Canadian Physical Activity, Fitness and Lifestyle Appraisal: CSEP's Plan for Healthy Active Living,* 2nd edition © 1998. Reprinted with permission from the Canadian Society for Exercise Physiology." Schematic developed by N. Gledhill and V. Jamnik of York University.

Examples of Moderate Amounts of Physical Activity

This list contains examples of moderate amounts of physical activity. (A moderate amount of physical activity is roughly that which uses approximately 150 kcal energy per day, or 1000 kcal per week. Some activities can be performed at various intensities; the suggested durations correspond to expected intensity of effort.) More vigorous activities, such as stair climbing and running, require less time (15 min). On the other hand, less vigorous activities, like washing and waxing the car, require more time (45 to 60 min).

Less Vigorous, More Time

- Washing and waxing a car for 45-60 min
- Washing windows or floors for 45-60 min
- Playing volleyball for 45 min
- Playing touch football for 30-45 min
- Gardening for 30-45 min
- Wheeling self in wheelchair for 30-40 min
- Walking 1.75 miles (2.8 km) in 35 min (20 min/mile pace)
- Basketball (shooting baskets) for 30 min
- Bicycling 5 miles (8.0 km) for 30 min
- Dancing fast (social) for 30 min
- Pushing a stroller 1.5 miles (2.4 km) for 30 min
- Raking leaves for 30 min
- Walking 2 miles (3.2 km) in 30 min (15 min/mile pace)
- Water aerobics for 30 min

More Vigorous, Less Time

- Swimming laps for 20 min
- Playing wheelchair basketball for 20 min
- Playing basketball for 15-20 min
- Bicycling 4 miles (6.4 km) in 15 min
- Jumping rope for 15 min
- Running 1.5 miles (2.4 km) in 15 min (10 min/mile pace)
- Shoveling snow for 15 min
- Stair walking for 15 min

Data from U.S. Dept. of Health and Human Services, 1996, *Physical Activity and Health: A Report of the Surgeon General—At a Glance* (Washington, D.C.: Author), 2.

physical activity participation needed for the same degree of relative improvement (%) varies among health benefit indicators. For example, to improve triglycerides from 0 to 40% requires 500 kcal/wk of physical activity compared to 1800 kcal/wk for the same relative improvement (0 to 40%) in high density lipoprotein (see figure 1.2). Likewise, different volumes of physical activity are needed to move between health benefit zones. To move from the "needs improvement" to the "fair" zone, for example, requires an increase in physical activity

participation of 500 kcal/wk, compared to the 800 kcal/wk increase that is needed to move between the "very good" and "excellent" health benefit zones for all health benefit indicators (Canadian Society for Exercise Physiology 1998). Additionally, you should note that too much physical activity (see Caution zone in figure 1.2), defined as engaging in 5 hr of structured high-intensity activity per week, may be associated with negative health consequences or overuse injuries. For extensive reviews of literature dealing with the dose-response relationship between physical activity and health, see *Medicine & Science in Sports & Exercise* (June 2001, Supplement).

The Exercise and Physical Activity Pyramid, developed by the Metropolitan Life Insurance Company (1995), illustrates a balanced plan of physical activity and exercise to promote a healthy lifestyle and improve physical fitness (see figure 1.3). You should encourage your clients to engage in physical activities around the home and workplace on a daily basis to establish a foundation (base of pyramid) for an active lifestyle. They should perform aerobic activities and flexibility exercises at least three to five days a week; they should do weight-resistance exercises and recreational, sport activities, two to three days a week (middle levels of pyramid). High-intensity training and competitive sports (top of pyramid) require a solid fitness base to prevent injury, and they offer relatively few health benefits. Most people should engage in these activities only sparingly. Later chapters contain more detailed information regarding exercise prescriptions for cardiovascular and musculoskeletal fitness.

CARDIOVASCULAR DISEASE

Cardiovascular diseases cause 12 million deaths worldwide each year. According to the World Health Organization (1993), **cardiovascular disease** (CVD) is the principal cause of mortality in Europe, accounting for more than 50% of all deaths in those older than 65 years. For developing countries in Africa, western Asia, and Southeast Asia, 15% to 20% of the annual deaths are due to CVDs

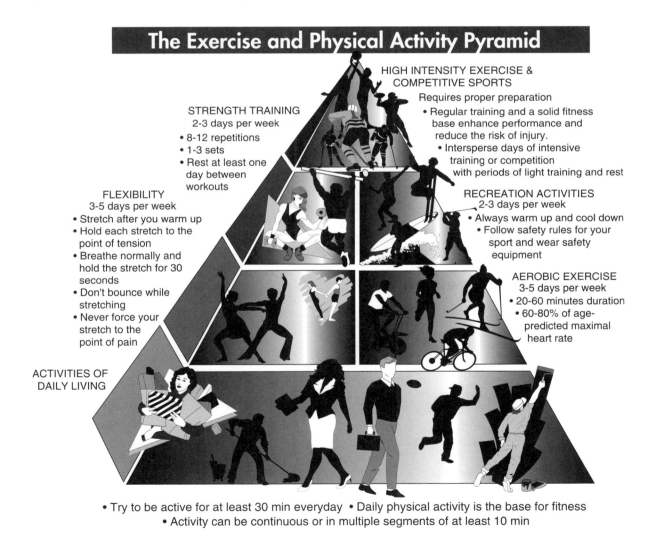

Figure 1.3 The Exercise and Physical Activity Pyramid.
Adapted from "Exercise and Activity Pyramid" Metropolitan Life Insurance Company, 1995.

(American Heart Association 2001). The proportion of deaths from CVD ranges from 25% for Latin American countries to 45% for eastern Mediterranean countries (American Heart Association 2001). In 1997, diseases of the heart and blood vessels claimed the lives of 953,110 people in the United States alone. It is estimated that CVD is responsible for more than 41% of all deaths in the United States and that one-sixth of all people dying from CVD are younger than 65 years. More than 59 million, or one out of every five, Americans has some form of CVD: hypertension (50.0 million), coronary heart disease (12.2 million), congestive heart failure (4.6 million), or stroke (4.4 million) (American Heart Association 1999). Other forms of CVD afflict millions more (see figure 1.1). Although the death rate from CVD in the United States declined almost 19% between 1987 and 1997, the actual number of deaths declined only 2.1% during this same 10-year period (American Heart Association 1999).

Coronary heart disease accounts for more deaths annually than any other disease, with more than 466,000 people dying each year from CHD (American Heart Association 1999). Among American adults 20 years of age or older, the estimated age-adjusted prevalence of CHD is higher for black and Hispanic men and women compared to white men and women (American Heart Association 1999).

Coronary heart disease (CHD) is caused by a lack of blood supply to the heart muscle (**myocardial ischemia**), resulting from a progressive, degenerative disorder known as atherosclerosis. **Atherosclerosis** involves a buildup and deposition of fat and fibrous plaques in the intima, or inner lining, of the coronary arteries. These plaques restrict the blood flow to the myocardium and may produce **angina pectoris,** which is a temporary sensation of tightening and heavy pressure in the chest and shoulder region. A **myocardial infarction,** or heart attack, can occur if a blood clot, or thrombus, obstructs the coronary blood flow. In this case, blood flow through the coronary arteries is usually reduced by over 80%. The portion of the myocardium supplied by the obstructed artery dies and is replaced eventually with scar tissue.

Coronary Heart Disease Risk Factors

Epidemiological research indicates that many factors are associated with the risk of CHD. The greater the number and severity of risk factors, the greater the probability of CHD. The positive risk factors for CHD are

- family history,
- hypercholesterolemia,
- hypertension,
- current cigarette smoking,
- impaired fasting glucose (diabetes mellitus),
- obesity, and
- physical inactivity.

An increased level of high-density lipoprotein cholesterol or **HDL-cholesterol** (HDL-C >60 mg·dl^{-1}) in the blood decreases CHD risk. If the HDL-C is high, you should subtract one risk factor from the sum of the positive factors when assessing your client's CHD risk.

Physical Activity and Coronary Heart Disease

As an exercise scientist, you must educate your clients about the benefits of physical activity and regular exercise for preventing CHD. Physically active people have lower incidences of myocardial infarction and mortality from CHD and tend to develop CHD at a later age compared to their sedentary counterparts (Berlin and Colditz 1990). Individuals who exercise regularly reduce their relative risk of developing CHD by a factor of 1.5 to 2.4 (American Heart Association 1999; Powell, Thompson, Casperson, and Kendrick 1987). Physical activity exerts its effect independently of smoking, hypertension, hypercholesterolemia, obesity, diabetes, or family history of CHD (Bouchard, Shephard, and Stephens 1994). Also, people who engage in regular exercise as part of their rehabilitation following a myocardial infarction have improved survival rates compared to individuals who do not exercise during their rehabilitation (O'Connor et al. 1989).

HYPERTENSION

Hypertension is a chronic, persistent elevation of blood pressure, affecting an estimated one out of every four (25%) adults in the United States. About 50 million Americans age 6 years and older have high blood pressure (American Heart Association 1999). In the United States, a higher percentage of men have hypertension compared to women, up to age 55 years. The percentage of women having high blood pressure progressively increases from

55 to 74 years of age. After age 74 years the percentage of women with hypertension is greater than that of men. Also, blacks have a greater prevalence of hypertension compared to Asians, American Indians, Hispanics, and whites in the United States (American Heart Association 1999).

In comparison, the prevalence of hypertension is estimated to be between 10% and 17% for eastern Mediterranean adults, 4% to 12% for adults in India, 8% for people age 15 years and older in China, and 5% to 12% for adults living in rural and urban areas of Africa (American Heart Association 2001). Table 1.1 summarizes the risk factors associated with developing hypertension.

Epidemiological studies indicate an inverse relationship between blood pressure and physical activity level in women and men (Fagard 1999; Hagberg 1990; Paffenbarger, Jung, Leung, and Hyde 1991; Reaven, Barrett-Connor, and Edelstein 1991). Regular aerobic exercise performed at an intensity of 40% to 60% of maximal oxygen uptake, three to five times a week, reduces systolic and diastolic blood pressure by about 10 mm Hg in hypertensive individuals; moreover, these reductions in blood pressure in overweight and normal-weight individuals are independent of weight loss (Fagard 1999; Hagberg 1990). The blood pressure-lowering effect depends on the initial blood pressure, but not on the body mass index or age of the individual (Fagard 1999). On average, the training-induced change in blood pressure is less for normotensive compared to hypertensive individuals (Fagard 1999; Fagard and Tipton 1994).

While endurance training substantially lowers blood pressure in men and women with mild to moderate hypertension (Hagberg 1990), resistance training also lowers blood pressure in both adolescents and adults with hypertension (Hagberg et al. 1984; Harris and Holly 1987). However, Cononie et al. (1991) reported no change in blood pressure in response to six months of resistance training among older men and women (70 to 79 years) with normal or slightly elevated blood pressures.

HYPERCHOLESTEROLEMIA AND DYSLIPIDEMIA

Hypercholesterolemia, an elevation of **total cholesterol** (TC) in the blood, is associated with increased risk of developing CVD. Hypercholesterolemia is also referred to as **hyperlipidemia,** which is an increase in blood lipid levels;

dyslipidemia refers to an abnormal blood lipid profile. About 40 million Americans have TC levels of 240 mg·dl^{-1} or higher, and a greater percentage of women ($\geq$50 years of age) have TC $\geq$200 mg·dl^{-1} compared to men (American Heart Association 1999). Compared to those in Western countries, the average TC levels are uniformly lower for adults in China, Japan, and Indonesia (average TC = 190 to 207 mg·dl^{-1}) (American Heart Association 2001). Risk factors for hypercholesterolemia are identified in table 1.1.

LDLs, HDLs, and TC

In the body, cholesterol and triglycerides are transported as lipoproteins (a lipid bound to a protein carrier). Low-density lipoproteins (LDL) are larger molecules that precipitate in the plasma and are actively transported into the vascular walls. Excess **LDL-cholesterol** (LDL-C) stimulates the formation of plaque on the intima of the coronary arteries. This reduces the cross-sectional area and obstructs blood flow through the coronary arteries, eventually producing a myocardial infarction.

The high-density lipoproteins (HDL) are smaller molecules that remain suspended in the plasma and are metabolized by the liver. High-density lipoprotein serves a protective function by picking up excess cholesterol from the arterial walls and removing it from the body. High-density lipoprotein cholesterol values exceeding 45 mg·dl^{-1} are desirable, and women tend to have higher HDL-C compared to men.

Individuals with low HDL-C and/or high TC levels (dyslipidemia) have a greater risk than others of heart attack. However, those with lower HDL-C ($\leq$37 mg·dl^{-1} for men; $\leq$47 mg·dl^{-1} for women) are at higher risk regardless of their TC level. This emphasizes the importance of screening for both TC and HDL-C levels in adults.

Physical Activity and Lipid Profiles

Regular physical activity, especially habitual aerobic exercise, positively affects lipid metabolism and lipid profiles (Despres and Lamarche 1994; Durstine and Thompson 2000). Cross-sectional comparisons of lipid profiles in physically active and sedentary women and men suggest that physical fitness is inversely related to TC and TC/HDL-C ratio (Despres and Lamarche 1994; Shoenhair and Wells 1995). Regular endurance exercise also lowers plasma triglycerides and sometimes reduces

Table 1.1 Summary of Factors Associated With Disease Risk

Factor	CHD	Diabetes	Hypertension	Hypercholesterolemia	Low back pain	Obesity	Osteoporosis
Age	↑	↑	↑	↑	↑	↑	↑
Gender	M>F[a]	F>M	F>M[b]	F>M[b]	F=M	F>M	F>M[b]
Race	B, H>A, AI, W	AI, B, H>A, W	B>A, AI, H, W	B, H, W>A, AI		AI, B, H, W>A	A, W>AI, B
Family history	↑	↑	↑	↑		↑	↑
SES	↓	↓	↓	↓	↓	↓	
Alcohol use			↑	↑			↑
Smoking	↑		↑	↑			↑
Nutrition							
Na intake			↑				
Ca intake							↓
Fat/cholesterol intake	↑		↑	↑		↑	
CHO intake		↑					
Intake>expenditure			↑			↑	
Physical activity	↓	↓		↓	↓	↓	↓
Exercise amenorrhea							↑
Flexibility					↓		
Muscular strength					↓		↓
Skeletal frame size							↓
Other diseases							
Anorexia nervosa							↑
Diabetes	↑						
Hypertension	↑						
Hypercholesterolemia	↑						
Obesity and overweight	↑	↑	↑	↑	↑		

↑ = Direct relationship; as factor increases, risk increases.

↓ = Indirect relationship; as factor increases, risk decreases.

[a] Males (M) at higher risk than females (F) up to age 55 years.

[b] Menopausal females at higher risk than males.

CHD = coronary heart disease; CHO = carbohydrate; A = Asian; AI = American Indian; B = black; H = Hispanic; W = white; Na = sodium; Ca = calcium; SES = socioeconomic status (reflects income and education levels).

TC and LDL-C levels in individuals with initially high levels (Bouchard and Despres 1995). High-density lipoprotein cholesterol increases in response to endurance training. This response appears to be related to the exercise training dose (interaction of intensity, frequency, and duration of each exercise session and the length of the training period) and is less dramatic in women than in men (Kokkinos and Fernhall 1999; Lokey and Tran 1989). Spate-Douglas and Keyser (1999) reported, however, that a moderate-intensity (60% of heart rate reserve) walking program is as effective as a high-intensity (80% of heart rate reserve) program for improving the HDL profile of women as long as the total training volume (2 miles, three times weekly) is similar.

Some researchers have reported improved lipid profiles following resistance training (Fripp and Hodgson 1987; Goldberg, Elliot, Schultz, and Kloster 1984; Hurley et al. 1988); but because of methodological flaws in the study design, such as the lack of a control group or the use of only one baseline blood sample, more research is needed to justify this claim. In fact, some researchers have observed that resistance training does not improve lipid profiles in men at risk for CHD (Kokkinos et al. 1991) and in obese women (Manning et al. 1991) when body weight remains stable. These findings suggest that changes in lipid profiles in response to resistance training may be partially dependent on weight loss and the total training volume (Manning et al. 1991).

CIGARETTE SMOKING

The World Health Organization estimates that about one-third of the global adult population smokes. Worldwide, nearly 47% of men and 7% of women smoke; however, in developed countries, 42% of men and 24% of women smoke. By 2020, it is estimated that tobacco will become the leading cause of death and disability worldwide, killing more than 10 million people per year (American Heart Association 2001). Since 1965, smoking has declined 42% among U.S. adults. Yet 430,700 Americans died of smoking-related diseases between 1990 and 1994, and every day approximately 3000 young people in the United States become smokers (American Heart Association 1999).

Cigarette smoking has been linked to lung cancer, pulmonary disorders, and CHD. Smokers have more than twice the risk of heart attack compared to nonsmokers. The nicotine contained in cigarette smoke produces an increase in heart rate and blood pressure and inhibits the anticlotting mechanisms of the blood.

When individuals stop smoking, the risk of CHD declines rapidly, regardless of how long or how much they have smoked. One year after quitting, the risk of CHD decreases by 50%; and within 15 years, the relative risk of dying from CHD is almost the same as that of a longtime nonsmoker (American Heart Association 1999).

DIABETES MELLITUS

Globally, the prevalence of diabetes in adults was 4% in 1995. By the year 2025, it is projected to be 5.4%, with the number of individuals having diabetes expected to increase 42% in developed countries and 170% in developing countries (American Heart Association 2001). Approximately 13 million people in the United States have diabetes; 90% to 95% of these individuals have **type 2**, or **non-insulin-dependent diabetes mellitus** (NIDDM) (Kriska, Blair, and Pereira 1994). **Type 1**, or **insulin-dependent diabetes mellitus**, usually occurs before the age of 30 years but can develop at any age. Compared to the value for white adults in the United States, the age-adjusted prevalence of diabetes and impaired fasting blood glucose levels of black, Hispanic, and Native American adults is higher (American Heart Association 1999). Risk factors for developing diabetes are presented in table 1.1.

Research suggests that regular physical activity reduces one's risk of developing NIDDM through its association with weight loss and the effects of exercise on insulin sensitivity and glucose tolerance (Kelley and Goodpaster 1999; Kriska, Blair, and Pereira 1994; Wells 1996). Manson et al. (1991) reported that women who engaged in vigorous exercise at least once a week have a reduced risk of diabetes. The reduction in diabetes risk, however, appears to be associated with the frequency of exercise. The risk of diabetes decreased 23%, 38%, and 42%, respectively, in male physicians who exercised vigorously one time, two to four times, and five or more times a week (Manson et al. 1992). Vigorous exercise was defined as physical activity of sufficient duration to produce sweating. Specific guidelines for prescribing exercise programs for people who have type 1 and type 2 diabetes are available elsewhere (ACSM and American Diabetes Association 1997; Campaigne 1998; Colberg 2001).

OBESITY AND OVERWEIGHT

In clinical guidelines established by the Obesity Education Initiative Task Force of the National Institutes of Health and National Heart, Lung, and Blood Institute (1998), **overweight** and **obesity** are classified using the **body mass index** (BMI = weight [kg]/height [m]^2). Individuals with a BMI between 25 and 29.9 kg/m^2 are classified as overweight; those with a BMI of 30 kg/m^2 or more are classified as obese.

Using these definitions, the overall average prevalence of obesity in adults for the year 2000 is 8.2% of the global population. The prevalence of obesity progressively increases with the degree of development of countries, as seen in the data for undeveloped countries (1.8%), developing countries (4.8%), countries in transition (17.1%), and developed countries (20.4%) (World Health Organization 2001). In Indonesia, 12.5% of adults ages 25 to 64 years are obese; a 1988-1989 survey indicated that 35.2% of men and 39.5% of women in Beijing, China, were overweight; and in Africa, 8.3% of the men and 36% to 50% of the women are obese (American Heart Association 2001). The prevalence of overweight and obesity in the United States since 1960 has increased across all age, gender, and ethnic groups (Flegal, Carroll, Kuczmarski, and Johnson 1998). According to the most recent National Health and Nutrition Examination Survey (NHANES III), almost 55% of American adults are overweight or obese (Flegal et al. 1998; Grundy et al. 1999). Also, the prevalence of overweight among young Americans is on the rise; more than one in every five children and adolescents is overweight (Troiano, Flegal, Kuczmarski, Campbell, and Johnson 1995). Table 1.1 summarizes factors associated with increased risk of obesity.

Excess body weight and fatness pose a threat to both the quality and quantity of one's life. Obese individuals have a shorter life expectancy and greater risks of CHD, hypercholesterolemia, hypertension, diabetes mellitus, certain cancers, and osteoarthritis (Grundy et al. 1999; National Institutes of Health and National Heart, Lung, and Blood Institute 1998). Although obesity is strongly associated with CHD risk factors such as hypertension, glucose intolerance, and hyperlipidemia, the contribution of obesity to CHD appears to be independent of the influence of obesity on these risk factors (Grundy et al. 1999). For a comprehensive report and roundtable discussion of the role of physical activity in the prevention and treat-

ment of obesity and its comorbidities, see the November 1999 supplement to *Medicine & Science in Sports & Exercise*.

Obesity may be caused by genetic and environmental factors. Although studies suggest that genetic factors contribute to some of the variation in body fatness, there has been no substantial change in the genotype of the American population over the past 30 years (Hill and Melanson 1999). Thus, the major cause of obesity in the United States may be linked to our environment. Over the past three decades, we have been exposed to an environment that strongly promotes not only the consumption of high-fat, energy-dense foods (increased energy intake), but also reliance on technology that discourages physical activity and reduces the amount of physical activity (decreased energy expenditure) needed for daily living (e.g., use of energy-saving devices and prepared foods) (Hill and Melanson 1999). As an exercise specialist, you play an important role in combating this major health problem by encouraging a physically active lifestyle and by planning exercise programs and scientifically sound diets for your clients, in consultation with trained nutrition professionals. Restricting caloric intake and increasing caloric expenditure through physical activity and exercise are effective ways of reducing body weight and fatness while normalizing blood pressure and blood lipid profiles.

MUSCULOSKELETAL DISEASES AND DISORDERS

Diseases and disorders of the musculoskeletal system, such as osteoporosis, osteoarthritis, bone fractures, connective tissue tears, and low back syndrome, are also related to physical inactivity and a sedentary lifestyle. A loss of bone mass due to aging and physical inactivity is characteristic of **osteoporosis** (see table 1.1 for osteoporosis risk factors). Approximately 25 million Americans have this disease, which increases the risk of bone fracture in both women and men. Adequate calcium intake and regular physical activity help counteract age-related bone loss. Epidemiological studies show that the incidence of bone fractures is lower in women with higher levels of physical activity. Although no data have demonstrated that exercise alone can prevent the loss of bone mass during and after menopause, ACSM (1995) recommends increasing physical activity, especially weight-bearing exercise and resistance training exercise, to counteract bone loss due to aging. However, exercise should not be substituted for hormone replacement therapy at menopause.

Low back pain afflicts millions of people each year. More than 80% of all low back problems are produced by muscular weakness or imbalance caused by a lack of physical activity (see table 1.1). If the muscles are not strong enough to support the vertebral column in proper alignment, poor posture results and low back pain develops. Excessive weight, poor flexibility, and improper lifting habits also contribute to low back problems. While gender and age are associated with low back pain and are not modifiable risks, lifestyle behaviors such as smoking, physical inactivity, flexibility, and muscular strength and endurance are all modifiable risk factors that are related to low back pain (Albert, Bonneau, Stevenson, and Gledhill 2001).

Because the origin of low back problems is often functional rather than structural, in many cases the problem can be corrected through an exercise program designed to develop strength and flexibility in the appropriate muscle groups. Also, people who remain physically active throughout life retain more bone, ligament, and tendon strength and are, therefore, less prone to bone fractures and connective tissue tears (Pollock, Wilmore, and Fox 1978).

KEY POINTS

- More than 60% of all Americans do not get the recommended amount of physical activity needed for health benefits.

- Major chronic diseases associated with a lack of physical activity are CVDs, diabetes, obesity, and musculoskeletal disorders.

- Cardiovascular diseases are responsible for 41% of all deaths in the United States and more than 50% of all deaths in Europeans older than 65 years.

- The positive risk factors for CHD are the following: family history, hypercholesterolemia, hypertension, cigarette smoking, glucose intolerance, obesity, and physical inactivity.

- The prevalence of obesity is on the rise, especially in developed countries; in the United States, one of every two adults and more than one of every five adolescents and children are overweight or obese.

- Osteoporosis and low back syndrome are musculoskeletal disorders afflicting millions of people each year.

- To benefit health and prevent disease, every adult should accumulate 30 min or more of moderate-intensity physical activity on most, preferably all, days of the week.

KEY TERMS

Learn the definition for each of the following key terms. Definitions of key terms can be found in "Glossary of Terms," page 349.

angina pectoris	LDL-cholesterol
atherosclerosis	low back pain
body mass index	myocardial infarction
cardiovascular disease	myocardial ischemia
coronary heart disease	obesity
dyslipidemia	osteoporosis
HDL-cholesterol	overweight
hypercholesterolemia	total cholesterol
hyperlipidemia	type 1 diabetes
hypertension	type 2 diabetes

REVIEW QUESTIONS

In addition to being able to define each of the key terms just listed, test your knowledge and understanding of the material by answering the following review questions.

1. What percentage of the American population does not get the recommended amount of physical activity for health benefits?

2. What is the recommended minimum amount of daily physical activity for health?

3. Give examples of moderate physical activity.

4. What percentage of Americans have some form of CVD?

5. Name four types of CVD. Which is most prevalent?

6. Explain the etiology of CHD.

7. Identify the positive and negative risk factors for CHD.

8. Explain how regular physical activity impacts each of the CHD risk factors, as well as overall CHD risk.

9. Define obesity and overweight relative to BMI.

10. What types of exercise are effective for counteracting bone loss due to aging?

11. Explain the relationship between physical inactivity and low back pain.

REFERENCES

Albert, W.J., Bonneau, J., Stevenson, J.M., and Gledhill, N. 2001. Back fitness and back health assessment considerations for the Canadian Physical Activity, Fitness and Lifestyle Appraisal. *Canadian Journal of Applied Physiology* 26: 291–317.

American College of Sports Medicine (ACSM). 1995. ACSM position stand on osteoporosis and exercise. *Medicine & Science in Sports & Exercise* 27: i–vii.

American College of Sports Medicine and American Diabetes Association. 1997. Joint position statement on diabetes mellitus and exercise. *Medicine & Science in Sports & Exercise* 27(12): i–vi.

American Heart Association. 1999. *2000 heart and stroke statistical update*. Dallas: Author.

American Heart Association. 2001. *International cardiovascular disease statistics*. Dallas: Author.

Berlin, J.A., and Colditz, G.A. 1990. A meta-analysis of physical activity in the prevention of coronary heart disease. *American Journal of Epidemiology* 132: 612–628.

Bouchard, C. 2001. Physical activity and health: Introduction to the dose-response symposium. *Medicine & Science in Sports & Exercise* 33 (Suppl.): S347–S350.

Bouchard, C., and Despres, J.P. 1995. Physical activity and health: Atherosclerotic, metabolic, and hypertensive diseases. *Research Quarterly for Exercise and Sport* 66: 268–275.

Bouchard, C., Shephard, R.J., and Stephens, T., eds. 1994. *Physical activity, fitness, and health. International proceedings and conference statement*. Champaign, IL: Human Kinetics.

Campaigne, B.N. 1998. Exercise and diabetes mellitus. In *ACSM's resource manual for guidelines for exercise testing and prescription*, ed. J.L. Roitman (3rd ed.), 267–274. Philadelphia: Lippincott Williams & Wilkins.

Colberg, S.R. 2001. *The diabetic athlete*. Champaign, IL: Human Kinetics.

Cononie, C.C., Graves, J.E., Pollock, M.L., Phillips, M.I., Sumners, C., and Hagberg, J.M. 1991. Effect of exercise training on blood pressure in 70- to 79-yr-old men and women. *Medicine & Science in Sports & Exercise* 23: 505–511.

Crespo, C.J., Ainsworth, B.E., Keteyian, S.J., Heath, G.W., and Smit, E. 1999. Prevalence of physical inactivity and its relation to social class in U.S. adults: Results from the Third National Health and Nutrition Examination Survey, 1988-1994. *Medicine & Science in Sports & Exercise* 31: 1821–1827.

Despres, J.P., and Lamarche, B. 1994. Low-intensity endurance training, plasma lipoproteins, and the risk of coronary heart disease. *Journal of Internal Medicine* 236: 7–22.

Durstine, J.L., and Thompson, R.W. 2000. Exercise modulates blood lipids and lipoproteins: A great explanation and exercise plan. *ACSM's Health & Fitness Journal* 4(4): 7–12.

Fagard, R.H. 1999. Physical activity in the prevention and treatment of hypertension in the obese. *Medicine & Science in Sports & Exercise* 31(Suppl.): S624–S630.

Fagard, R.H., and Tipton, C.M. 1994. Physical activity, fitness, and hypertension. In *Physical activity, fitness, and health*, ed. C. Bouchard, R.J. Shephard, and T. Stephens, 633–655. Champaign, IL: Human Kinetics.

Flegal, K.M., Carroll, M.D., Kuczmarski, R.J., and Johnson, C.L. 1998. Overweight and obesity in the United States: Prevalence and trends, 1960-1994. *International Journal of Obesity* 22: 39–47.

Fripp, R.R., and Hodgson, J.L. 1987. Effect of resistance training on plasma lipid and lipoprotein levels in male adolescents. *Journal of Pediatrics* 111: 926–931.

Goldberg, L.S., Elliot, L., Schultz, W., and Kloster, F.E. 1984. Changes in lipid and lipoprotein levels after weight training. *Journal of the American Medical Association* 252: 504–506.

Grundy, S., Blackburn, G., Higgins, M., Lauer, R., Perri, M., and Ryan, D. 1999. Roundtable consensus statement: Physical activity in the prevention and treatment of obesity and its comorbidities: Evidence report of independent panel to assess the role of physical activity in the treatment of obesity and its comorbidities. *Medicine & Science in Sports & Exercise* 31(Suppl.): S502–S508.

Hagberg, J.M. 1990. Exercise, fitness, and hypertension. In *Exercise, fitness, and health: A consensus of current knowledge*, ed. C. Bouchard, R.J. Shephard, T. Stephens, J.R. Sutton, and B.D. McPherson, 455–466. Champaign, IL: Human Kinetics.

Hagberg, J.M., Ehsani, A.A., Goldring, D., Hernandez, A., Sinacore, D.R., and Holloszy, J.O. 1984. Effect of weight training on blood pressure and hemodynamics in hypertensive adolescents. *Journal of Pediatrics* 104: 147–151.

Harris, K.A., and Holly, R.G. 1987. Physiological response to circuit weight training in borderline, hypertensive subjects. *Medicine & Science in Sports & Exercise* 19: 246–252.

Health Canada and Canadian Society for Exercise Physiology. 1998. *Canada's physical activity guide to healthy active living.* Ontario: Health Canada.

Hill, J.O., and Melanson, E.L. 1999. Overview of the determinants of overweight and obesity: Current evidence and research issues. *Medicine & Science in Sports & Exercise* 31(Suppl.): S515–S521.

Hurley, B.F., Hagberg, J.M., Goldberg, A.P., Seals, D.R., Ehsani, A.A., Brennan, R.E., and Holloszy, J.O. 1988. Resistive training can reduce coronary risk factors without altering VO_2max or percent body fat. *Medicine & Science in Sports & Exercise* 20: 150–154.

Kelley, D.E., and Goodpaster, B.H. 1999. Effects of physical activity on insulin action and glucose tolerance in obesity. *Medicine & Science in Sports & Exercise* 31(Suppl.): S619–S623.

Kesaniemi, Y.K., Danforth, E., Jensen, M.D., Kopelman, P.G., Lefebvre, P., and Reeder, B.A. 2001.

Dose-response issues concerning physical activity and health: An evidenced-based symposium. *Medicine & Science in Sports & Exercise* 33 (Suppl.): S351–S358.

Kokkinos, P.F., and Fernhall, B. 1999. Physical activity and high density lipoprotein cholesterol levels: What is the relationship? *Sports Medicine* 28: 307–314.

Kokkinos, P.F., Hurley, B.F., Smutok, M.A., Farmer, C., Reece, C., Shulman, R., Charabogos, C., Patterson, J., Will, S., Devane-Bell, J., and Goldberg, A.P. 1991. Strength training does not improve lipoprotein–lipid profiles in men at risk for CHD. *Medicine & Science in Sports & Exercise* 23: 1134–1139.

Kriska, A.M., Blair, S.N., and Pereira, M.A. 1994. The potential role of physical activity in the prevention of non-insulin dependent diabetes mellitus: The epidemiological evidence. In *Exercise and Sport Sciences Reviews,* ed. J.O. Holloszy, 22: 121–143.

Lokey, E.A., and Tran, Z.V. 1989. Effects of exercise training on serum lipids and lipoprotein concentrations in women: A meta-analysis. *International Journal of Sports Medicine* 10: 424–429.

Manning, J.M., Dooly-Manning, C.R., White, K., Kampa, I., Silas, S., Kessellhaut, M., and Ruoff, M. 1991. Effects of a resistance training program on lipoprotein-lipid levels in obese women. *Medicine & Science in Sports & Exercise* 23: 1222–1226.

Manson, J.E., Nathan, D.M., Krolewski, A.S., Stampfer, M.J., Willett, W.C., and Hennekens, C.H. 1992. A prospective study of exercise and incidence of diabetes among US male physicians. *Journal of the American Medical Association* 268: 63–67.

Manson, J.E., Rimm, E.B., Stampfer, M.J., Rosner, B., Hennekens, C.H., Speizer, F.E., Colditz, G.A., Willett, W.C., and Krolewski, A.S. 1991. Physical activity incidence of non-insulin dependent diabetes mellitus in women. *Lancet* 338: 774–778.

Metropolitan Life Insurance Company. 1995. *Your guide to physical activity for health.* New York: Author.

National Institutes of Health and National Heart, Lung, and Blood Institute. 1998. Clinical guidelines on the identification, evaluation, and treatment of overweight and obesity in adults: The evidence report. *Obesity Research* 6 (Suppl. 2): S51–S209.

O'Connor, G., Buring, J., Yusuf, S., Goldhaber, S., Olmstead, E., Paffenbarger, R., and Hennekens, C. 1989. An overview of randomized trials of rehabilitation with exercise after myocardial infarction. *Circulation* 80: 234–244.

Paffenbarger, R.S., Jung, D.L., Leung, R.W., and Hyde, R.T. 1991. Physical activity and hypertension: An epidemiological view. *Annuals of Medicine* 23: 319–327.

Pate, R.R., Pratt, M., Blair, S.N., Haskell, W.L., Macera, C.A., Bouchard, C., Buchner, D., Ettinger, W., Heath, G.W., and King, A.C. 1995. Physical activity and public health: A recommendation from the Centers for Disease Control and Prevention and the American College of Sports Medicine. *Journal of the American Medical Association* 273: 402–407.

Pollock, M.L., Wilmore, J.H., and Fox, S.M. III. 1978. *Health and fitness through physical activity.* New York: Wiley.

Powell, K.E., Thompson, P.D., Casperson, C.J., and Kendrick, J.S. 1987. Physical activity and the incidence of coronary heart disease. *Annual Review of Public Health* 8: 253–287.

Pratt, M., Macera, C., and Blanton, C. 1999. Levels of physical activity and inactivity in children and adults in the United States: Current evidence and research issues. *Medicine & Science in Sports & Exercise* 31(Suppl.): S526–S533.

Reaven, P.D., Barrett-Connor, E., and Edelstein, S. 1991. Relation between leisure-time physical activity and blood pressure in older women. *Circulation* 83: 559–565.

Shoenhair, C.L., and Wells, C.L. 1995. Women, physical activity, and coronary heart disease: A review. *Medicine, Exercise, Nutrition and Health* 4: 200–206.

Spate-Douglas, T., and Keyser, R.E. 1999. Exercise intensity: Its effect on the high-density lipoprotein profile. *Archives of Physical Medicine and Rehabilitation* 80: 691–695.

Troiano, R.P., Flegal, K.M., Kuczmarski, R.J., Campbell, S.M., and Johnson, C.L. 1995. Overweight prevalence and trends for children and adolescents. The National Health and Nutrition Examination Surveys 1963-1991. *Archives of Pediatric and Adolescent Medicine* 149: 1085–1091.

U.S. Department of Health and Human Services. 1996. *Physical activity and health: A report of the Surgeon General—At a glance.* Atlanta: U.S. Department of Health and Human Services, Centers for Disease Control and Prevention, National Center for Chronic Disease Prevention and Health Promotion.

U.S. Department of Health and Human Services. 2000. *Healthy people 2010—conference edition: Physical activity and fitness (22).* Atlanta: Author.

Wells, C.L. 1996. Physical activity and women's health. In *Physical Activity and Fitness Research Digest,* ed. C. Corbin and B. Pangrazi, series 2, no. 5, 1–6. Washington, D.C.: President's Council on Physical Fitness and Sports.

World Health Organization. 1993. World health statistics. *World Health Statistics Quarterly* 46(2).

World Health Organization. 2001. Global database on obesity and body mass index (BMI) in adults. **Http://www.who.int/nut/db_bmi**.

chapter 2

Preliminary Health Screening and Risk Classification

- What are the major components of the health evaluation, and how is this information used to screen clients for exercise testing and participation?

- What factors do I need to focus on when evaluating the client's medical history and lifestyle characteristics?

- How is the client's disease risk classified?

- Do all clients need a physical examination and medical clearance from their physician before taking an exercise test?

- What are the standards for classifying blood cholesterol levels?

- How is blood pressure measured and evaluated? Are automated blood pressure devices accurate?

- How is heart rate measured? Are heart rate monitors accurate?

- What is an ECG, and does every client need to have one before taking an exercise test?

- Is it safe to give a graded exercise test to all clients? When does a physician need to be present?

- What are the major components of the lifestyle evaluation, and how can this information be used?

- What are the purposes of informed consent?

Before assessing your client's physical fitness profile, it is important to classify the person's health status and lifestyle. You will use information from the initial health and lifestyle evaluations to screen clients for physical fitness testing. You also will use this information to identify individuals with medical contraindications to exercise, with disease symptoms and risk factors, and with special needs.

This chapter discusses the components of a comprehensive health evaluation, including a coronary risk factor profile, medical history questionnaire, lifestyle evaluation, and informed consent. It also presents guidelines and standards for classifying blood cholesterol levels, blood pressures, and disease risk, along with techniques and procedures for measuring heart rate and blood pressure at rest and during exercise and for conducting a resting 12-lead electrocardiogram (ECG).

PRELIMINARY HEALTH EVALUATION

The purpose of the health evaluation is to detect the presence of disease and to assess the initial disease risk classification of your clients. The components of a comprehensive health evaluation are listed in table 2.1. To evaluate the client's health status, information from questionnaires and data from clinical tests are analyzed. Minimally, for pretest health screening of clients for exercise testing and exercise program participation, you should

- administer the Physical Activity Readiness Questionnaire (PAR-Q),
- identify signs and symptoms of diseases,
- analyze the coronary risk profile, and
- classify the disease risk of your clients.

Step-by-step procedures for conducting a comprehensive health evaluation are listed in "Procedures for Comprehensive Pretest Health Screening."

Questionnaires and Screening Forms

Appendix A provides questionnaires and forms that may be used to obtain information for the preliminary health screening and evaluation of your clients. The client should complete the PAR-Q, medical history questionnaire, lifestyle evaluation, and the informed consent form. You will interview your client to gather information about signs/symptoms of disease, analyze your client's coronary heart disease (CHD) risk factors, and determine your client's disease risk classification. For some clients, it may be necessary to obtain a medical clearance from their physician.

Physical Activity Readiness Questionnaire

The PAR-Q has seven questions designed to identify individuals who need medical clearance from their physicians before taking any physical fitness tests or starting an exercise program (see appen-

---

Table 2.1 Components of a Comprehensive Health Evaluation

Component	Purpose
Questionnaires/screening forms	
PAR-Q	To determine client's readiness for physical activity
Signs and symptoms of disease and medical clearance	To identify individuals in need of medical referral and to obtain evidence of physician approval for exercise testing and participation
Coronary risk factor analysis	To determine the number of CHD risk factors for client
Disease risk classification	To categorize clients as low, moderate, or high risk
Medical history	To review client's past and present personal and family health history, focusing on conditions requiring medical referral and clearance
Lifestyle evaluation	To obtain information about the client's living habits
Informed consent	To explain the purpose, risks, and benefits of physical fitness tests and to obtain your client's consent for participation in these tests
Clinical tests	
Physical examination	To detect signs and symptoms of disease
Blood chemistry profile	To determine if client has normal values for selected blood values; values of blood cholesterol are used in the coronary risk factor analysis
Blood pressure assessment	To determine if client is hypertensive; these values are also used in the coronary risk factor analysis
12-lead ECG	To evaluate cardiac function and detect cardiac abnormalities that are contraindications to exercise
Graded exercise test	To assess functional aerobic capacity and to detect cardiac abnormalities due to exercise stress
Additional laboratory tests (e.g., angiograms, echocardiograms, pulmonary tests)	To provide a more in-depth assessment of clients' health status, particularly those with known disease

Procedures for Comprehensive Pretest Health Screening

Here are step-by-step procedures you should follow when conducting a comprehensive health evaluation:

- Greet the client.
- Explain the purpose of the health evaluation and lifestyle evaluation.
- Obtain the client's informed consent for health screening.
- Administer and evaluate the PAR-Q; refer client to physician if needed.
- Administer and evaluate client's medical history, focusing on signs, symptoms, and diseases; refer client to physician if needed.
- Evaluate client's lifestyle profile.
- Evaluate and classify the client's cholesterol and lipoprotein levels if test results are available.
- Measure and classify the client's resting blood pressure and heart rate.
- Assess the client's coronary risk factors.
- Classify the client's disease risk.
- Evaluate the client's blood chemistry profile if test results are available.

If so requested by the client's physician, you may do the following:

- Explain the purpose of and answer any questions about the 12-lead resting ECG and graded exercise test (GXT).
- Obtain the client's informed consent for these tests.
- Prepare the client and administer the 12-lead resting ECG.
- Have a physician interpret the results of the 12-lead resting ECG.
- Use the client's disease risk classification to determine whether a maximal or submaximal GXT should be administered and whether a physician needs to be present during this test.
- Assess the client's resting blood pressure and heart rate.
- Administer the GXT.
- Assess and classify the client's functional aerobic capacity.

dix A.1, "Physical Activity Readiness Questionnaire (Par-Q)," p. 260). If clients answer "yes" to any of these questions, they should be referred to their physicians to obtain medical clearance before engaging in physical activity. Also, older clients and those who are not used to regular physical activity should always check with their physicians before starting an exercise program.

Medical History Questionnaire

You should require your clients to complete a comprehensive medical history questionnaire that includes questions concerning personal and family health history (appendix A.2, "Medical History Questionnaire," p. 262). Use the questionnaire to

- examine the client's record of personal illnesses, surgeries, and hospitalizations (section A);

- assess previous medical diagnoses and signs and symptoms of disease that have occurred within the past year or are currently present (section B); and
- analyze your client's family history of diabetes, heart disease, stroke, and hypertension (section C).

Also, when reviewing the medical history, you should carefully focus on conditions that require medical referral (see "Absolute and Relative Contraindications to Exercise Testing" [Gibbons et al. 1997] on p. 18). If any of these conditions are noted, refer your client to a physician for a physical examination and medical clearance prior to exercise testing or starting an exercise program. It is also important to note the types of medication being used by the client. Drugs such as digitalis, beta-blockers, bronchodilators, vasodilators, diuretics, and insulin may alter the individual's heart rate, blood pressure, ECG, and exercise capacity. If your client reports a medical condition or drug that is unfamiliar to you, be certain to consult medical references or a physician to obtain more information before conducting any exercise tests or allowing the client to participate in an exercise program.

Signs and Symptoms of Disease and Medical Clearance

As part of the pretest health screening, you should ask your clients if they have any of the conditions or symptoms listed in appendix A.3, "Checklist for Signs and Symptoms of Disease," page 264. Feel free to reproduce and use this checklist.

Clients with any of the signs or symptoms on the checklist should be referred to their physicians to obtain a signed medical clearance prior to any exercise testing or participation. The Physical Activity Readiness Medical Examination (PARmed-X) was designed for this purpose (Canadian Society for Exercise Physiology 1998). The PARmed-X is a physical activity-specific checklist (see Appendix A.4, page 266) that is used by the physician to assess and convey medical clearance for physical activity participation or to make a referral to a medically-supervised exercise program for individuals who answered "yes" to one of the questions in the Physical Activity Readiness Questionnaire (PAR-Q). For definitions of specific medical terms used, refer to "Glossary of Terms" (p. 349).

Absolute and Relative Contraindications to Exercise Testing[a]

Absolute Contraindications

1. Recent significant change in resting ECG suggesting significant ischemia, recent myocardial infarction (within 2 days), or other acute cardiac events
2. Unstable angina
3. Uncontrolled cardiac arrhythmias causing symptoms or hemodynamic compromise
4. Uncontrolled symptomatic heart failure
5. Acute infections
6. Severe symptomatic aortic stenosis
7. Suspected or known dissecting aneurysm
8. Acute myocarditis or pericarditis
9. Acute pulmonary embolus or pulmonary infarction

Relative Contraindications

1. Left main coronary stenosis
2. Moderate stenotic valvular heart disease
3. Known electrolyte abnormalities (hypokalemia, hypomagnesemia)
4. Severe arterial hypertension; resting diastolic BP > 110 mm Hg and/or resting systolic BP > 200 mm Hg
5. Tachyarrhythmias or bradyarrhythmias
6. Hypertrophic cardiomyopathy and other forms of outflow tract obstruction
7. High-degree atrioventricular block
8. Ventricular aneurysm
9. Uncontrolled metabolic disease (e.g., diabetes, thyrotoxicosis, or myxedema)
10. Chronic infectious disease (e.g., mononucleosis, hepatitis, AIDS)
11. Neuromuscular, musculoskeletal, or rheumatoid disorders that are exacerbated by exercise

[a]For definitions of specific medical terms, refer to "Glossary of Terms," page 349.

From Gibbons, R.J. et al. 1997. ACC/AHA Guidelines for exercise testing. A report of the American College of Cardiology/American Heart Association Task Force on Practice Guidelines (Committee on Exercise Testing). *Journal of the American College of Cardiology* 30: 260-311.

Coronary Risk Factor Analysis

To assess your client's coronary risk profile, evaluate each item in table 2.2 carefully. Guidelines for classification of blood pressure and blood cholesterol levels in adults are presented in tables 2.3 and 2.4, respectively. If your client's high-density lipoprotein cholesterol (HDL-C) equals or exceeds 60 mg·dl⁻¹, subtract 1 from the total number of positive risk factors. This information is especially helpful in classifying the individual for exercise testing and in designing safe exercise programs.

Table 2.2 Coronary Heart Disease Risk Factors

Positive risk factors	Criteria
1. Family history	Myocardial infarction, coronary revascularization, or sudden death before 55 years of age for father or other first-degree male relative (brother or son); or before 65 years of age in mother or other first-degree female relative (sister or daughter)
2. Cigarette smoking	Current cigarette smoking, or smoking cessation within previous 6 months
3. Hypertension	Systolic BP $\geq$140 mm Hg *or* diastolic BP $\geq$90 mm Hg measured on two separate occasions, or individual taking antihypertensive medication
4. Hypercholesterolemia	TC $\geq$200 mg·dl⁻¹, HDL-C <40 mg·dl⁻¹, LDL-C $\geq$130 mg·dl⁻¹ or on lipid-lowering medication
5. Impaired fasting glucose	Fasting blood glucose $\geq$110 mg·dl⁻¹, measured on two separate occasions
6. Obesity	Body mass index $\geq$30 kg/m² or waist circumference >100 cm (40 in.) for men and >88 cm (35 in.) for women
7. Physical inactivity	Not participating in regular exercise program or not meeting the minimum physical activity recommendations from the U.S. Surgeon General's report (accumulating 30 min or more of moderate physical activity on most days of the week)

Negative risk factor[a]

High HDL-C	Serum HDL-C $\geq$60 mg·dl⁻¹

[a]If HDL-C is high, subtract one risk factor from the sum of the positive risk factors.

Data from National Cholesterol Education Program Committee (2001) "Executive Summary of the Third Report of the National Cholesterol Education Program (NCEP) Expert Panel on Detection, Evaluation, and Treatment of High Blood Cholesterol in Adults (Adult Treatment Panel III)," *Journal of the American Medical Association* 285(19): 2486–2497.

Table 2.3 Classification of Blood Pressure for Adults, 18 Years or Older[a]

Systolic BP (mm Hg)[b]	Category	Diastolic BP (mm Hg)
<120	Optimal[c]	<80
120-129	Normal	80-84
130-139	High normal	85-89
140-159	Stage I hypertension	90-99
160-179	Stage II hypertension	100-109
$\geq$180	Stage III hypertension	$\geq$110

[a]For individuals not taking antihypertensive medication and not acutely ill. Based on average of two or more readings on two or more occasions.

[b]When systolic and diastolic pressures fall into different categories, use the higher category for classification.

[c]Optimal BP with respect to cardiovascular risk is below 120/80 mm Hg. However, unusually low readings should be evaluated for clinical significance.

Data from *The Sixth Report of the Joint National Committee on Detection, Evaluation, and Treatment of High Blood Pressure,* by the Joint National Committee, Public Health Service, National Institutes of Health, National Heart, Lung, and Blood Institute, NIH Publication No. 98-4080, November 1997.

Table 2.4 Classification of TC, LDL-C, Triglycerides, and HDL-C (mg·dl⁻¹)

Total cholesterol, low-density lipoprotein cholesterol, and triglycerides

Classification	TC	LDL-C	Triglycerides
Optimal or desirable	<200	<100	<150
Near or above optimal	———	100-129	———
Borderline high	200-239	130-159	150-199
High	≥240	160-189	200-499
Very high	———	≥190	≥500

High-density lipoprotein cholesterol

Classification	HDL-C
Low	<40
Normal	40-59
High	≥60

Data from National Cholesterol Education Program Committee (2001) "Executive Summary of the Third Report of the National Cholesterol Education Program (NCEP) Expert Panel on Detection, Evaluation, and Treatment of High Blood Cholesterol in Adults (Adult Treatment Panel III)," *Journal of the American Medical Association* 285(19): 2487.

Disease Risk Classification

On the basis of the results from the coronary risk factor analysis, you should classify individuals as low, moderate, or high risk (see table 2.5). According to ACSM (2000), the **low CHD risk** category comprises younger men (<45 years) and women (<55 years) who are asymptomatic with no more than one major risk factor (see table 2.2). Older individuals (men ≥45 years and women ≥55 years) or those having two or more risk factors are classified as **moderate CHD risk** The **high CHD risk** category includes individuals who have one or more signs/symptoms of cardiovascular and pulmonary disease or individuals with known cardiovascular, pulmonary, or metabolic disease (see p. 264).

Lifestyle Evaluation

Planning a well-rounded physical fitness program for an individual requires that you obtain information concerning the client's living habits. The lifestyle assessment provides useful information regarding the individual's risk factor profile. Factors such as smoking, lack of physical activity, and

Table 2.5 ACSM Risk Stratification (ACSM 2000)

Classification	Criteria
Low risk	Younger individuals (men <45 years and women <55 years) who are asymptomatic and have no more than one risk factor (see table 2.2)
Moderate risk	Older individuals (men ≥45 years and women ≥55 years) *or* individuals of any age having two or more risk factors (see table 2.2)
High risk	Individuals with one or more signs/symptoms of cardiovascular and/or pulmonary disease *or* individuals with known cardiovascular, pulmonary, or metabolic disease (see appendix A.3)

Reprinted, by permission, from American College of Sports Medicine, 2000, *ACSM's guidelines for exercise testing and prescription*, 6th ed. (Philadelphia: Lippincott Williams & Wilkins).

diets high in saturated fats or cholesterol increase the risk of CHD, atherosclerosis, and hypertension. These factors can be used to pinpoint patterns and habits that need modification and to assess the likelihood of the client's adherence to the exercise program. You can obtain a lifestyle profile for your clients by using either the Lifestyle Evaluation form or the Fantastic Lifestyle Checklist provided in appendix A.5, page 270. The Fantastic Lifestyle Checklist is a self-administered tool designed to assess your client's present health-related behaviors (Canadian Society for Exercise Physiology 1998).

Informed Consent

Before conducting any physical fitness tests or exercise programs, you should see that each participant signs the informed consent (see appendix A.6, "Informed Consent," p. 274). This form explains the purpose and nature of each physical fitness test, any inherent risks in the testing, and the expected benefits of these tests. The informed consent also assures your clients that test results will remain confidential and that their participation is strictly voluntary. If your client is underage (<18 years), a parent or guardian must also sign the informed consent. All consent forms should be approved by your institutional review board or legal counsel.

Clinical Tests

For a comprehensive health screening, you will need to evaluate information and data obtained from the physician's medical examination and clinical tests. Clinical tests provide data about your client's blood chemistry, blood pressure, cardiopulmonary function, and aerobic capacity.

Physical Examination

Your prospective exercise program participants should obtain a physical examination and a signed medical clearance from a physician (appendix A.4, "PARmed-X," p. 267), especially if they are

- men ≥ 45 years of age or women ≥ 55 years of age;
- individuals of any age with two or more major risk factors;
- individuals of any age with one or more signs/symptoms of cardiovascular or pulmonary disease; or
- individuals of any age with known cardiovascular, pulmonary, or metabolic disease.

The physical examination should focus on signs and symptoms of CHD and should include an evaluation of body weight; orthopedic problems; edema; acute illness; pulse rate; cardiac regularity; blood pressure (supine, sitting, and standing); and auscultation of the heart, lungs, and major arteries. The physical examination and medical history may reveal signs or symptoms of CHD particularly if accompanied by shortness of breath, chest pains, leg cramps, or high blood pressure. Clients with these symptoms must obtain a signed medical clearance (p. 267) from their physician prior to exercise testing or exercise participation.

Blood Chemistry Profile

Information obtained from a complete blood analysis is used to assess your client's overall health status and readiness for exercise. Table 2.6 provides normal values for selected blood variables. If any of these values fall outside of the normal range, refer your clients to their physician. Pay special attention to your client's fasting blood glucose and blood lipid values.

Table 2.6 Normal Values for Selected Blood Variables	
Variable	Ideal or typical values
Triglycerides	<150 mg·dl^{-1}
Total cholesterol	<200 mg·dl^{-1}
LDL-cholesterol	<100 mg·dl^{-1}
HDL-cholesterol	≥40 mg·dl^{-1}
TC/HDL-cholesterol	<3.5
Blood glucose	60-109 mg·dl^{-1}
Hemoglobin	13.5-17.5 g·dl^{-1} (men) 11.5-15.5 g·dl^{-1} (women)
Hematocrit	40-52% (men) 36-48% (women)
Potassium	3.5-5.5 meq·dl^{-1}
Blood urea nitrogen	4-24 mg·dl^{-1}
Creatinine	0.3-1.4 mg·dl^{-1}
Iron	40-190 μg·dl^{-1} (men) 35-180 μg·dl^{-1} (women)
Calcium	8.5-10.5 mg·dl^{-1}

Recently, the National Cholesterol Education Program (NCEP) (2001) updated its guidelines for classifying lipoprotein levels and major risk factors that modify low-density lipoprotein cholesterol (LDL-C) treatment goals. For adults aged 20 years or older, NCEP (2001) recommends that a fasting lipoprotein profile (i.e., total cholesterol, LDL-C, HDL-C, and triglycerides) be obtained every five years. To classify your client's lipoprotein values, use the NCEP (2001) guidelines (see table 2.4). For nonfasting lipoprotein tests, only the total cholesterol (TC) and HDL-C values can be evaluated. If your client's TC is borderline high (200 to 239 mg·dl^{-1}) or high (≥240 mg·dl^{-1}), and the HDL-C level is less than 40 mg·dl^{-1}, a follow-up fasting lipoprotein test will be needed to assess LDL-C. Refer clients to their physicians for an extensive clinical evaluation and dietary therapy if they have high (160 to 189 mg·dl^{-1}) or very high (>190 mg·dl^{-1}) LDL-C values. Treatment goals for lowering LDL-C depend on the number of major risk factors (exclusive of LDL-C) that the client has. To determine your client's risk category, focus on the following risk factors in table 2.2: cigarette smoking, hypertension, low HDL-C, family history of premature CHD, and age (men ≥45 years; women ≥55 years). Table 2.7 is NCEP's listing of three risk categories that modify LDL-C treatment goals. The NCEP (2001) dietary therapy guidelines for individuals with high LDL-C are included in table 9.2, page 204.

Table 2.7 Three Risk Categories That Modify LDL-C Goals (NCEP 2001)

Risk category	LDL-C goal (mg·dl^{-1})
CHD and CHD risk equivalents[a]	<100
Multiple (2+) risk factors[b]	<130
0-1 risk factor	<160

[a]CHD risk equivalents include diabetes and atherosclerotic disease (i.e., peripheral arterial disease, abdominal aortic aneurysm, and symptomatic carotid artery disease).

[b]Risk factors include cigarette smoking, hypertension, low high-density lipoprotein cholesterol, family history of premature CHD, and age.

In addition to TC and lipoproteins, you can evaluate your client's triglyceride value and the ratio of TC to HDL-C. Clients with triglyceride levels of ≥150 mg·dl^{-1} or TC/HDL-C ratios >5.0 are at higher risk for CHD.

Resting Blood Pressure

Blood pressure (BP) is a measure of the force or pressure exerted by the blood on the arteries. The highest pressure (systolic blood pressure) reflects the pressure in the arteries during systole of the heart when myocardial contraction forces a large volume of blood into the arteries. Following systole, the arteries recoil and the pressure drops during diastole, or the filling phase of the heart. Diastolic blood pressure is the lowest pressure in the artery during the cardiac cycle. Resting systolic BP usually varies between 110 and 140 mm Hg, and diastolic BP between 60 and 80 mm Hg. Usually a person is not classified as hypertensive unless the BP remains elevated (systolic BP ≥ 140 or diastolic BP ≥ 90 mm Hg) on two occasions (see table 2.3). The difference between the systolic and diastolic BPs is known as the pulse pressure. The pulse pressure creates a pulse wave that can be palpated at various sites in the body to determine pulse rate and to estimate BP.

Effective treatments are available for hypertension. A sodium-restricted diet, weight reduction, restricted alcohol intake, and exercise may help to lower BP in people with mild hypertension. Many antihypertensive drugs are also available to lower BP:

- Diuretics rid the body of excess salt and fluids.
- Beta-blockers reduce heart rate and cardiac output.
- Sympathetic nerve inhibitors prevent constriction of arterioles.
- Vasodilators induce relaxation in smooth muscles of arterial walls.
- Angiotensin-converting enzyme inhibitors disrupt the body's production of angiotensin, which constricts arterioles.

Additional Clinical Tests

For individuals with known or suspected CHD, additional tests may be indicated. These may include a resting 12-lead ECG, angiogram, echocardiogram, and a physician-monitored graded exercise test. A chest X-ray, comprehensive blood chemistry, and complete blood count should also be obtained (ACSM 2000). For clients with known pulmonary disease, ACSM (2000) recommends a chest X-ray, pulmonary function tests, and specialized pulmonary tests (e.g., blood gas analysis).

Graded Exercise Test

Coronary heart disease often is not detectable from the resting ECG, and abnormalities may not appear until the individual engages in relatively strenuous exercise. The client's physician may recommend administration of a graded exercise test as part of the health evaluation to assess functional aerobic capacity of some individuals. Graded exercise tests should be administered only by trained, professionally certified personnel such as exercise scientists, physicians, and nurses.

Use the client's risk classification to determine whether the test should be a maximal or a submaximal exercise test and whether a physician needs to be present during the exercise testing (table 2.8). Also, you need to be familiar with medical conditions that are absolute and relative contraindications to exercise testing in an out-of-hospital setting (see "Absolute and Relative Contraindications to Exercise Testing" on p. 18). For definitions of the medical terms included in this list, refer to "Glossary of Terms" (p. 349).

The ACSM (2000) recommends a maximal exercise test for older men (≥45 years) and women (≥55 years) before they begin a vigorous (>6 METs [metabolic equivalents] or >60% of functional aerobic capacity) exercise program (see table 2.8). These maximal exercise tests should be administered with physician supervision. For low-risk individuals of any age, submaximal exercise testing can be done without physician supervision. However, the exercise tests should be conducted by exercise specialists, who are preferably ACSM certified and who are well trained and experienced in monitoring exercise tests and handling emergencies (ACSM 2000). The results from these tests provide a basis for prescription of exercise for healthy and coronary-prone individuals, as well as for cardiopulmonary patients.

TESTING PROCEDURES FOR BLOOD PRESSURE, HEART RATE, AND ELECTROCARDIOGRAM

One of your major responsibilities as an exercise scientist is to become proficient at measuring BP, heart rate, and ECGs during rest and exercise. During a graded exercise test, you will expected to be able to obtain accurate and precise measurements of BP and heart rate while the client is exercising. Because of their importance and complexity, this section is devoted to a thorough discussion of these procedures.

Measuring Blood Pressure

The "gold standard" for assessing BPs is the direct measurement of intra-arterial BP. This method

Table 2.8   ACSM Guidelines for Medical Examination and Exercise Testing Prior to Participation Based on Risk Classification (ACSM 2000)[a]

	Low risk	Moderate risk	High risk
Medical exam and exercise test recommended prior to participation in:			
Moderate exercise (3-6 METs or 40-60% $\dot{V}O_2$max)	0[b]	0	+[c]
Vigorous exercise (>6 METs or >60% $\dot{V}O_2$max)	0	+	+
Physician supervision recommended during exercise test[d]			
Submaximal test	0	0	+
Maximal test	0	+	+

[a]For definitions of low, moderate, or high risk, see table 2.5.

[b]0 indicates that item is not necessary; however, it should not be viewed as inappropriate.

[c]+ indicates that item is recommended.

[d]For physician supervision—this suggests that a physician be in close proximity and readily available should there be an emergent need.

is invasive and requires catheterization. Therefore, in clinical or field settings, BP is typically measured indirectly by auscultation using a stethoscope and **sphygmomanometer** consisting of a BP cuff and either an aneroid or mercury column manometer. A mercury column manometer is preferable because aneroid manometers lose their calibration more easily. Technicians with hearing impairments can use an anesthesiologist's stethoscope, which magnifies sound. Alternatively, you can measure resting BP using automated BP devices. The validity of these devices for measuring exercise BPs has not yet been firmly established (Griffin, Robergs, and Heyward 1997). Also, you can obtain an estimate of resting BP using the palpation method described later. These estimates are generally within 10 mm Hg of auscultatory values (Reeves 1995).

To check the accuracy of an aneroid manometer against a mercury unit, follow the procedures suggested by Reeves (1995):

- Disconnect the bulbs of both cuffs and reconnect the bulb and dial of the aneroid unit to the cuff of the mercury unit.
- Roll the cuff up loosely, securing the Velcro strips, and hold the cuff steadily while gradually inflating it.
- Hold the dial of the aneroid manometer close to the mercury column, and compare the two

readings at several pressures throughout the range of the measurement scale (e.g., 40 to 220 mm Hg). If the aneroid and mercury manometer pressures differ by more than 2 to 3 mm Hg, send the aneroid manometer to the manufacturer for adjustment.

Blood Pressure Measurement Techniques

Measure resting BP in the supine and exercise (sitting or standing) positions prior to testing (ACSM 2000). The client should be wearing a short-sleeved or sleeveless garment and should be seated in a quiet room. Take BP measurements rapidly, and completely deflate the cuff for at least 30 sec between consecutive readings. For more accurate results, obtain two or three determinations of pressure from each arm.

Proper cuff size is important, because a large cuff on a small arm causes low readings. Cuffs for average-sized adults are usually 12 to 14 cm (4.7 to 5.5 in.) wide and 30 cm (11.8 in.) in length. Smaller cuffs for children and larger cuffs for obese persons are also available. You should use the larger cuff to measure BP of individuals with well-developed arm musculature.

It takes a great deal of practice to become proficient at measuring BPs. When you are first learning this method, it is highly recommended that

RESTING BLOOD PRESSURE MEASUREMENT

To measure resting BP (seated position), use the following recommended procedures (Reeves 1995):

1. Seat the client in a quiet room for at least 5 min. The client's bare arm should be resting on a table so that the middle of the arm is at the level of the heart.
2. Estimate the client's arm circumference or measure it at the midpoint between the acromion process of the shoulder and the olecranon process of the elbow (see appendix D.5, "Standardized Sites for Circumference Measurements," p. 318, for description of measuring arm circumference) using an anthropometric tape measure. The bladder of the cuff should encircle 80% of an adult's arm and 100% of a child's arm.
3. Palpate the brachial artery pulse on the anteromedial aspect of the arm below the belly of the biceps brachii and 2 to 3 cm (1 in.) above the antecubital fossa. Wrap the deflated cuff firmly around the upper arm so

that the midline of the cuff is over the brachial artery pulse. The lower edge of the cuff should be approximately 2.5 cm (1 in.) above the antecubital fossa. If the cuff is too loose, BP will be overestimated. Avoid placing the cuff over clothing; and if the shirt sleeve is rolled up, make certain that it is not occluding the circulation.

4. Position the manometer so that the center of the mercury column or dial is at eye level and the cuff's tubing is not overlapping or obstructed.
5. Locate and palpate the radial pulse (see p. 26 for anatomical description of this site), close the valve of the BP unit completely by screwing it away from you, and rapidly inflate the cuff to 70 mm Hg. Then slowly increase the pressure in 10-mm Hg increments while palpating the radial pulse, and note when the pulse disappears (estimate of systolic BP). Partially open the valve by unscrewing it to-

ward you to slowly release the pressure at a rate of 2 to 3 mm Hg/sec and note when the pulse reappears (estimate of diastolic BP). Fully open the valve to completely release the pressure in the cuff. The estimate of systolic BP from the palpatory method is then used to determine how much the cuff needs to be inflated for measuring BP by means of the auscultatory technique. In this way, you can avoid over- or underinflating the cuff for clients with low or high BPs, respectively.

6. Position the earpieces of the stethoscope so that they are aligned with the auditory canals (i.e., angled anteriorly).

7. Place the head (bell) of the stethoscope over the brachial pulse (about 1 cm superior and medial to the antecubital fossa). Make certain that the entire head of the stethoscope is contacting the skin. To avoid extraneous noise, do not place any part of the head of the stethoscope underneath the cuff.

8. Close the valve, and quickly and steadily inflate the cuff pressure to about 20 to 30 mm Hg above the estimated systolic pressure previously determined by palpation.

9. Partially open the valve to slowly release the pressure at a rate of 2 to 3 mm Hg/sec. Note when you hear the first sharp thud caused by the sudden rush of blood as the artery opens. This is known as the first Korotkoff sound and corresponds to the systolic pressure (Phase I).

10. Continue reducing the pressure slowly (no more than 2 mm Hg/sec), noting when the metallic tapping sound becomes muffled (Phase IV diastolic pressure) and when the sound disappears (Phase V diastolic pressure). Typically, the Phase V value is used as the index of diastolic pressure. However, both Phase IV and V diastolic pressures should be noted. During rhythmic exercise, the Phase V pressure tends to decrease because of reduction in peripheral resistance. In some cases, it may even drop to zero.

11. After noting the Phase V pressure, continue deflating the cuff for at least 10 mm Hg, making certain that no additional sounds are heard. Then rapidly and completely deflate the cuff.

12. Record all three BP values (Phase I, IV, and V) to the nearest 2 mm Hg. Wait at least 30 sec and repeat the measurement. Use the average of the two measurements for each of the three values.

you practice with a trained BP technician, using a dual- or multiple-head stethoscope so that you can listen simultaneously and compare BP readings for the same trial.

Measuring BP during exercise is much more difficult than during rest. You should not attempt to measure exercise BP until you have demonstrated competency and have confidence in your ability to measure resting BP. It is particularly difficult to obtain accurate BP measurements when the client is running on the treadmill, because of extraneous noise and movement of the arms during running. Sometimes you will not be able to determine diastolic BP because of the noise and vibration during exercise. Novice BP technicians should practice taking BPs during bicycle ergometer exercise first and then try measuring BP during treadmill exercise. See "Exercise Blood Pressure Precautions" for tips on obtaining accurate readings while measuring BP during exercise.

Sources of Measurement Error

Sources of error in measuring BP are numerous (Reeves 1995). You need to be aware of the fol-

Exercise Blood Pressure Precautions

When you are measuring exercise BP, extra precautions are necessary to ensure accurate readings:

- Instruct the client to refrain from grasping the handlebars or handrails of the exercise apparatus during the BP measurement.
- Limit arm movement during the BP measurement; stabilize the client's arm during the measurement by placing and holding it firmly between your arm and trunk.
- Inflate the cuff well above the anticipated value or reading obtained during the previous stage of the graded exercise test, keeping in mind that systolic BP increases with exercise intensity.

lowing sources of error and do as much as possible to control them:

- Inaccurate sphygmomanometer

- Improper cuff width or length
- Cuff not centered, too loose, or over clothing
- Arm unsupported or elbow lower than heart level
- Poor auditory acuity of technician
- Improper rate of inflation or deflation of the cuff pressure
- Improper stethoscope placement or pressure
- Expectation bias and inexperience of the technician
- Slow reaction time of the technician
- Parallax error in reading the manometer
- Background noise
- Client holding treadmill handrails or cycle ergometer handlebars

Measuring Heart Rate

The average resting heart rate for adults is 60 to 80 beats per minute (bpm), with the average resting heart rate of women typically 7 to 10 bpm higher than that of men. Heart rates as low as 28 to 40 bpm have been reported for highly conditioned endurance athletes, whereas poorly trained, sedentary individuals may have heart rates that exceed 100 bpm.

Before you measure resting heart rate, your client should rest for 5 to 10 min in either a supine or a seated position. It is important that you measure resting heart rate carefully because this value is sometimes used in the calculation of target exercise heart rates for submaximal exercise tests, as well as for exercise prescriptions. You can measure heart rate using auscultation, palpation, heart rate monitors, or ECG recordings.

Auscultation

When measuring resting heart rate by **auscultation,** place the bell of the stethoscope over the third intercostal space to the left of the sternum. The sounds arising from the heart are counted for 30 or 60 sec. The 30-sec count is multiplied by 2 to convert it to beats per minute.

Palpation

With use of the **palpation** technique for determining heart rate, the pulse is palpated at one of the following sites:

- Brachial artery—on the anteromedial aspect of the arm below the belly of the biceps

brachii, approximately 2 to 3 cm (1 in.) above the antecubital fossa
- Carotid artery—in the neck just lateral to the larynx
- Radial artery—on the anterolateral aspect of the wrist directly in line with the base of the thumb
- Temporal artery—along the hairline of the head at the temple

For precautions necessary to be sure your measurement is accurate, refer to "Heart Rate Determination by Palpation."

Heart Rate Determination by Palpation

Follow these procedures when determining heart rate by palpation:

- Use the tips of the middle and index fingers. Do not use your thumb; it has a pulse of its own and may produce an inaccurate count.
- When palpating the carotid site, do not apply heavy pressure to the area. Baroreceptors in the carotid arteries detect this pressure and cause a reflex slowing of the heart rate.
- If you start the stopwatch simultaneously with the pulse beat, count the first beat as zero. If the stopwatch is running, count the first beat as 1. Continue counting either for a set period of time (6, 10, 15, 30, or 60 sec) or for a set number of beats. When the heart rate is counted for less than 1 min, use the following multipliers to convert the count to beats per minute: 6-sec count times 10; 10-sec count times 6; 15-sec, 4; 30-sec, 2. Typically, shorter time intervals (i.e., 6- or 10-sec counts) are used to measure exercise and postexercise heart rates during and immediately following exercise. Because there is a rapid and immediate decline in heart rate when a person stops exercising, the 6- or 10-sec count reflects the individual's actual exercise heart rate more accurately than the longer counts do.

Heart Rate Monitors and Electrocardiogram (ECG) Recordings

Heart rate can be also be measured using heart rate monitors or an ECG monitoring system. Generally, heart rate monitors are designed to detect either the pulse or the ECG electrical signal from the heart, and provide a digital display of the heart rate. Pulse monitors use infrared sensors attached to the client's fingertip or earlobe to detect pulsations in blood flow during the cardiac cycle. Chest-strap wire and wireless ECG-type monitors tend to be more accurate and reliable than pulse monitors, especially during vigorous exercise. However, the accuracy of wireless chest-strap monitors may be affected by electrical equipment (such as some treadmills, stair climbers, rowing machines, and video screens) generating radio or magnetic interference.

Most ECG monitoring systems provide a continuous digital display of the heart rate. This value is usually recorded at the top of the ECG strip recording. If your equipment does not provide a digital readout, you can use a heart rate ruler that converts the distance of two cardiac cycles to beats per minute. Alternatively, you can count the heart rate by measuring the distance between four consecutive beats (R-R intervals) using a millimeter ruler. Convert the distance to beats per minute based on the paper speed of the recorder (usually 25 mm·sec^{-1}). For example, if the distance for four beats is 60 mm and the distance for 1 min is 1500 mm (i.e., 25 mm $\times$ 60 sec), the per minute heart rate is determined by setting up the following equation and solving for x:

$$4 \text{ beats}/60 \text{ mm} = x(\text{bpm})/1500 \text{ mm}$$

Cross-multiplying, $60x = 6000$; then $x = 100$ bpm. You can use the sample ECG recordings in appendix A.7, "Sample Electrocardiogram Tracings" (p. 276), to practice measuring heart rates using this method.

No matter which technique is used to measure heart rate, you should be aware that heart rate fluctuates easily due to temperature, anxiety, exercise, stress, eating, smoking, drinking coffee, time of day, and body position. In a supine position, the resting heart rate is lower than in either a sitting or a standing position.

Do not use resting heart rate as a measure of cardiorespiratory fitness. There is wide variability in resting heart rate within the population, and a low resting heart rate is not always indicative of cardiorespiratory fitness level. In some cases, a low resting heart rate indicates a diseased heart (McArdle, Katch, and Katch 1996). The following general guidelines may be used to classify resting heart rate:

1. <60 bpm = **bradycardia** (slow rate)
2. 60 to 100 bpm = normal rate
3. >100 bpm = **tachycardia** (fast rate)

Twelve-Lead Electrocardiogram

The **electrocardiogram** is a composite record of the electrical events in the heart during the cardiac cycle. As the heart depolarizes and repolarizes during contraction, an electrical impulse spreads to the tissues surrounding the heart. Electrodes placed on opposite sides of the heart transmit the electrical potential to an ECG recorder.

In addition to providing baseline data, the resting ECG is used to detect such contraindications to exercise testing as evidence of previous myocardial infarction, ischemic ST-segment changes, conduction defects, and left ventricular hypertrophy. The reading and interpretation of ECGs require a high degree of skill and practice. As an exercise technician you can administer the resting 12-lead ECG, but a qualified physician should interpret the results. This chapter includes only basic information about administering an ECG. You should consult other references for more detailed information concerning the reading and interpretation of ECG abnormalities (Adamovich 1984; Conover 1992; Dubin 1980; Goldberger and Goldberger 1981; Goldman 1982).

Electrocardiogram Basics

A typical normal ECG (figure 2.1) is composed of a **P wave** that represents depolarization of the atria. The **PR interval** indicates the delay in the impulse at the atrioventricular node. Electrical currents generated during ventricular depolarization and contraction produce the **QRS complex.** The **T wave** and **ST segment** correspond to ventricular repolarization.

A lead is a pair of electrodes placed on the body and connected to an ECG recorder. An axis is an imaginary line connecting the two electrodes. A standard 12-lead ECG consists of three limb leads, three augmented unipolar leads, and six chest leads. Each of the 12 ECG leads records a different view of the heart's electrical activity. Thus, the tracings from the various leads differ from one another.

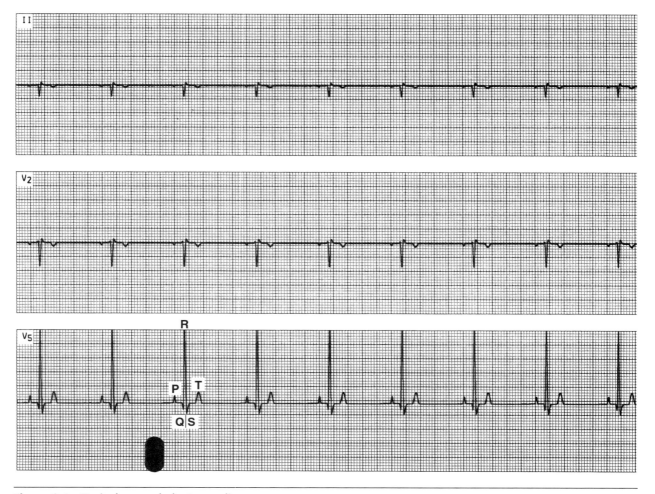

Figure 2.1 Typical normal electrocardiogram.

Resting 12-Lead Electrocardiogram Procedures

To measure the 12 leads, 10 electrodes are used. The electrodes for the three **limb leads** (I, II, and III) are placed on the right arm, left arm, and left leg. A ground electrode is placed on the right leg. This is electronically equivalent to placing the electrodes at the shoulders and the symphysis pubis. Limb lead I measures the voltage differential between the left and right arm electrodes. Limb leads II and III measure the voltage between the left leg and right (lead II) and left (lead II) arms. Figure 2.2 shows the three limb leads and three augmented unipolar leads.

The three **augmented unipolar leads** are aVF (feet), aVL (left), and aVR (right). The augmented unipolar lead compares the voltage across one of the limb electrodes with the average voltage across the two opposite electrodes. Lead aVL, for

example, records the voltage across an electrode placed on the left arm and the average voltage across the other two limb electrodes (see figure 2.2).

The six **chest leads** (V_1 to V_6) measure the voltage across a specific area of the chest, with the average voltage across the other three limb leads. Figure 2.3 illustrates electrode placement for the chest leads, V_1 through V_6.

During the resting ECG, the client should lie quietly in a supine position on a table. The electrode sites should be shaved if hair is present and should be cleaned with alcohol. Remove the superficial layer of skin at each site by rubbing it with fine-grain emery paper or a gauze pad. Disposable electrodes contain electrode gel and adhesive disks. After applying the electrode, tap it firmly to test for noisy leads. You should always calibrate the ECG recorder prior to use by recording the standard 1-mV deflection per centimeter.

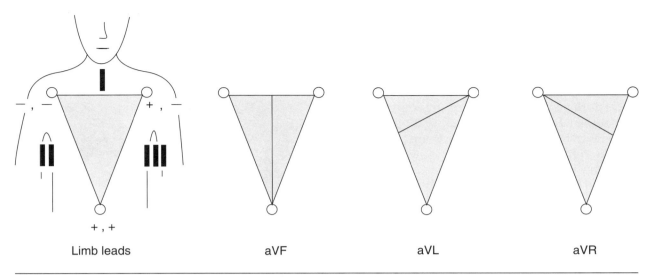

| Limb leads | aVF | aVL | aVR |

Figure 2.2 Three limb leads and three augmented unipolar leads.

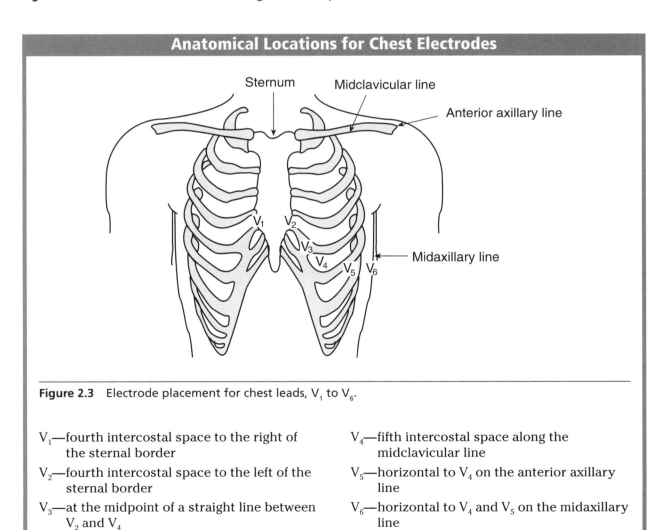

Anatomical Locations for Chest Electrodes

Figure 2.3 Electrode placement for chest leads, V_1 to V_6.

V_1—fourth intercostal space to the right of the sternal border

V_2—fourth intercostal space to the left of the sternal border

V_3—at the midpoint of a straight line between V_2 and V_4

V_4—fifth intercostal space along the midclavicular line

V_5—horizontal to V_4 on the anterior axillary line

V_6—horizontal to V_4 and V_5 on the midaxillary line

Also, to standardize the time base for the ECG, set the paper speed to 25 mm/sec.

The Twelve-Lead Exercise ECG

To avoid poor ECG tracings caused by moving limbs during exercise, the electrode configuration is modified slightly for an exercise 12-lead ECG. The right and left arm electrodes are placed below the right and left clavicles, respectively. The right and left leg electrodes are attached to the right and left sides of the trunk, below the rib cage on the anterior axillary line. The six chest electrodes are positioned as previously described (see figure 2.4).

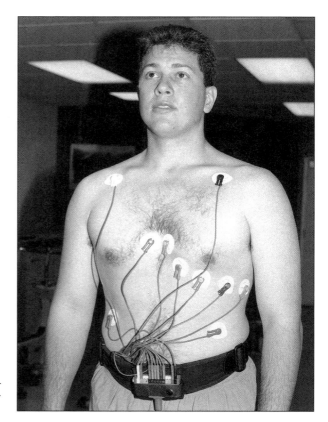

Figure 2.4 Electrode placement for 12-lead exercise electrocardiogram.

SOURCES FOR EQUIPMENT

Product	Manufacturer's Address
Aneroid or mercury sphygmomanometer and blood pressure cuffs	W.A. Baum Co. 620 Oak St. Copiague, NY 11726 (888) 281-6061 www.wabaum.com
Electrocardiograph	GE Marquette Medical Systems P.O. Box 414 Milwaukee, WI 53201 www.gemedicalsystems.com
Heart rate monitors	Creative Health Products 7621 East Joy Rd. Ann Arbor, MI 48105 www.chponline.com

KEY POINTS

- The purpose of the health evaluation is to detect disease and to assess disease risk.

- Important components of the health evaluation are a medical history, CHD risk factor analysis, physical examination, clinical tests, and medical clearance.

- The lifestyle evaluation includes information about the diet, tobacco and alcohol use, physical activity, and psychological stress levels of the individual.

- All clients are required to sign an informed consent prior to taking any physical fitness tests or participating in an exercise program.

- The resting evaluation of cardiorespiratory function includes heart rate, BP, and a 12-lead ECG that is interpreted by a qualified physician.

- Resting BP can be assessed using auscultation, palpation, or automated BP devices.

- Heart rate may be taken using auscultation, palpation, heart rate monitors, or ECG recordings.

- The 12-lead ECG includes three limb leads (I, II, III), three augmented unipolar leads (aVF, aVR, aVL), and six chest leads (V_1 through V_6).

- A graded maximal exercise test is the best way to assess functional aerobic capacity.

- Unless contraindications to exercise are observed, a maximal exercise test is recommended for men 45 years or older and women 55 years or older before they begin a vigorous exercise program.

KEY TERMS

Learn the definition for each of the following key terms. Definitions of key terms can be found in "Glossary of Terms," page 349.

augmented unipolar leads	palpation
auscultation	PR interval
bradycardia	pulse pressure
chest leads	P wave
diastolic blood pressure	QRS complex
electrocardiogram	sphygmomanometer
high CHD risk	ST segment
limb leads	systolic blood pressure
low CHD risk	tachycardia
moderate CHD risk	T wave

REVIEW QUESTIONS

In addition to being able to define each of the key terms, test your knowledge and understanding of the material by answering the following review questions.

1. Identify the purpose of each component of the comprehensive health evaluation.

2. At minimum, a pretest health screening should include four items. Name these.

3. Identify cardiovascular, pulmonary, metabolic, and musculoskeletal diseases and/or disorders that warrant referral to a physician for medical clearance (name three signs or symptoms for each category).

4. Identify the positive and negative risk factors for CHD. Specify the criteria for each of these risk factors.

5. Identify the cutoff values for classifying resting BPs.

6. Identify the cutoff values for classifying TC, LDL-C, HDL-C, and triglycerides.

7. List the three ACSM risk stratification categories and the criterion for each category.

8. Describe the criteria used to determine whether or not an individual needs a physical examination and medical clearance prior to exercise testing or exercise participation.

9. Name three methods for measuring BP. Which one is considered to be the "gold standard" method?

10. Name three sources of error in measurement of BP.

11. Describe three things you should do to ensure accurate BP readings during exercise.

12. Name three methods for measuring heart rate.

13. Identify the component parts of a typical normal ECG tracing. What does each component represent relative to the cardiac cycle?

14. Describe the anatomical locations for placement of the 10 electrodes used to obtain a 12-lead ECG recording.

15. Identify ACSM's guidelines for medical examinations and exercise testing for low-, moderate-, and high-risk individuals.

16. Name three absolute and three relative contraindications to exercise testing.

REFERENCES

Adomovich, D.R. 1984. *The heart*. East Moriches, NY: Sports Medicine Books.

American College of Sports Medicine (ACSM). 2000. *ACSM's guidelines for exercise testing and prescription*, 6th ed. Philadelphia: Lippincott Williams & Wilkins.

Canadian Society for Exercise Physiology. 1998. *The Canadian physical activity, fitness and lifestyle appraisal*. 2d ed. Ottawa, ON: author.

Conover, M.B. 1992. *Understanding electrocardiography*. St. Louis: Mosby Year Book.

Dubin, D. 1980. *Rapid interpretation of EKGs*. Tampa: Cover.

Gibbons, R.J., Balady, G.J., Beasley, J.W., Bricker, J.T., Duvernoy, W.F., Froelicher, V.F., Mark, D.B., Marwick, T.H., McCallister, B.D., Thompson, P.D., Winters, W.L., Yanowitz, F.G., Ritchie, J.L., Gibbons, R.J., Cheitlin, M.D., Eagle, K.A., Gardner, T.J., Garson, A., Lewis, R.P., O'Rourke, R.A., and Ryan, T.J. 1997. ACC/AHA Guidelines for exercise testing. A report of the American College of Cardiology/American Heart Association Task Force on Practice Guidelines (Committee on Exercise Testing). *Journal of the American College of Cardiology* 30: 260–311.

Goldberger, A.L., and Goldberger, E. 1981. *Clinical electrocardiography: A simplified approach*. St. Louis: Mosby.

Goldman, M.J. 1982. *Principles of clinical electrocardiography*. Cambridge, MD: Lange Medical.

Griffin, S., Robergs, R., and Heyward, V. 1997. Assessment of exercise blood pressure: A review. *Medicine & Science in Sports & Exercise* 29: 149–159.

Joint National Committee on Detection, Evaluation, and Treatment of High Blood Pressure. 1997. *The sixth report of the Joint National Committee on detection, evaluation, and treatment of high blood pressure (JNC VI)*. Washington, D.C.: Public Health Service, National Institutes of Health, National Heart, Lung, and Blood Institute, November, NIH publication no. 98–4080.

McArdle, W.D., Katch, F.I., and Katch, V.L. 1996. *Exercise physiology: Energy, nutrition and human performance*, 4th ed. Baltimore: Williams & Wilkins.

National Cholesterol Education Program (NCEP). 2001. Executive summary of the second report of the National Cholesterol Education Program (NCEP) expert panel on detection, evaluation, and treatment of high blood cholesterol in adults (Adult Treatment Panel III). *Journal of the American Medical Association* 285: 2486–2497.

Reeves, R.A. 1995. Does this patient have hypertension? How to measure blood pressure. *Journal of the American Medical Association* 273: 1211–1218.

chapter 3

Principles of Assessment, Prescription, and Exercise Program Adherence

KEY QUESTIONS

- What are the essential components of a physical fitness profile?

- What are the purposes of physical fitness tests and how can I use the results?

- Several physical fitness tests are available; how do I select the best test for my client?

- Are field tests as good as laboratory tests for measuring physical fitness?

- What is the best way to interpret test results for my client?

- What are the essential elements of an exercise prescription?

- Is one type of exercise better than others for improving each component of physical fitness?

- Does high-intensity exercise improve physical fitness faster than low-intensity exercise?

- Is it safe to exercise every day?

- When should I increase the frequency, intensity, and duration in an exercise prescription? Can these elements be increased simultaneously?

- Do older people benefit as much from exercise as younger people?

- How can I get my clients to stick with their exercise programs?

- Do I need to be professionally certified or licensed in order to work in this field?

Health/fitness professionals need to master the basic principles of physical fitness assessment and exercise prescription. You must know how to use the results of physical fitness tests to plan scientifically sound exercise programs that are individualized to meet your client's needs, interests, and abilities. With your knowledge, leadership, and guidance, your clients can reduce their risk of disease and improve their health and physical fitness levels safely and effectively.

As an exercise specialist, you will have diverse responsibilities, such as

- educating clients about the positive benefits of regular physical activity;

- conducting pretest health evaluations to screen clients for exercise participation (see chapter 2);

- selecting, administering, and interpreting tests designed to assess each component of physical fitness;

- designing individualized exercise programs;

- leading exercise classes;

- analyzing your clients' exercise performance and correcting performance errors;
- educating your clients about the "do's and don'ts" of exercise; and
- motivating your clients to improve their adherence to exercise.

Exercise specialists play many roles: educator, leader, technician, and artist. To be effective in these roles, you must integrate knowledge from many disciplines such as anatomy, physiology, chemistry, nutrition, education, and psychology, as well as refine your exercise testing, prescription, and leadership skills.

This chapter presents principles of exercise testing and prescription, along with information about exercise program adherence and the importance of professional certification for individuals in the field of exercise science.

PHYSICAL FITNESS TESTING

There are several areas that you must understand in order to plan and administer physical fitness tests. These comprise

- the components of physical fitness to be tested;
- purposes of physical fitness testing;
- testing order and the testing environment;
- test validity, reliability, and objectivity;
- prediction equation evaluation; and
- test administration and interpretation.

Components of Physical Fitness

Physical fitness is the ability to perform occupational, recreational, and daily activities without becoming unduly fatigued. As an exercise specialist, one of your primary responsibilities is to assess each of the following physical fitness components:

1. **Cardiorespiratory endurance. Cardiorespiratory endurance** is the ability of the heart, lungs, and circulatory system to supply oxygen and nutrients efficiently to working muscles. Exercise physiologists measure the **maximum oxygen consumption** ($\dot{V}O_2max$), or the rate of oxygen utilization of the muscles during aerobic exercise, in order to assess cardiorespiratory endurance and functional aerobic capacity. Physical fitness evaluations should include a test of cardiorespiratory

function during rest and exercise. Graded exercise tests (GXTs) are used for this purpose. Improved cardiorespiratory endurance is one of the most important benefits of aerobic exercise training programs. Chapters 4 and 5 present detailed information about graded exercise testing and aerobic exercise programs.

2. **Musculoskeletal fitness. Musculoskeletal fitness** refers to the ability of the skeletal and muscular systems to perform work. This requires muscular strength, muscular endurance, and bone strength. **Muscular strength** is the maximal force or tension level that can be produced by a muscle group; **muscular endurance** is the ability of a muscle to maintain submaximal force levels for extended periods; **bone strength** is directly related to the risk of bone fracture and is a function of the mineral content and density of the bone tissue. Resistance training is one of the most effective ways to improve the strength of muscles and bones and to develop muscular endurance. Chapters 6 and 7 provide detailed information about assessing musculoskeletal fitness and designing resistance training programs.

3. **Body weight and body composition. Body weight** refers to the size or mass of the individual. **Body composition** refers to body weight in terms of the absolute and relative amounts of muscle, bone, and fat tissues. Aerobic exercise and resistance training are effective in altering body weight and composition. Chapters 8 and 9 discuss body composition assessment techniques and exercise programs for weight management.

4. **Flexibility. Flexibility** is the ability to move a joint or series of joints fluidly through the complete range of motion. Flexibility is limited by factors such as bony structure of the joint and the size and strength of muscles, ligaments, and other connective tissues. Daily stretching can greatly improve flexibility. Chapter 10 gives more information about assessing flexibility and designing stretching programs.

5. **Neuromuscular relaxation. Neuromuscular relaxation** refers to the ability to reduce or eliminate unnecessary tension or contraction in a muscle group. Progressive relaxation exercise and tai chi are examples of effective techniques for decreasing stress and neuromuscular tension levels. Chapter 11 provides additional information about neuromuscular tension and stress assessment, as well as about the use of regular physical activity as a stress management technique.

Purposes of Physical Fitness Testing

As mentioned in chapter 2, it is imperative that you carefully screen your clients for exercise testing, classify their disease risk, identify any contraindications to exercise testing, and obtain their informed consent before conducting any physical fitness tests. You can use laboratory and field tests to assess each component of physical fitness and to develop physical fitness profiles for your clients. Results from these tests enable you to identify strengths and weaknesses and to set realistic and attainable goals for your clients. Data from specific tests (e.g., heart rates from a GXT) will help you make accurate and precise exercise prescriptions for each client. Also, you can use baseline and follow-up data to evaluate the progress of exercise program participants.

Testing Order and the Testing Environment

When you administer a complete battery of physical fitness tests in a single session, ACSM (2000) recommends using the following test sequence to minimize the effects of previous tests on subsequent test performance:

- Resting blood pressure and heart rate
- Body composition
- Cardiorespiratory endurance
- Muscular fitness
- Flexibility

If your physical fitness test battery includes an evaluation of neuromuscular tension and stress levels, these tests should follow the resting evaluation of heart rate and blood pressure.

Often clients are apprehensive about taking physical fitness tests. Test anxiety may affect the validity and reliability of test results. Therefore, you should put your client at ease by establishing good rapport; projecting a sense of relaxed confidence; and creating a testing environment that is friendly, quiet, private, safe, and comfortable. Room temperature should be maintained at 70° to 74° F (21° to 23° C), and the relative humidity should be controlled whenever possible. For pretest health screening and interpretation of the client's test results, the room should have comfortable chairs and a table for completing questionnaires and paperwork, as well as an examina- tion table or bed for the resting evaluation of heart rate, blood pressure, and the 12-lead electrocardiogram. All equipment used for physical testing should be carefully calibrated and prepared before your client arrives for testing. This will ensure valid test data and efficient use of time.

Test Validity, Reliability, and Objectivity

To accurately assess your client's physical fitness status, you must select tests that are valid, reliable, and objective. It is necessary to understand these basic concepts fully in order to evaluate the relative worth of specific physical fitness tests and prediction equations.

Test Validity

With regard to physical fitness testing, test **validity** is the ability of a test to *measure accurately*, with minimal error, a specific physical fitness component. **Reference** or **criterion methods** are used to obtain *direct* measures of physical fitness components. However, some physical fitness components cannot be measured directly, requiring the use of *indirect* measures for estimation of the value of the reference measure. For example, exercise physiologists consider the direct measurement of $\dot{V}O_2$max (i.e., collection and analysis of expired gas samples) during maximal exercise to be the criterion measure of cardiorespiratory fitness. Direct measurement of $\dot{V}O_2$max, however, requires expensive equipment and considerable technical expertise. Therefore in the laboratory setting, $\dot{V}O_2$max is usually estimated using formulas to convert the amount of work output during a GXT to oxygen consumption (see chapter 4). In field settings, prediction equations are used to estimate $\dot{V}O_2$max from a combination of physiological, demographic, and performance predictor variables. Because field tests and conversion formulas indirectly measure the physical fitness component, these equations have prediction errors.

One way in which researchers quantify the validity of physical fitness tests is by calculating the relationship between predicted scores (y') and the criterion scores (y) using correlation coefficients ($r_{y,y'}$). This value, $r_{y,y'}$, is known as the **validity coefficient.** The magnitude of the validity coefficient cannot exceed 1.0. The closer the value is to 1.0, the stronger the validity of the test. Valid physical fitness field tests and prediction equations typically have validity coefficients in excess of $r_{y,y'} = 0.80$.

Test Reliability

Reliability is the ability of a test to yield *consistent* and *stable* scores across trials and over time. For example, the skinfold test is considered to be reliable because a trained skinfold technician obtains similar skinfold values when taking duplicate measurements on the same person. Researchers quantify reliability by calculating the relationship between trial 1 and trial 2 test scores or day 1 and day 2 test scores. This value, $r_{x1,x2}$, is known as the **reliability coefficient**. The magnitude of the reliability coefficient cannot exceed 1.0. In general, physical fitness tests have high reliability coefficients, typically exceeding $r_{x1,x2} = 0.90$.

It is important to know that test reliability affects test validity. Tests with poor reliability also have poor validity because unreliable tests fail to produce consistent test scores. It is possible, however, for a test to have excellent reliability ($r_{x1,x2} > 0.90$) but poor validity. Even when a test yields stable and precise values across trials or between days, it may not validly measure a specific physical fitness component. For example, researchers reported high test-retest reliability ($r_{x1,x2} = 0.99$) for the sit-and-reach test, but also noted that this test has poor validity ($r_{y,y'} = 0.12$) as a measure of low back flexibility in women (Jackson and Langford 1989).

Test Objectivity

Objectivity is also known as intertester reliability. Objective tests yield similar test scores for a given individual when the same test is administered by different technicians. Objectivity is quantified by calculating the correlation between pairs of test scores measured on the same individuals by two different technicians. This value, $r_{1,2}$, is known as the **objectivity coefficient**. As with validity and reliability coefficients, the magnitude of the objectivity coefficient cannot exceed 1.0. Most physical fitness tests have high objectivity coefficients ($r_{1,2} > 0.90$), especially when technicians are highly trained, practice together, and carefully follow standardized testing procedures.

Prediction Equation Evaluation

Although reference measures obtained in the laboratory setting provide the most valid assessment of each physical fitness component, these tests are expensive and time consuming and require considerable technical expertise. In field and clinical settings, you can obtain estimates of these reference measures by selecting valid field tests and prediction equations that have good predictive accuracy. Table 3.1 provides an overview of the types of tests used in laboratory and field settings to assess each physical fitness component.

To select the most appropriate tests for measuring your client's physical fitness, it is important to be able to evaluate the relative worth of the fitness tests and their prediction equations. To do this, you should ask the following questions:

■ *What reference measure was used to develop the prediction equation?*

As mentioned earlier, the reference or criterion measure of a specific physical fitness component is obtained by directly measuring the component. Reference measures are used as the "gold standard" to validate field tests and to develop prediction equations that accurately estimate the reference measure. For example, skinfold prediction equations are developed and cross-validated through comparison of the estimated body density, calculated from the skinfold equation, to the reference measure of body density typically obtained from hydrodensitometry (underwater weighing). Similarly, the validity of the sit-and-reach test for measuring low back flexibility was tested by comparing sit-and-reach scores to range-of-motion values (reference measure) directly measured by X-ray or goniometric methods. Table 3.1 describes reference measures that experts commonly use to assess each physical fitness component. Field tests and prediction equations developed using indirect methods instead of reference methods as a criterion have questionable validity.

■ *How large was the sample used to develop the prediction equation?*

Large randomly selected samples ($N = 100$ to 400 subjects) generally are needed to ensure that the data are representative of the population for whom the prediction equation was developed. Also, equations based on large samples tend to have more stable regression weights for each predictor variable in the equation.

■ *What is the ratio of sample size to the number of predictor variables in the equation?*

In multiple regression, the correlation between the reference measure of the physical fitness component and the predictors in the equation is represented by the **multiple correlation coefficient** (R_{mc}). The larger the R_{mc} (up to maximum value of

Table 3.1 Direct (Reference) and Indirect (Field) Measures of Physical Fitness Components

Physical fitness component	Reference measure	Laboratory or reference method	Indirect measures or field tests	Prediction error (SEE)	Chapter
Cardiorespiratory endurance	Direct measurement of $\dot{V}O_2$ max (ml·kg⁻¹·min⁻¹)	Maximal GXT	Submaximal GXT, distance run/walk tests, step tests	<5.0 ml·kg⁻¹·min⁻¹	4
Body composition	Db (g·cc⁻¹), FFM (kg), or %BF	Hydrodensitometry or dual-energy X-ray absorptiometry	Bioimpedance, skinfold, anthropometry	<0.0080 g·cc⁻¹ <3.5 kg FFM (men) <2.8 kg FFM (women) <3.5 %BF	8
Muscular strength	Maximal force (kg) or torque (Nm)	Isokinetic or 1-RM tests	Submaximal tests (2- to 10-RM value)	<2.0 kg	6
Bone strength	Bone mineral content and bone density	Dual-energy X-ray absorptiometry	Anthropometric measures of bony width	NR	8
Flexibility	ROM at joint (degrees)	X-ray or goniometry	Linear measures of ROM	<6°	10
Neuromuscular relaxation	Electrical activity in resting muscles	Electromyography	Rathbone manual tension test	NR	11

Db = total body density; FFM = fat-free mass; %BF = relative body fat; SEE = standard error of estimate;
GXT = graded exercise test; ROM = range of motion; RM = repetition maximum; NR = not reported; Nm = newton-meter.

1.00), the stronger the relationship. The size of R_{mc} will be artificially inflated if there are too many predictors in the equation compared to the total number of subjects. Statisticians recommend that there should be a minimum of 10 to 20 subjects per predictor variable. For example, if a skinfold (SKF) prediction equation has three predictors (e.g., triceps SKF, calf SKF, and age), then the minimum sample size needs to be 30 to 60 subjects. Prediction equations that are based on small samples or that have a poor subject-to-predictor ratio are suspect and should not be used.

- **What were the sizes of the R_{mc} and the standard error of estimate for the prediction equation?**

In general, the R_{mc} for equations predicting physical fitness components exceeds 0.80. This means that at least 64% [$R^2 = 0.80^2 \times 100$] of variance in the reference measure can be accounted for by the predictors in the equation. As you can easily see, the larger the R_{mc}, the greater the amount of shared variance between the reference measure and predictor variables. When you evaluate the relative worth of a prediction equation, it is more important to note the size of the prediction error (*SEE*) than that of the R_{mc} because the magnitude of R_{mc} is greatly affected by sample size and variability of the data. The **standard error of estimate** (*SEE*) reflects the degree of deviation of individual data points (participants' scores) around the line of best fit through the entire sample's data points. The **line of best fit** is the **regression line** that depicts the linear relationship

between the reference measure and the predictors. The closer the individual data points fall to the regression line, the smaller the *SEE* or prediction error (see figure 3.1). Table 3.1 presents standards for evaluating prediction errors of physical fitness prediction equations.

- **To whom is the prediction equation applicable?**

To answer this question, you need to pay close attention to the physical characteristics of the sample used to derive the equation. Factors such as age, gender, race, fitness level, and body fatness need to be examined carefully. Prediction equations are either **population specific** or **generalized**. Population-specific equations are intended only for individuals from a specific homogeneous group. For example, separate skinfold equations have been developed for prepubescent boys and girls (see table 8.3, p. 166). Population-specific equations are likely to systematically over- or underestimate the physical fitness component if they are applied to individuals who do not belong to that population subgroup. On the other hand, there are generalized prediction equations that can be applied to individuals who differ greatly in physical characteristics. Generalized equations are developed using diverse, heterogeneous samples and account for differences in physical characteristics by including these variables as predictors in the equation. For example, the prediction equation for the Rockport walking test (see chapter 4) is a generalized equation because gender and age are predictors in this equation.

- **How were the variables measured by the researchers who developed the prediction equation?**

It is important to know not only which variables are included in a prediction equation, but also how each one of these predictors was measured by the researchers developing the equation. Although it is highly recommended that standardized procedures be used for all physical fitness testing, this is not always done. For example, the suprailiac skinfold used in the skinfold equations developed by Jackson, Pollock, and Ward (1980) is measured above the iliac crest at the anterior axillary line. In contrast, the *Anthropometric Standardization Reference Manual* (Lohman, Roche, and Martorell 1988) recommends that the suprailiac skinfold be measured above the iliac crest at the midaxillary line. For most individuals, there will be a difference between skinfold thicknesses measured at these two sites. Thus, larger-than-expected pre-

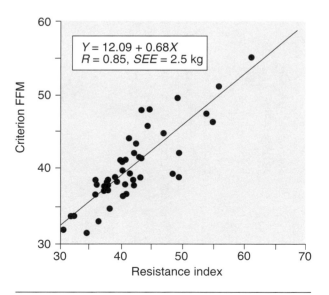

Figure 3.1 Line of best fit and *SEE* (prediction error).

diction errors may result if physical fitness variables are not measured according to the descriptions provided by the researchers who developed the equation.

■ *Was the prediction equation cross-validated on another sample from the population?*

An equation must be tested on other samples from the population before its validity or predictive accuracy can be determined. For example, the Rockport 1.0-mile walking test was originally developed to assess the cardiorespiratory fitness of women and men ages 20 to 69 years (Kline et al. 1987). Other researchers cross-validated this equation to establish its predictive accuracy for women 65 years of age or older (Fenstermaker, Plowman, and Looney 1992). In general, prediction equations that have not been cross-validated on the original study sample or on additional samples in other studies should not be used.

■ *What was the size of the correlation $(r_{y,y'})$ between the reference measure (y) and predicted (y') scores (validity coefficient)? What was the size of the prediction error (SEE) when this equation was applied to the cross-validation sample?*

As already noted, an equation with good predictive accuracy should yield a moderately high validity coefficient ($r_{y,y'}$ >0.80) and an acceptable *SEE* (see table 3.1). Keep in mind that the *SEE* represents the degree of deviation of individual scores from the regression line (see figure 3.1).

Physical Fitness Tests: Administration and Interpretation

To obtain good test results, it is important to prepare your clients for physical fitness testing by giving them appropriate instructions at least one day before the scheduled exercise tests.

Pretest Instructions

Give the client directions to the testing facility and make special arrangements if the facility requires a parking pass. Make sure the client has the following instructions in preparation for the test:

■ Wear comfortable clothing, socks, and athletic shoes if available.

■ Drink plenty of fluids during the 24-hr period before the test.

■ Refrain from eating, smoking, and drinking alcohol or caffeine for 3 hr prior to the test.

■ Do not engage in strenuous physical activity the day of the test.

■ Get adequate sleep (6 to 8 hr) the night before the test.

Test Administration

Later chapters give detailed procedures for administering laboratory and field tests for each physical fitness component. Your technical skills and expertise in administering these tests are directly related to your mastery of standardized testing procedures and the amount of time you spend practicing testing techniques. For example, to become a proficient skinfold technician, you probably should practice on at least 50 to 100 people (Jackson and Pollock 1985). You also need a great deal of practice in order to measure exercise blood pressures and heart rates accurately and to coordinate the timing of these measurements during a GXT on the treadmill or bicycle ergometer. Remember that you cannot obtain valid test scores if you do not follow the standardized testing procedures.

Test Interpretation

After collecting the test data, you must analyze and interpret the results for your client. Computer software programs are available that display and compare the client's test results to normative data. Some graphs display the individual's physical fitness profile so that you and your client can easily pinpoint strengths, as well as physical fitness components in need of improvement.

To classify your client's physical fitness status, you should compare test scores to established norms. For this purpose, age-gender norms are provided for many of the cardiorespiratory fitness, muscular fitness, body composition, and flexibility tests included in this book. For some tests, percentile rankings are used to classify a client's performance. To illustrate the interpretation of a percentile ranking, let's use the example of a 35-year-old male client whose sit-and-reach score ranks in the 60th percentile. This ranking means that his score is better than 60% of the scores of all males the same age taking this test.

When interpreting results for clients, use lay language, rather than highly technical terms and jargon, to explain their test scores. Whenever possible, try to phrase poor results in positive terms. For example, if a female client's body fat level is classified as obese, do not embarrass and alarm her by saying: "Your underwater weighing test indicates that you are obese and need to lose at least

20 pounds to achieve a healthy body fat level in order to reduce your risk of diseases linked to obesity. You need to decrease your caloric intake and increase your caloric expenditure by dieting and exercising. The sooner you start a weight management program, the better."

Instead, you should use a more positive and less intimidating approach when interpreting this result. The following approach is more appropriate, especially for clients with low self-efficacy or motivation to initiate and adhere to an exercise program: "People with more than 32% body fat are at risk for disease. If you wish, I will evaluate your daily calorie intake and suggest healthy foods you like to eat that are low in fat. Also, we can discuss ways to increase your physical activity level. I think we can find some activities that you will enjoy and have time for, so that you'll burn more calories each day. With these changes, you should be able to lower your body fat to a healthy level in a reasonable amount of time."

BASIC PRINCIPLES FOR EXERCISE PROGRAM DESIGN

A number of basic training principles apply to all types of exercise programs, whether they are designed to improve cardiorespiratory fitness, musculoskeletal fitness, body composition, or flexibility.

- **Specificity-of-Training Principle.** The **specificity principle** states that the body's physiological and metabolic responses and adaptations to exercise training are specific to the type of exercise and the muscle groups involved. For example, physical activities requiring continuous, dynamic, and rhythmical contractions of large muscle groups are best suited for stimulating improvements in cardiorespiratory endurance; stretching exercises develop range of joint motion and flexibility; and resistance exercises are effective for improving muscular strength and muscular endurance. Furthermore, the gains in muscular fitness are specific to the exercised muscle groups, type and speed of contraction, and training intensity.

- **Overload Training Principle.** To promote improvements in physical fitness components, the physiological systems of the body must be taxed using loads that are greater (**overload principle**) than those to which the individual is accustomed. Overload can be achieved through increases in the frequency, intensity, and duration of aerobic exercise. Muscle groups can be effectively over-loaded through increases in the number of repetitions, sets, or exercises in programs designed to improve muscular fitness and flexibility.

- **Principle of Progression.** Throughout the training program, you must progressively increase the training volume, or overload, to stimulate further improvements (i.e., **progression principle**). The progression needs to be gradual because "doing too much, too soon" may cause musculoskeletal injuries and is a major reason why some individuals drop out of exercise programs.

- **Principle of Initial Values.** Individuals with low initial physical fitness levels will show greater relative (%) gains and a faster rate of improvement in response to exercise training than individuals with average or high fitness levels (**initial values principle**). For example, during the first month of an aerobic exercise program, the $\dot{V}O_2$max of a client with poor cardiorespiratory endurance capacity may improve 12% or more, whereas a highly trained endurance athlete may improve only 1% or less.

- **Principle of Interindividual Variability.** Individual responses to a training stimulus are quite variable and depend on a number of factors such as age, initial fitness level, and health status (i.e., **interindividual variability principle**). You therefore must design exercise programs with the specific needs, interests, and abilities of each client in mind and develop personalized exercise prescriptions that take into account individual differences and preferences.

- **Principle of Diminishing Returns.** Each person has a genetic ceiling that limits the extent of improvement that is possible due to exercise training. As individuals approach their genetic ceiling, the rate of improvement in physical fitness slows and eventually levels off (i.e., **diminishing return principle**).

- **Principle of Reversibility.** The positive physiological effects and health benefits of regular physical activity and exercise are reversible. When individuals discontinue their exercise programs (detraining), exercise capacity diminishes quickly, and within a few months most of the training improvements are lost (i.e., **reversibility principle**).

The Art and Science of Exercise Prescription

Traditionally, some exercise specialists have focused on rigidly applying scientific principles of exercise prescription and devoted little or no attention to the *art* of exercise prescription. As an exercise programming artist, you need to be creative, flexible, and able to modify the exercise prescription based on your client's goals, behaviors, and responses to the exercise. Using both a scientific and an artistic approach will enable you to personalize the exercise prescription, increasing the probability of your clients' making long-term commitments to including physical activity and exercise as an indispensable part of their lifestyles.

Basic Elements of the Exercise Prescription

Although prescriptions are individualized for each client, there are basic elements common to all exercise prescriptions. These basic elements include mode, intensity, duration, frequency, and progression.

Mode

As mentioned earlier, the specificity-of-training principle implies that certain types of exercise training are better suited than others to developing specific components of physical fitness. Table 3.2 presents types of training and examples of exercise modes that optimize improvements for each physical fitness component.

To promote changes in body composition, bone health, neuromuscular tension, and stress levels, many experts recommend using more than one type of exercise training. For body composition changes, you should prescribe a combination of aerobic exercise to reduce body fat and resistance exercise to build muscle and bone. Similarly, weight-bearing, aerobic activities and resistance training are both effective for building bone mass for improved bone health. Although many different kinds of physical activity can be used to reduce neuromuscular tension and stress levels (see chapter 11), some experts favor using exercise modes that require focusing on specific muscle groups during the activity to induce a state of relaxation (e.g., progressive relaxation techniques and tai chi).

Intensity

Exercise intensity dictates the specific physiological and metabolic changes in the body during exercise training. As mentioned previously, the initial exercise intensity in the exercise prescription depends on the client's program goals, age, capabilities, preferences, and fitness level and should stress, but not overtax, the cardiopulmonary and musculoskeletal systems (ACSM 2000). Later chapters provide detailed information and guidelines on selecting exercise intensities for the

---

Table 3.2 Types of Training and Exercise Modes for Improving Physical Fitness Components

Physical fitness component	Type of training	Exercise modes
Cardiorespiratory endurance	Aerobic exercise	Walking, jogging, cycling, rowing, stair climbing, simulated cross-country skiing, aerobic dance, and step aerobics
Muscular strength and muscular endurance	Resistance exercise	Free weights and exercise machines
Bone strength	Weight-bearing aerobic exercise and resistance exercise	Walking, jogging, aerobic dance, step aerobics, stair climbing, simulated cross-country skiing, free weights, and exercise machines
Body composition	Aerobic exercise and resistance exercise	Same modes as listed for cardiorespiratory endurance and muscular strength
Flexibility	Stretching exercise	Static stretches and PNF stretches
Neuromuscular relaxation	Relaxation exercises requiring mild physical exertion and concentration	Progressive relaxation exercise and tai chi

PNF = proprioceptive neuromuscular facilitation.

development of each physical fitness component, as well as for the progression of exercise intensity.

Duration

Duration and intensity of exercise are inversely related; the higher the intensity, the shorter the duration of the exercise. Exercise duration depends not only on the intensity of exercise but also on the client's health status, initial fitness level, functional capability, and program goals. For improved health benefits, ACSM and the Centers for Disease Control and Prevention (CDC) recommend that every individual should accumulate 30 min or more of moderate physical activity on most, but preferably all, days of the week (Pate et al. 1995). This amount of physical activity can be achieved in either one continuous bout of exercise or in multiple bouts of shorter duration throughout the day (e.g., 10-min bouts, three times a day), depending on the client's functional capacity and time constraints.

As the client adapts to the exercise training, the duration of exercise may be slowly increased about every two to three weeks. For older and less fit individuals, ACSM (2000) recommends increasing exercise duration, rather than intensity, in the initial stages of the exercise program. For most clients, the duration of aerobic, resistance, and flexibility exercise workouts should not exceed 60 min (ACSM 2000). This will lessen the chance of overuse injuries and exercise "burnout."

Frequency

Frequency typically refers to the total number of weekly exercise sessions. Research shows that exercising three days a week on alternate days is sufficient to improve various components of physical fitness. However, frequency is related to the duration and intensity of exercise and varies depending on the client's program goals and preferences, time constraints, and functional capacity. Sedentary clients with poor initial fitness levels may exercise more than once a day. When improved health is the primary goal of the exercise program, ACSM and CDC recommend daily physical activity of moderate intensity. Therefore, when you prescribe daily physical activity for an apparently healthy client, it is important to vary the type of exercise (i.e., aerobic, resistance, and flexibility exercises) or exercise mode (e.g., walking, cycling, and weightlifting) to lessen the risk of overuse injuries to the bones, joints, and muscles.

Progression of Exercise

Throughout the exercise program, physiological and metabolic changes enable the individual to perform more work. For continued improvements, the cardiopulmonary and musculoskeletal systems must be progressively overloaded through periodic increases in the frequency, intensity, and duration of the exercise.

When applying the principle of progression to an exercise prescription, you should increase the frequency, intensity, and duration gradually, and you should do so one element at a time. A simultaneous increase in frequency, intensity, and duration, or in any combination of these elements, may overtax the individual's physiological systems, thereby increasing the risk of exercise-related injuries and exercise burnout. Generally, for older and less fit clients, it is better to increase exercise duration, instead of exercise intensity, especially during the initial stage of their exercise prescriptions.

Stages of Progression in the Exercise Program

Most individualized exercise programs include initial conditioning, improvement, and maintenance stages. The **initial conditioning stage** typically lasts four weeks and serves as a primer to familiarize the client with exercise training. During this stage, you should prescribe stretching exercises, light calisthenics, and low-intensity aerobic or resistance exercises. Have your clients progress slowly by increasing exercise duration first, followed by small increases in exercise intensity. The initial stage of the exercise program may be skipped for some physically active individuals provided that their initial fitness level is good to excellent and that they are accustomed to the exercise modes prescribed for their programs.

The **improvement stage** of the exercise program typically lasts four to five months, and the rate of progression is more rapid than in the initial conditioning stage. During this stage, the frequency, intensity, and duration are systematically and slowly advanced, one element at a time, until the client's fitness goal is reached.

The **maintenance stage** of the exercise program is designed to maintain the level of fitness achieved by the client at the end of the improvement stage. This stage usually begins six months after the beginning of the exercise program and should continue on a regular, long-term basis. The amount of exercise required to maintain the client's physical fitness level is less than that needed to improve specific fitness components. Thus, the frequency of a specific mode of exercise used to develop any given fitness component can be decreased and that mode replaced with other types of physical activities. By the end of the improvement stage, for example, a client may be jogging five days a week. For maintenance, jogging may be reduced to two or three days a week, and different aerobic activities (e.g., rollerblading and stair climbing) or other types of exercise and sport activities (e.g., weightlifting or tennis) may be substituted the other three days. Including a variety of enjoyable physical activities during this stage helps to counteract boredom and to maintain the client's interest level.

EXERCISE PROGRAM ADHERENCE

Exercise professionals face the challenge of convincing individuals to start exercising and getting them to make a lifelong commitment to a physically active lifestyle. More than three of every five adults (>60%) in the United States do not get the recommended amount of physical activity, and 25% of the adult population report no physical activity at all (U.S. Department of Health and Human Services 1996). Exercise specialists play an important role in educating the public about why regular physical activity is absolutely essential for good health and how to exercise safely and effectively.

Of those individuals starting an exercise program, almost 50% will drop out within one year (ACSM 2000). As an exercise specialist, you must help the client to develop a positive attitude toward physical activity and to make a firm commitment to the exercise program. To increase adherence, you need to be aware of factors related to exercise attrition.

Adherence to an exercise program is related to biological, psychological, behavioral, social, and environmental factors. Predictors of exercise program adherence are listed in "Factors Related to Exercise Program Adherence."

The most critical factors characterizing exercise program dropouts are as follows (Martin and Dubbert 1985):

- Overweight
- Low self-motivation
- Anxiety about exercise
- Lack of spousal support
- The feeling that the exercise facility is inconvenient

Factors Related to Exercise Program Adherence

Biological Factors
Relative body fat
Overweight

Psychological Factors
Self-motivation
Self-efficacy
Attainment of goals
Depression/anxiety/introversion

Social Factors
Family support
Family problems
Exercise/job conflicts
Income and education

Behavioral Factors
Smoking
Leisure time
Credit rating
Type A behavior proneness

Program Factors
Social support (group vs. individual exercise)
Location and convenience of facility
Exercise leadership and supervision
Initial exercise intensity
Variety of exercise modes and activities
Program costs

- Perception that exercise intensity is too high
- Lack of social support during and after exercise

As an exercise specialist, you also need to understand and implement psychological theories related to successful behavior change. These theories are as follows:

- Behavior modification
- Social cognitive theory
- Stages of readiness theory

With use of the **behavior modification theory**, clients become actively involved in the change process by setting realistic short- and long-term goals, developing a plan to achieve these goals, and signing a contract that describes each goal and how it may be achieved. Throughout the exercise program, you should provide your client with feedback and revise the plan as needed. You can help your clients adopt physical activity into their lifestyle by implementing behavior counseling strategies such as having clients keep a diary of their physical activity and developing a social support system for a client. Sometimes it can be effective to give rewards such as T-shirts, certificates, emblems, and pins to recognize the attainment of specific goals, such as walking a total of 50 miles (80.5 km) in one month. Help your client set both short-term and long-term goals that are attainable. For this purpose, you can periodically reevaluate your client's fitness levels to assess improvement. You can state goals in performance or physiological terms. An example of a short-term performance goal is to complete a 3-mile (4.8 km) fun run in less than 33 min. A long-term physiological goal might be to increase maximum oxygen uptake ($\dot{V}O_2$max) by 15% in four months. As the exercise specialist, you must help each individual set realistic goals.

The **social cognitive theory**, developed by Bandura (1982), is based on the concepts of self-efficacy and outcome expectation. The likelihood that people will engage in a specific behavior, like exercising regularly, depends on their **self-efficacy** or perception of their ability to perform the task, as well as their confidence in making the behavioral change (Grembowski et al. 1993). To assess self-efficacy, have your clients rate, on a scale of 0% to 100%, their confidence in making the specific behavior change (ACSM 2000). Individuals with high self-efficacy ratings ($\geq$70%) believe they have the knowledge and skill to exercise successfully. As a result, they are more likely to succeed in making a long-term behavior change. To increase self-efficacy, you should educate your clients so that they fully understand their beliefs and should help them identify specific barriers to engaging in physical activity (Stuhr 1998). Techniques to improve your client's exercise self-efficacy include performance mastery (e.g., teach your clients scientifically sound and safe exercise principles and techniques and allow them to practice these techniques); modeling (e.g., give clients an opportunity to observe role models who are performing the exercise successfully); positive reinforcement (e.g., compliment clients when they perform activities correctly or improve a specific physical fitness component); and emotional arousal (e.g., educate clients about the health benefits of physical activity and exercise). Schlicht, Godin, and

Camaione (1999) provide more detailed descriptions of how you can incorporate these techniques into your clients' exercise programs.

The **readiness for change theory** (Prochaska and DiClemente 1982) has been used successfully to facilitate long-term changes in health behaviors such as smoking, weight management, dietary modifications, and stress management (Riebe and Niggs 1998). This theory states that your clients' ability to make a long-term behavioral change is based on their emotional and intellectual readiness. The following example illustrates the five stages of readiness in terms of making a change in exercise behavior:

1. **Precontemplation:** Client does not exercise and does not intend to start exercising.
2. **Contemplation:** Client is not exercising but intends to start.
3. **Preparation:** Client is exercising but is not meeting the recommended amount of physical activity.
4. **Action:** Client has been performing the recommended amount of exercise regularly for less than six months.
5. **Maintenance:** Client has been exercising regularly at the recommended amount for six months or longer.

As an exercise specialist, you need to integrate principles from each of these theories and implement strategies to improve your clients' exercise program adherence. The ACSM (2000) recommends program modifications and motivational strategies to increase long-term adherence to an exercise program (see "Strategies to Increase Exercise Program Adherence"). The key to increasing exercise program adherence lies in the leadership, education, and motivation that you provide. First, you must be a positive role model. You also must be knowledgeable, able to educate clients about exercise and fitness, and able to provide motivation and encourage social support.

CERTIFICATION AND LICENSURE

Exercise specialists need to have extensive knowledge and technical skills in order to be effective. Historically, individuals working in exercise settings, such as health or fitness clubs, were not necessarily required to have specialized education and training in exercise science. Often, the only prerequisites for employment as a health/fitness in-

Strategies to Increase Exercise Program Adherence

- Recruiting physician support of the exercise program
- Prescribing moderate-intensity exercise to minimize injury and complications
- Advocating exercising with others
- Offering a variety of exercise and fitness activities that are enjoyable
- Providing positive reinforcement through periodic testing
- Recruiting support of the program from clients' families and friends
- Adding optional recreational games to the conditioning program
- Using progress charts to record exercise achievements
- Establishing a reward system to recognize participant accomplishments
- Providing qualified, exercise professionals who are well trained, innovative, and enthusiastic

structor or exercise leader were personal experience with exercise and a lean or muscular body. Over the past 20 years, however, professional organizations such as ACSM have increased public awareness about all aspects of exercise and fitness, including the importance of dealing with highly trained and qualified exercise professionals.

Professional certification and licensure are two ways to ensure the competency of professionals working in the exercise science field. Although many professional organizations offer certification programs for exercise professionals, Louisiana was the first state in the United States to pass a law requiring licensure of all clinical exercise physiologists (Herbert 1995). This requirement places clinical exercise physiologists on a par with other allied health professionals (e.g., nurses, nutritionists, physical therapists, and occupational therapists) who in many states are required to have licenses to practice. In the future, it is highly probable that other states will pass legislation requiring licensure of exercise professionals.

A number of professional organizations (e.g., ACSM, American Society of Exercise Physiologists, National Strength and Conditioning Association, the YMCA of the USA, and the Canadian Society for Exercise Physiology) offer certification workshops and examinations for health/fitness instructors, exercise physiologists, exercise leaders, personal trainers, strength and conditioning specialists, and health/fitness directors working with healthy populations. Appendix A.9 (see p. 288) lists Web site addresses for selected professional organizations. Clinical-track workshops and certifications are also available for exercise specialists and program directors who are working with higher-risk individuals enrolled in exercise rehabilitation programs. Some of these professional certifications require an undergraduate or graduate degree in exercise science or a closely allied field, as well as experience working in health/fitness or clinical settings. Your career goals will dictate which type of professional certification is best for you.

Many advantages are associated with obtaining either state licensure or certification by professional organizations. You will have a better chance of finding a job in the health/fitness field because many employers are now hiring only professionally certified health/fitness instructors. Certification by reputable, professional organizations upgrades the quality of the typical person working in the field and assures employers and their clientele that employees have mastered the knowledge and skills needed to be competent exercise science professionals. Hence, the likelihood of lawsuits resulting from negligence or incompetence may be lessened. Also, certification and licensure help to validate exercise specialists as health professionals who are equally deserving of the respect afforded to professionals in other allied health professions.

KEY POINTS

- The essential components of physical fitness are cardiorespiratory endurance, musculoskeletal fitness, body composition, flexibility, and neuromuscular relaxation.
- Valid, reliable, and objective laboratory and field tests have been developed to assess each fitness component.
- Test validity refers to the ability of a physical fitness test to accurately measure a specific fitness component.

- Test reliability is the ability of a test to yield consistent and stable scores across trials and over time.
- Objective tests give similar test scores when different technicians administer the test to the same client.
- To obtain valid and reliable test results, one must follow standardized testing procedures and have technical skills.
- Established norms for most tests are available and are used to classify physical fitness status based on the client's test scores.
- When interpreting test results to clients, one needs to be positive and to use simple, nontechnical terms.
- To design an effective exercise program, it is necessary to understand and apply training principles. These principles include specificity, overload, progression, initial values, interindividual variability, diminishing returns, and reversibility.
- The basic elements of an exercise prescription are mode, intensity, duration, and frequency.

- The exercise prescription should be individualized to meet the needs, interests, and abilities of the client.
- The three stages of an exercise program are initial conditioning, improvement, and maintenance.
- Throughout the improvement stage of an exercise program, the frequency, intensity, and duration of exercise are increased, one at a time.
- Exercise adherence is related to biological, psychological, behavioral, social, environmental, and program factors.
- When developing strategies for increasing exercise program adherence, it is important to integrate principles and concepts from the behavior modification, social cognitive, and readiness for change theories.
- Professional certification and licensure are two ways to ensure competency of professionals working in the exercise science field.

KEY TERMS

Learn the definition for each of the following terms. Definitions of key terms can be found in "Glossary of Terms," page 349.

behavior modification theory
body composition
body weight
bone strength
cardiorespiratory endurance
criterion method
diminishing return principle
flexibility
generalized equations
improvement stage
initial conditioning stage
initial values principle
interindividual variability principle
line of best fit
maintenance stage
maximum oxygen consumption
multiple correlation coefficient
muscular endurance
muscular strength

musculoskeletal fitness
neuromuscular relaxation
objectivity
objectivity coefficient
overload principle
physical fitness
population-specific equations
progression principle
readiness for change theory
reference method
regression line
reliability
reliability coefficient
reversibility principle
self-efficacy
social cognitive theory
specificity principle
standard error of estimate
validity
validity coefficient

REVIEW QUESTIONS

In addition to being able to define the key terms, test your knowledge and understanding of the material by answering the following review questions.

1. Define physical fitness. Name and define the five components of physical fitness.

2. What is the recommended sequence of testing for administering a complete physical fitness test battery?

3. Identify the reference or criterion method for each of the five components of physical fitness.

4. Which is more important: test validity or test reliability? Explain your choice.

5. Select one physical fitness component and explain how you can determine the relative worth or predictive accuracy of a field test developed to assess this component.

6. Select one physical fitness component and give an example of how each of the seven training principles can be applied to this component.

7. Identify exercise modes suitable to develop each of the five components of fitness.

8. Identify the three elements of an exercise prescription. For older or less fit clients, which of the elements should be increased first during the initial stage of their exercise programs?

9. Name the three stages of an exercise program. On average, how long should each stage last?

10. Identify three of the most critical factors characterizing exercise program dropouts.

11. Choose one of the psychological theories related to successful behavior change and give specific examples of how this theory could be applied to a client undertaking a resistance training program to develop muscular fitness.

12. What are the advantages of becoming a professionally certified exercise scientist?

REFERENCES

American College of Sports Medicine (ACSM). 2000. *ACSM's guidelines for exercise testing and prescription*. Philadelphia: Lippincott Williams & Wilkins.

Bandura, A. 1982. Self-efficacy mechanism in human agency. *American Psychologist* 37: 122–147.

Fenstermaker, K., Plowman, S., and Looney, M. 1992. Validation of the Rockport walking test in females 65 years and older. *Research Quarterly for Exercise and Sport* 63: 322–327.

Grembowski, D., Patrick, D., Diehr, P., Durham, M., Beresford, S., Kay, E., and Hecht, J. 1993. Self-efficacy and health behavior among older adults. *Journal of Health and Social Behavior* 34(6): 89–104.

Herbert, D.L. 1995. First state licenses exercise physiologists. *Fitness Management,* October, 26–27.

Jackson, A.S., and Pollock, M.L. 1985. Practical assessment of body composition. *The Physician and Sportsmedicine* 13: 76–90.

Jackson, A.S., Pollock, M.L., and Ward, A. 1980. Generalized equations for predicting body density of women. *Medicine & Science in Sports & Exercise* 12: 175–182.

Jackson, A.W., and Langford, N.J. 1989. The criterion-related validity of the sit-and-reach test: Replica-

tion and extension of previous findings. *Research Quarterly for Exercise and Sport* 60: 384–387.

Kline, G.M., Porcari, J.P., Hintermeister, R., Freedson, P.S., Ward, A., McCarron, R.F., Ross, J. and Rippe, J.M. 1987. Estimation of $\dot{V}O_2$max from a one-mile track walk, gender, age, and body weight. *Medicine & Science in Sports & Exercise* 19: 253–259.

Lohman, T.G., Roche, A.F., and Martorell, R., eds. 1988. *Anthropometric standardization reference manual*. Champaign, IL: Human Kinetics.

Martin, J.E., and Dubbert, P.M. 1985. Adherence to exercise. In *Exercise and Sport Sciences Reviews,* ed. R.L. Terjung, 13: 137–167. New York: Academic Press.

Pate, R.R., Pratt, M., Blair, S.N., Haskell, W.L., Macera, C.A., Bouchard, C., Buchner, D., Ettinger, W., Heath, G.W., and King, A.C. 1995. Physical activity and public health: A recommendation from the Centers for Disease Control and Prevention and the American College of Sports Medicine. *Journal of the American Medical Association* 273: 402–407.

Prochaska, J.O., and DiClemente, C.C. 1982. Transtheoretical therapy: Toward a more integrative model of change. *Psychotherapy: Theory, Research, and Practice* 19: 276–288.

Riebe, D., and Niggs, C. 1998. Setting the stage for healthy living. *ACSM's Health & Fitness Journal* 2(3): 11–15.

Schlicht, J., Godin, J., and Camaione, D.C. 1999. How to help your client stick with an exercise program: Build self-efficacy to promote exercise adherence. *ACSM's Health & Fitness Journal* 3(6): 27–31.

Stuhr, R.M. 1998. Strategies for beating the barriers to exercise in women. *ACSM's Health & Fitness Journal* 2(5): 20–29, 51.

U.S. Department of Health and Human Services. 1996. *Physical activity and health: A report of the Surgeon General.* Atlanta: U.S. Department of Health and Human Services, Centers for Disease Control and Prevention, National Center for Chronic Disease Prevention and Health Promotion.

Assessing Cardiorespiratory Fitness

One of the most important components of physical fitness is cardiorespiratory endurance. **Cardiorespiratory endurance** is the ability to perform dynamic exercise involving large muscle groups at moderate-to-high intensity for prolonged periods (ACSM 2000). Every physical fitness evaluation should include an assessment of cardiorespiratory function during both rest and exercise.

This chapter presents guidelines for graded exercise testing, as well as maximal and submaximal exercise test protocols and procedures. Although many of the graded exercise test protocols presented in this chapter were developed years ago, these classic protocols are still widely used in research and clinical settings. In addition, each of these protocols meets the current ACSM (2000) guidelines for graded exercise tests. The chapter also addresses graded exercise testing for children and older adults and includes a discussion of car-

diorespiratory field tests. All of the test protocols included in this chapter are summarized in appendix B.1, "Summary of Graded Exercise Test and Cardiorespiratory Field Test Protocols," on page 290.

DEFINITION OF TERMS

Exercise physiologists consider directly measured **maximum oxygen uptake ($\dot{V}O_2$max)** or **peak $\dot{V}O_2$** the most valid measure of functional capacity of the cardiorespiratory system.

The **$\dot{V}O_2$max,** or rate of oxygen uptake during maximal aerobic exercise, reflects

1. the capacity of the heart, lungs, and blood to transport oxygen to the working muscles; and

2. the utilization of oxygen by the muscles during exercise.

Maximal and submaximal $\dot{V}O_2$ is expressed in absolute or relative terms. **Absolute** $\dot{V}O_2$ is measured in liters per minute ($L \cdot min^{-1}$) or milliliters per minute ($ml \cdot min^{-1}$) and provides a measure of energy cost for non-weight-bearing activities such as leg or arm cycle ergometry. Absolute $\dot{V}O_2$ is directly related to body size; thus men typically have a larger absolute $\dot{V}O_2$max than women.

To compare individuals who differ in body size, $\dot{V}O_2$ is expressed relative to body weight, that is, as $ml \cdot kg^{-1} \cdot min^{-1}$. **Relative** $\dot{V}O_2$ is used to estimate the energy cost of weight-bearing activities such as walking, running, aerobic dancing, stair climbing, and bench stepping. Sometimes $\dot{V}O_2$ is expressed relative to the individual's fat-free mass (see chapter 8), that is, as $ml \cdot kg \cdot FFM^{-1} \cdot min^{-1}$. For example, your client's improvement in relative $\dot{V}O_2$max following a 16-week aerobic exercise program may reflect both improved capacity of the cardiorespiratory system (increase in absolute $\dot{V}O_2$max) and weight loss (increase in relative $\dot{V}O_2$ expressed as $ml \cdot kg^{-1} \cdot min^{-1}$ due to a decrease in body weight). Thus, expressing $\dot{V}O_2$max relative to fat-free mass, instead of body weight, provides you with an estimate of cardiorespiratory endurance that is independent of changes in body weight.

The rate of oxygen consumption can also be expressed as a **gross** $\dot{V}O_2$ or **net** $\dot{V}O_2$. Gross $\dot{V}O_2$ is the total rate of oxygen consumption and reflects the caloric costs of both rest and exercise (gross $\dot{V}O_2$ = resting $\dot{V}O_2$ + exercise $\dot{V}O_2$). On the other hand, net $\dot{V}O_2$ represents the rate of oxygen consumption in excess of the resting $\dot{V}O_2$ and is used to describe the caloric cost of the exercise. Both gross and net $\dot{V}O_2$ can be expressed in either absolute (e.g., $L \cdot min^{-1}$) or relative ($ml \cdot kg^{-1} \cdot min^{-1}$) terms. Unless specified as a net $\dot{V}O_2$, the $\dot{V}O_2$ values reported throughout this book refer to gross $\dot{V}O_2$.

GRADED EXERCISE TESTING: GUIDELINES AND PROCEDURES

Exercise scientists and physicians use exercise tests to evaluate functional aerobic capacity ($\dot{V}O_2$max) objectively. The $\dot{V}O_2$max, determined from graded maximal or submaximal exercise tests, is used to classify the cardiorespiratory fitness level of your client (see table 4.1). You can use baseline and follow-up data to evaluate the progress of exercise program participants and to set realistic goals for your clients. You can use the heart rate (HR) and oxygen uptake data obtained during the graded exercise test to make accurate, precise exercise prescriptions.

As discussed in chapter 2, before the start of a vigorous (>60% $\dot{V}O_2$max) exercise program, ACSM

Table 4.1   Cardiorespiratory Fitness Classification: Maximal Oxygen Uptake ($ml \cdot kg^{-1} \cdot min^{-1}$)

Age (years)	Poor	Fair	Good	Excellent	Superior
Women					
20-29	≤31	32-34	35-37	38-41	42+
30-39	≤29	30-32	33-35	36-39	40+
40-49	≤27	28-30	31-32	33-36	37+
50-59	≤24	25-27	28-29	30-32	33+
60+	≤23	24-25	26-27	28-31	32+
Men					
20-29	≤37	38-41	42-44	45-48	49+
30-39	≤35	36-39	40-42	43-47	48+
40-49	≤33	34-37	38-40	41-44	45+
50-59	≤30	31-34	35-37	38-41	42+
60+	≤26	27-30	31-34	35-38	39+

The Physical Fitness Specialist Certification Manual, The Cooper Institute for Aerobics Research, Dallas, TX, revised 1997.

(2000) recommends a graded **maximal exercise test** for

- older men (≥45 years) and women (≥55 years),
- individuals of any age with moderate risk (two or more coronary heart disease risk factors),
- high-risk individuals with one or more signs/symptoms of cardiovascular and pulmonary disease, and
- high-risk individuals with known cardiovascular, pulmonary, or metabolic disease.

However, you may use **submaximal exercise tests** for low-risk individuals, as well as clients with moderate risk, if they are starting a moderate (40% to 60% $\dot{V}O_2$max) exercise program (ACSM 2000). For medical conditions that are absolute and relative contraindications to exercise testing, see chapter 2, page 18.

General Guidelines for Exercise Testing

You may use a maximal or submaximal **graded exercise test** (GXT) to assess the cardiorespiratory fitness of the individual. The selection of a maximal or submaximal GXT depends on

- your client's age and risk stratification (low risk, moderate risk, or high risk),
- your reasons for administering the test (physical fitness testing or clinical testing), and
- the availability of appropriate equipment and qualified personnel.

In clinical and research settings, $\dot{V}O_2$max is typically measured directly and requires expensive equipment and experienced personnel. Although $\dot{V}O_2$max can be predicted from maximal exercise intensity with a fair degree of accuracy, submaximal tests also provide a reasonable estimate of your client's cardiorespiratory fitness level and are less costly, time consuming, and risky. Submaximal exercise testing, however, is considered less sensitive as a diagnostic tool for coronary heart disease (CHD).

In either case, the exercise test should be a multistage, graded test. This means that the individual exercises at gradually increasing submaximal workloads. Many commonly used exercise test protocols require that each workload be performed for 3 min. The GXT measures maximum aerobic capacity ($\dot{V}O_2$max) when the oxygen uptake plateaus and does not increase by more than 150 ml·min^{-1} with a further increase in workload. Other criteria (ACSM 2000) used to indicate the attainment of $\dot{V}O_2$max are the following:

- Failure of the HR to increase with increases in exercise intensity
- Venous lactate concentration exceeding 8 mmol/L
- **Respiratory exchange ratio** (RER) greater than 1.15
- Rating of perceived exertion greater than 17 using the original Borg scale (6-20)

During GXTs, many individuals are unable to attain a true plateau in $\dot{V}O_2$ (Robergs and Roberts 2000). If the test is terminated before the person reaches a plateau in $\dot{V}O_2$ and an RER greater than 1.15, the GXT is a measure of $\dot{V}O_2$peak rather than $\dot{V}O_2$max. Children, older adults, sedentary individuals, and clients with known disease are more likely than other groups to attain a $\dot{V}O_2$peak rather than a $\dot{V}O_2$max. For CHD screening and classification purposes, bringing a person to at least 85% of the age-predicted maximal HR is desirable, because some electrocardiogram (ECG) abnormalities do not appear until the HR reaches this level of intensity (Pollock, Wilmore, and Fox 1978).

Evidence suggests that maximal exercise tests are no more dangerous than submaximal tests (Pollock et al. 1978; Rochmis and Blackburn 1971; Shephard 1977), provided you carefully follow guidelines for exercise tolerance testing and monitor the physiological responses of the exercise participant continuously. Shephard (1977) predicted one fatality in every 10 to 20 years for a population of 5 million middle-aged Canadians who undergo maximal exercise testing. For high-risk patients, he estimated 1 fibrillation per 5000 submaximal exercise tests and 1 fibrillation per 3000 maximal exercise tests. For clinical testing, the risk of an exercise test being fatal is approximately 0.4 to 0.5 per 10,000 tests (Atterhog, Jonsson, and Samuelsson 1979; Rochmis and Blackburn 1971), and the risk of myocardial infarction is estimated to be 4 per 10,000 tests (Thompson 1993). The risk for apparently healthy individuals (without known disease) is very low, with no complications occurring in 380,000 exercise tests done on young individuals (Levine, Zuckerman, and Cole 1998).

General Procedures for Cardiorespiratory Fitness Testing

At least one day before the exercise test, you should give your client pretest instructions (see chapter 3, p. 39). Prior to graded exercise testing, the client should read and sign the informed consent and complete the PAR-Q; see appendix A.1, "Physical Activity Readiness Questionnaire (Par-Q)," p. 260).

Step-by-step procedures, as recommended by ACSM (2000), for administering a GXT are listed below.

Pretest, exercise, and recovery HRs can be measured using the palpation or auscultation techniques (see chapter 2) if a heart rate monitor or ECG recorder is unavailable. Because of extraneous noise and vibration during exercise, it may be difficult to obtain accurate measurements of BP, especially when your client is running on the treadmill. To become proficient at taking exercise BP, you need to practice as much as possible.

To obtain **ratings of perceived exertions** during exercise testing, you can use either the original (6 to 20) or revised (0 to 10) RPE scale (see table 4.2). These scales allow clients to rate their degree of exertion subjectively during exercise and are highly related to exercise HRs and $\dot{V}O_2$. Both RPE scales take into account the linear rise in HR and $\dot{V}O_2$ during exercise. The revised scale also reflects nonlinear changes in blood lactate and ventilation during exercise. Ratings of 10 on the revised scale and 19 on the original scale usually correspond with the maximal level of exercise. Ratings of perceived exertion are useful in determining the end points of the GXT, particularly for patients who are taking beta-blockers or other medications that may alter the HR response to exercise. You can teach your clients how to use the RPE scale to monitor relative intensities during aerobic exercise programs.

Test Termination

In a maximal or submaximal GXT, the exercise usually continues until the client voluntarily terminates the test or a predetermined end point is reached. As an exercise technician, however, you must be acutely aware of all indicators for stopping a test. If you notice any of the signs or symptoms listed on page 54, you should stop the exercise test prior to the client's reaching $\dot{V}O_2$max (for a maximal GXT) or the predetermined end point (for a submaximal GXT).

General Procedures for Clinical Exercise Testing

You can use a maximal GXT for diagnostic and functional testing in order to determine safe levels of exercise for clients with or without heart

---

PROCEDURES FOR ADMINISTERING A GRADED EXERCISE TEST

- Measure the client's resting HR and blood pressure (BP) (see chapter 2 for these procedures).

- Begin the GXT with a 2- to 3-min warm-up to familiarize clients with the exercise equipment and prepare them for the first stage of the exercise test.

- During the test, monitor HR, BP, and ratings of perceived exertion (RPEs) at regular intervals. Measure exercise HR at least two times during each stage of the test, near the end of the minute. Assess exercise BP and RPE near the end of each exercise stage. Throughout the exercise test, continuously monitor the client's physical appearance and symptoms.

- Discontinue the GXT when the test termination criteria are reached, if the client requests stopping the test, or if any of the indications for stopping an exercise test are apparent (see p. 54).

- Have the client cool down by exercising at a low work rate that does not exceed the intensity of the first stage of the exercise test (e.g., walking on the treadmill at 2 mph [53.6 m·min^{-1}] and 0% grade or cycling on the bicycle ergometer at 50 to 60 revolutions per minute [rpm] and zero resistance). Active recovery reduces the risk of hypotension from venous pooling in the extremities.

- During recovery, continue measuring postexercise HR, BP, and RPE every 1 to 2 min for at least 4 min, or longer if there are any abnormal responses. The HR and BP during active recovery should be stable but may be higher than pre-exercise levels. Continue monitoring the client's physical appearance during recovery.

- If your client has signs of discomfort or if an emergency occurs, use a passive cool-down with the client in a sitting or supine position.

Table 4.2   Ratings of Perceived Exertion Scale and Category-Ratio Scale

RPE scale		CR10 scale		
6	No exertion at all	0	Nothing at all	"No P"
7		0.3		
	Extremely light	0.5	Extremely weak	Just noticeable
8		1	Very weak	
9	Very light	1.5		
10		2	Weak	Light
11	Light	2.5		
12		3	Moderate	
13	Somewhat hard	4		
14		5	Strong	Heavy
15	Hard (heavy)	6		
16		7	Very strong	
17	Very hard	8		
18		9		
19	Extremely hard	10	Extremely strong	"Max P"
20	Maximal exertion	11		
	Borg RPE scale © Gunnar Borg, 1970, 1985, 1994, 1998	●	Absolute maximum	Highest possible
			Borg CR10 scale © Gunnar Borg, 1981, 1982, 1998	

For correct instruction and administration see Borg's book: Borg, G. (1998), *Borg's Perceived Exertion and Pain Scales*, Champaign, IL: Human Kinetics.

disease. For clinical testing, measure both the BP and 12-lead ECG (see chapter 2 for these procedures) in the supine and exercise postures prior to exercise testing. During exercise, monitor and record the 12-lead ECG during the last 15 sec of each exercise stage and at peak exercise. Monitor the exercise BP and RPE at regular intervals as previously described for physical fitness testing. In addition, whenever symptoms or ECG changes occur during exercise, record the 12-lead ECG, HR, BP, and RPE (ACSM 2000). If you notice any of the signs or symptoms listed in "Absolute and Relative Indications for Termination of a Clinical Graded Exercise Test"on page 54, the exercise test should be stopped immediately. ST-segment elevation with a horizontal or downward slope is indicative of severe CHD or coronary spasm. Horizontal or downsloping ST-segment depression (>2

mm) reflects myocardial ischemia. The onset, duration, and magnitude of the ST-segment depression are related to the severity of the ischemia. Failure of systolic BP to rise, or a significant drop in systolic BP (20 mm Hg) during the exercise test, is an indicator of CHD or heart failure (Hanson 1988).

Immediately following exercise, record a 10-sec ECG. Then monitor and record the ECG every 1 to 2 min for at least 5 min. Measure BP immediately after exercise and then every 1 to 2 min until it stabilizes near baseline levels. If your clients are having difficulty breathing, they should sit down. Even though an active cool-down may decrease hypotension, it is not recommended following a GXT that is given for diagnostic purposes because active cool-down may increase the magnitude of ST-segment depression.

Absolute and Relative Indications for Termination of a Clinical Graded Exercise Test[a]

Absolute Indications

1. Moderate-to-severe angina
2. Drop in systolic blood pressure of ≥10 mm Hg from baseline blood pressure despite an increase in workload, when accompanied by other evidence of ischemia
3. Increasing nervous system symptoms (e.g., ataxia, dizziness, or near syncope)
4. Signs of poor perfusion (cyanosis or pallor)
5. Technical difficulties monitoring the electrocardiogram or systolic blood pressure
6. Client's desire to stop
7. Sustained ventricular tachycardia
8. ST elevation (≥1.0 mm) in leads without diagnostic Q waves (other than V_1 or aVR)

Relative Indications

1. Drop in systolic blood pressure of ≥10 mm Hg from baseline blood pressure despite an increase in workload, in the absence of other evidence of ischemia
2. Increasing chest pain
3. Fatigue, shortness of breath, wheezing, leg cramps, or claudication
4. Hypertensive response (systolic blood pressure >250 mmHg and/or diastolic blood pressure >115 mmHg)
5. Arrhythmias other than sustained ventricular tachycardia, including multifocal preventricular contractions (PVCs), triplets of PVCs, supraventricular tachycardia, heart block, or bradyarrhythmias
6. Development of bundle-branch block or intraventricular conduction delay that cannot be distinguished from ventricular tachycardia
7. ST or QRS changes such as excessive ST-segment depression (>2 mm horizontal or downsloping ST-segment depression) or marked axis shift

[a]For definitions of specific terms, refer to "Glossary of Terms," page 349.

From Gibbons, R.J. et al. 1997. ACC/AHA Guidelines for exercise testing. A report of the American College of Cardiology/American Heart Association Task Force on Practice Guidelines (Committee on Exercise Testing). *Journal of the American College of Cardiology* 30: 260-311.

MAXIMAL EXERCISE TEST PROTOCOLS

Many maximal exercise test protocols have been devised to assess aerobic capacity. As the exercise technician, you must be able to select an exercise mode and test protocol that is suitable for your clients given their age, gender, and health and fitness status. Commonly used modes of exercise are treadmill walking or running and stationary cycling. Arm ergometry is useful for persons with paraplegia and clients who have limited use of the lower extremities. Bench stepping is not highly recommended but could be useful in field situations when large groups need to be tested. Whichever mode of exercise you choose, be sure to adhere to "General Principles of Exercise Testing" (see p. 55).

The exercise test may be continuous or discontinuous. A continuous test is performed with no rest between work increments. Continuous exercise tests can vary in the duration of each exercise stage and the magnitude of the increment in exercise intensity between stages. The total test duration should be between 8 and 12 min to increase the probability of the individual's reaching $\dot{V}O_2$max. For most continuous exercise test protocols, the exercise intensity is increased gradually (2 to 3 METs for low-risk individuals) throughout the test, and the duration of each stage is usually 2 to 3 min. In contrast, ramp protocols continuously increase intensity each minute during the exercise test and are individually designed to

GENERAL PRINCIPLES OF EXERCISE TESTING

1. Typically, you will use either a treadmill or stationary bicycle ergometer for graded exercise testing (GXT). All equipment should be calibrated before use.

2. Begin the GXT with a 2- to 3-min warm-up to orient the client to the equipment and prepare the client for the first stage of the GXT.

3. The initial exercise intensity should be considerably lower than the anticipated maximal capacity.

4. Exercise intensity should be increased gradually throughout the stages of the test. Work increments may be 2 METs or greater for apparently healthy individuals and as small as 0.5 MET for patients with disease.

5. Closely observe contraindications for testing and indications for stopping the exercise test. When in any doubt about the safety or benefits of testing, do not perform the test at that time.

6. Monitor the heart rate at least two times, but preferably each minute, during each stage of the GXT. Heart rate measurements should be taken near the end of each minute. If the heart rate does not reach steady state (two heart rates within ±5-6 bpm), extend the work stage an additional minute, or until the heart rate stabilizes.

7. Measure blood pressure and RPE once during each stage of the GXT, in the later portion of the stage.

8. Continually monitor client appearance and symptoms.

9. For submaximal GXTs, terminate the test when the client's heart rate reaches 70% HRR or 85% HRmax, unless the protocol specifies a different termination criterion. Also, stop the test immediately if there is an emergency situation, if the client fails to conform to the exercise protocol, or if the client experiences signs of discomfort.

10. The test should include a cool-down period of at least 4 min, or longer if abnormal heart rate and blood pressure responses are observed. During recovery, heart rate and blood pressure should be monitored each minute. For active recovery, the workload should be no more than that used during the first stage of the GXT. A passive recovery is used in emergency situations and when clients experience signs of discomfort and cannot perform an active cool-down.

11. Exercise tolerance in METs should be estimated for the treadmill or ergometer protocol used, or directly assessed if oxygen uptake is measured during the GXT.

12. The testing area should be quiet and private. The room temperature should be 21 to 23 °C (70 to 72 °F) or less and the humidity 60% or less if possible.

ensure that the total duration of the exercise test does not exceed 12 min for each client. To design an individualized ramp protocol, you need to estimate your client's maximal exercise intensity based on his training history to determine how much the workload needs to be increased each minute during the test (Robergs and Roberts 2000). For discontinuous tests, the client is given a 5- to 10-min rest interval between workloads. On average, discontinuous tests take five times longer to administer than continuous tests.

McArdle, Katch, and Pechar (1973) compared the $\dot{V}O_2$max scores as measured by six commonly used continuous and discontinuous treadmill and bicycle ergometer tests. They noted that the $\dot{V}O_{2vv}$max scores for the bike ergometer tests were approximately 6% to 11% lower than for the treadmill tests. Many subjects identified local discomfort and fatigue in the thigh muscles as the major factors limiting further work on both the continuous and discontinuous bicycle ergometer tests. For the treadmill tests, subjects indicated windedness and general fatigue as the limiting factors and complained of localized fatigue and discomfort in the calf muscles and lower back.

Treadmill Maximal Exercise Tests

The exercise is performed on a motor-driven treadmill with variable speed and incline (see figure 4.1). Speed varies up to 25 mph, and incline is measured in units of elevation per 100 horizontal units and

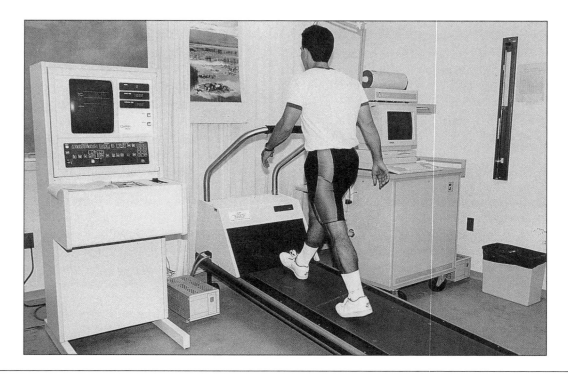

Figure 4.1 Treadmill.

is expressed as a percentage. The workload on the treadmill is raised through increases in the speed or incline or both. Workload is usually expressed in miles per hour and percent grade.

It is difficult and expensive to measure the oxygen consumption during exercise. Therefore, ACSM (2000) has developed equations (table 4.3) to estimate the metabolic cost of exercise ($\dot{V}O_2$). These equations provide a valid estimate of $\dot{V}O_2$ for steady-state exercise only. When used to estimate the maximum rate of energy expenditure ($\dot{V}O_2$max), the measured $\dot{V}O_2$ will be less than the estimated $\dot{V}O_2$ if steady state is not reached. Also, because maximal exercise involves both aerobic and anaerobic components, the $\dot{V}O_2$max will be overestimated since the contribution of the anaerobic component is not known.

Before using any of the ACSM metabolic equations to estimate $\dot{V}O_2$, make certain that all units of measure match those in the equation (see p. 57).

The ACSM metabolic equations in table 4.3 are useful in clinical settings for estimating the total rate of energy expenditure (gross $\dot{V}O_2$) during steady-state treadmill walking or running. The total energy expenditure, in ml·kg⁻¹·min⁻¹, is a function of three components: *speed, grade,* and *resting energy expenditures.* For treadmill walking, the oxygen cost of raising one's body mass against

CONVERTING UNITS OF MEASURE

- Convert body mass (M) in pounds to kilograms (1 kg = 2.2 lb). For example, 170 lb/2.2 = 77.3 kg.
- Convert treadmill speed (S) in miles per hour to meters per minute (1 mph = 26.8 m/min). For example, 5.0 mph × 26.8 = 134.0 m·min⁻¹.
- Convert treadmill grade (G) from percent to decimal form by dividing by 100. For example, 12%/100 = 0.12.
- Convert METs to ml·kg⁻¹·min⁻¹ by multiplying (1 MET = 3.5 ml·kg⁻¹·min⁻¹). For example, 6 METs × 3.5 = 21.0 ml·kg⁻¹·min⁻¹.
- Convert kgm·min⁻¹ to watts (W) (1 W = 6 kgm·min⁻¹) by dividing. For example, 900 kgm·min⁻¹/6 = 150 W.
- Convert step height in inches to meters (1 in. = 0.0254 m) by multiplying. For example, 8 in. × 0.0254 = 0.2032 m.

gravity (vertical work) is approximately 1.8 ml·kg⁻¹·m⁻¹, and 0.1 ml·kg⁻¹·m⁻¹ of oxygen is needed to move the body horizontally. For treadmill running, the oxygen cost for vertical work is one-half that for treadmill walking (0.9 ml·kg⁻¹·m⁻¹), whereas the

Table 4.3   Metabolic Equations for Estimating Gross $\dot{V}O_2$ (ACSM 2000)

Exercise mode Gross $\dot{V}O_2$ (ml·kg⁻¹·min⁻¹)	Resting $\dot{V}O_2$ (ml·kg⁻¹·min⁻¹)	Comments
Walking $\dot{V}O_2$ $= S^a \times 0.1 + S \times G^b \times 1.8$	+ 3.5	1. For speeds of 50-100 m·min⁻¹ (1.9-3.7 mph) 2. 0.1 ml·kg⁻¹·m⁻¹ = O_2 cost of walking horizontally 3. 1.8 ml·kg⁻¹·m⁻¹ = O_2 cost of walking on incline (% grade of treadmill)
Running $\dot{V}O_2$ $= S^a \times 0.2 + S \times G^b \times 0.9$	+ 3.5	1. For speeds >134 m·min⁻¹ (>5.0 mph) 2. If truly jogging (not walking), this equation can also be used for speeds of 80-134 m·min⁻¹ (3-5 mph) 3. 0.2 ml·kg⁻¹·m⁻¹ = O_2 cost of running horizontally 4. 0.9 ml·kg⁻¹·m⁻¹ = O_2 cost of running on incline (% grade of treadmill)
Leg ergometry $\dot{V}O_2$ $= W^c/M^d \times 10.8 + 3.5$	+ 3.5	1. For work rates between 50 and 200 W (300-1200 kgm·min⁻¹) 2. kgm·min⁻¹ = kg × m/rev × rev/min 3. Monark and Bodyguard = 6 m/rev; Tunturi = 3 m/rev 4. 10.8 ml·kg⁻¹·W⁻¹ = O_2 cost of cycling against external load (resistance) 5. 3.5 ml·kg⁻¹·min⁻¹ = O_2 cost of cycling with zero load
Arm ergometry $\dot{V}O_2$ $= W^c/M^d \times 18.0 + None$	+ 3.5	1. For work rates between 25 and 125 W (150-750 kgm·min⁻¹) 2. kgm·min⁻¹ = kg × m/rev × rev/min 3. 18.0 ml·kg⁻¹·W⁻¹ = O_2 cost of cycling against external load (resistance) 4. None = due to small mass of arm musculature, no special term for unloaded (zero load) cycling is needed
Stepping $\dot{V}O_2$ $= F^e \times 0.2 + F \times ht^f \times 1.8 \times 1.33$	+ 3.5	1. Appropriate for stepping rates between 12 and 30 steps/min and step heights between 0.04 m (1.6 in.) and 0.40 m (15.7 in.) 2. 0.2 ml·kg⁻¹·m⁻¹ = O_2 cost of moving horizontally 3. 1.8 ml·kg⁻¹·m⁻¹ = O_2 cost of stepping up (bench height) 4. 1.33 includes positive component of stepping up (1.0) + negative component of stepping down (0.33)

ᵃS = speed of treadmill in m·min⁻¹; 1 mph = 26.8 m·min⁻¹.

ᵇG = grade (% incline) of treadmill in decimal form; e.g., 10% = 0.10.

ᶜW = power output in watts; 1 W = 6 kgm·min⁻¹.

ᵈM = body mass in kilograms; 1 kg = 2.2 lb.

ᵉF = frequency of stepping in steps per minute.

ᶠht = bench height in meters; 1 in. = 0.0254 m.

energy expenditure for running on the treadmill (0.2 ml·kg⁻¹·m⁻¹) is twice that for walking. See page 58 for an example of how to take these three factors into account when figuring $\dot{V}O_2$.

The $\dot{V}O_2$ estimated from the ACSM walking equation (see table 4.3) is reasonably accurate for walking speeds between 50 and 100 m·min⁻¹ (1.9 to 3.7 mph). However, since the equation is more accurate for walking up a grade than on the level, $\dot{V}O_2$ may be underestimated as much as 15% to 20% during walking on the level (ACSM 2000). For the ACSM running/jogging equations, the $\dot{V}O_2$ estimates are relatively accurate for speeds exceeding 134 m·min⁻¹ (5 mph) and speeds as low as 80

ACSM WALKING EQUATION

To calculate the gross $\dot{V}O_2$ for a 70-kg subject who is walking on the treadmill at a speed of 3.5 mph and a grade of 10%, follow these steps:

$\dot{V}O_2$ = speed + (grade $\times$ speed)
+ resting $\dot{V}O_2$ (ml·kg^{-1}·min^{-1})
= [speed (m·min^{-1}) $\times$ 0.1] + [grade (decimal) $\times$ speed (m·min^{-1}) $\times$ 1.8] + 3.5

1. Convert the speed in mph to m·min^{-1}; 1 mph = 26.8 m·min^{-1}.

$$3.5 \text{ mph} \times 26.8 = 93.8 \text{ m·min}^{-1}$$

2. Calculate the speed component (S).

S = speed (m·min^{-1}) $\times$ 0.1
= 93.8 m·min^{-1} $\times$ 0.1
= 9.38 ml·kg^{-1}·min^{-1}

3. Calculate the grade $\times$ speed component (G $\times$ S). Convert % grade into a decimal by dividing by 100.

G $\times$ S = grade (decimal) $\times$ speed $\times$ 1.8
= 0.10 $\times$ (93.8 m·min^{-1}) $\times$ 1.8
= 16.88 ml·kg^{-1}·min^{-1}

4. Calculate the total gross $\dot{V}O_2$ in ml·kg^{-1}·min^{-1} by adding the speed, grade $\times$ speed, and resting $\dot{V}O_2$ (R).

$\dot{V}O_2$ = S + (S $\times$ G) + R
= (9.38 + 16.88 + 3.5) ml·kg^{-1}·min^{-1}
= 29.76 ml·kg^{-1}·min^{-1}

m·min^{-1} (3 mph) provided that the client is jogging and not walking (ACSM 2000).

Figure 4.2 illustrates commonly used treadmill exercise test protocols. These protocols conform to the general guidelines for maximal exercise testing. Some of the protocols are designed for a specific population, such as well-conditioned athletes or high-risk cardiac patients. The exercise intensity for each stage of the various treadmill test protocols can be expressed in METs. The MET estimations for each stage of some commonly used treadmill protocols are listed in table 4.4.

Population-specific and generalized equations have been developed to estimate $\dot{V}O_2$max from exercise time for some treadmill protocols (see table 4.5). It is important for exercise technicians to keep in mind that the initial workload in some of the protocols designed for highly trained athletes is too intense (exceeding 2 to 3.5 METs) for the average individual. The Balke and Bruce protocols are well suited for low-risk individuals, and the Bruce protocol is easily adapted for high-risk individuals using an initial workload of 1.7 mph at 0% to 5% grade.

Balke Treadmill Protocol

To administer the Balke and Ware (1959) exercise test protocol (see figure 4.2), set the treadmill speed at 3.4 mph (91.1 m·min^{-1}) and the initial grade of the treadmill at 0% during the first minute of exercise. Maintain a constant speed on the treadmill throughout the entire exercise test. At the start of the second minute of exercise, increase the grade to 2%. Thereafter, at the beginning of every additional minute of exercise, increase the grade by only 1%.

Use the prediction equation for the Balke protocol in table 4.5 to estimate your client's $\dot{V}O_2$max from exercise time. Alternatively, you can use a nomogram (see figure 4.3) developed for the Balke treadmill protocol to calculate the $\dot{V}O_2$max of your client. To use this nomogram, locate the time corresponding to the last complete minute of exercise during the protocol along the vertical axis labeled "Balke time," and draw a horizontal line from the time axis to the oxygen uptake axis. Be certain to plot the exercise time of women and men in the appropriate column when using this nomogram.

Bruce Treadmill Protocol

The Bruce, Kusumi, and Hosmer (1973) exercise test is a multistaged treadmill protocol (see figure 4.2). The workload is increased by changing both the treadmill speed and percent grade. During the first stage (minutes 1 to 3) of the test, the normal individual walks at a 1.7 mph pace at 10% grade. At the start of the second stage (minutes 4 to 6), increase the grade by 2% and the speed to 2.5 mph (67 m·min^{-1}). In each subsequent stage of the test, increase the grade 2% and the speed by either 0.8 or 0.9 mph (21.4 or 24.1 m·min^{-1}) until the client is exhausted. Prediction equations for this protocol have been developed to estimate the $\dot{V}O_2$max of active and sedentary women and men, cardiac patients, and people who are elderly (see table 4.5). As an alternative, you may use the nomogram (see figure 4.4) developed for the Bruce protocol. Plot the client's exercise time for this protocol along the vertical axis labeled "Bruce time," and draw a horizontal line from the time axis to the oxygen uptake. Again, be certain to use the appropriate column for men and women.

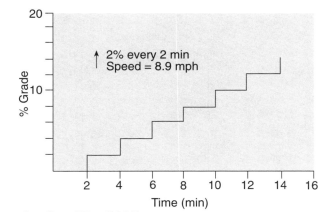

Costill and Fox (1969)
For: highly trained
Warmup: 10-min walk or run
Initial work load: 8.9 mph, 0%, 2 min

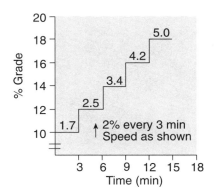

Bruce et al. (1973)
For: normal and high risk
Initial work load: 1.7 mph, 10%, 3 min = normal
                   1.7 mph, 0-5%, 3 min = high risk

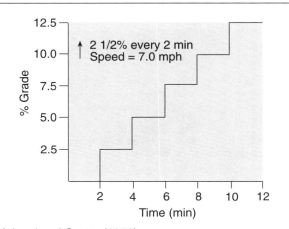

Maksud and Coutts (1971)
For: highly trained
Warmup: 10-min walking 3.5 mph, 0%
Initial work load: 7 mph, 0%, 2 min

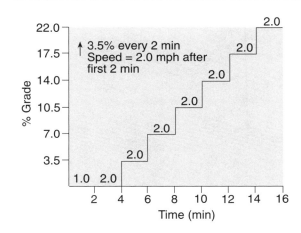

Naughton et al. (1964)
For: cardiac and high risk
Initial work load: 1.0 mph, 0%, 2 min

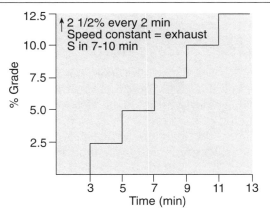

Modified Åstrand (Pollock et al. 1978)
For: highly trained
Warmup: 5-min walk or jog
Initial work load: 5-8 mph, 0%, 3 min

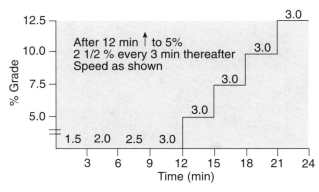

Wilson et al. (1978)
For: cardiac and high risk
Initial work load: 1.5 mph, 0%, 3 min

(continued)

Figure 4.2 Treadmill exercise test protocols.

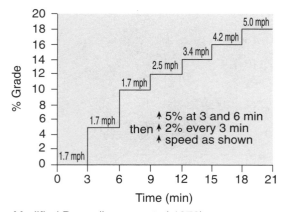

Modified Bruce (Lerman et al.1976)
For: normal and high risk
Initial workload: 1.7 mph, 0%, 3 min

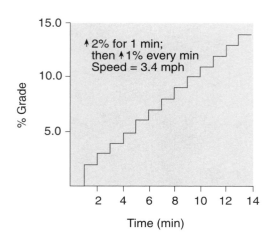

Balke and Ware (1959)
For: normal risk
Initial work load: 3.4 mph. 0%, 1 min

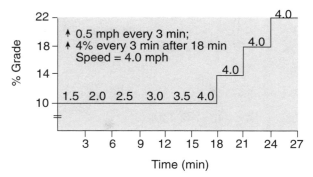

Kattus (1967)
For: cardiac and high risk
Initial work load: 1.5 mph, 10%, 3 min

Figure 4.2 *(continued)*

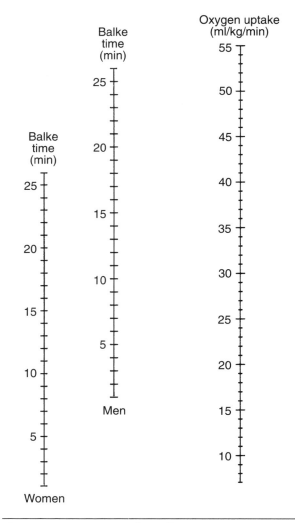

Figure 4.3 Nomogram for Balke graded exercise test.
From N. Ng: *Metcalc,* (p. 30), Human Kinetics, Champaign, 1995. Reproduced by permission.

Modified Bruce Protocol

The modified Bruce protocol (see figure 4.2) is more suitable than the Bruce protocol for high-risk and elderly individuals. However, with the exception of the first two stages, this protocol is similar to the standard Bruce protocol. Stage 1 starts at 0% grade and a 1.7 mph walking pace. For stage 2, the % grade is increased to 5%. McInnis and Balady (1994) compared physiological responses to the standard and modified Bruce protocols in patients with CHD and reported similar HR and BP responses at matched exercise stages despite the additional 6 min of low-intensity exercise performed using the modified Bruce protocol.

Table 4.4 MET Estimations for Each Stage of Commonly Used Treadmill Protocols

Stage[a]	Bruce	Modified Bruce[b]	Balke	Naughton
1	4.6	2.3	3.6	1.8
2	7.0	3.5	4.5	3.5
3	10.2	4.6	5.0	4.5
4	12.1	7.0	5.5	5.4
5	14.9	10.2	5.9	6.4
6	17.0	12.1	6.4	7.4
7	19.3	14.9	6.9	8.3

[a]Percent grade and speed for each stage are illustrated in figure 4.2.

[b]Stage 1 = 0% grade, 1.7 mph; Stage 2 = 5% grade, 1.7 mph.

Table 4.5 Population-Specific and Generalized Equations for Treadmill Protocols

Protocol	Population	Reference	Equation
Balke	Active and sedentary men	Pollock et al. 1976	$\dot{V}O_2max = 1.444(time) + 14.99$ $r = 0.92$, *SEE* = 2.50 ml·kg^{-1}·min^{-1}
	Active and sedentary women[a]	Pollock et al. 1982	$\dot{V}O_2max = 1.38(time) + 5.22$ $r = 0.94$, *SEE* = 2.20 ml·kg^{-1}·min^{-1}
Bruce[b]	Active and sedentary men;	Foster et al. 1984	$\dot{V}O_2max = 14.76 - 1.379(time) + 0.451(time^2) - 0.012(time^3)$ $r = 0.98$, *SEE* = 3.35 ml·kg^{-1}·min^{-1}
	Active and sedentary women	Pollock et al. 1982	$\dot{V}O_2max = 4.38(time) - 3.90$ $r = 0.91$, *SEE* = 2.7 ml·kg^{-1}·min^{-1}
	Cardiac patients and elderly persons[c]	McConnell and Clark 1987	$\dot{V}O_2max = 2.282(time) + 8.545$ $r = 0.82$, *SEE* = 4.9 ml·kg^{-1}·min^{-1}
Naughton	Male cardiac patients	Foster et al. 1983	$\dot{V}O_2max = 1.61(time) + 3.60$ $r = 0.97$, *SEE* = 2.60 ml·kg^{-1}·min^{-1}

[a]For women, the Balke protocol was modified: speed 3.0 mph; initial workload 0% grade for 3 min, increasing 2.5% every 3 min thereafter.

[b]For use with the standard Bruce protocol, *not* modified Bruce protocol.

[c]This equation is used only for treadmill walking while holding the handrails.

SEE = standard error of estimate.

Note that the prediction equations for the Bruce protocol (see table 4.5) can be used for only the standard, not the modified, Bruce protocol. To estimate $\dot{V}O_2$ for the modified Bruce protocol, use the ACSM metabolic equation for walking (see table 4.3).

Bicycle Ergometer Maximal Exercise Tests

The bicycle ergometer is a widely used instrument for assessing cardiorespiratory fitness. On a friction-type bicycle ergometer (see figure 4.5),

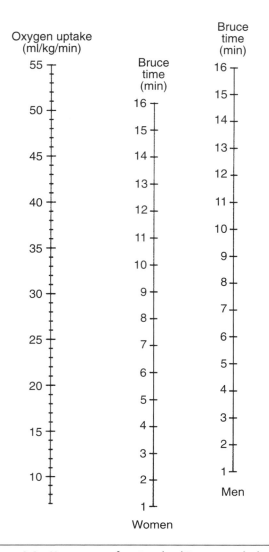

Figure 4.4 Nomogram for standard Bruce graded exercise test.

From N. Ng: *Metcalc,* (p. 32), Human Kinetics, Champaign, 1995. Reproduced by permission.

resistance is applied against the flywheel using a belt and weighted pendulums. The handwheel adjusts the workload by tightening or loosening the brake belt. The workload on the bicycle ergometer is raised through increases in the resistance on the flywheel. The power output is usually expressed in kilogram-meters per minute (kgm·min⁻¹) or watts (1 W = 6 kgm·min⁻¹) and is easily measured using the equation:

$$\text{power} = \text{force} \times \text{distance/time}$$

where force equals the resistance or tension setting on the ergometer (kilograms) and distance is the distance traveled by the flywheel rim for each revolution of the pedal times number of revolu-

tions per minute. On the Monark and Bodyguard bicycle ergometers, the flywheel travels 6 m per pedal revolution. Therefore, if a resistance of 2 kg is applied and the pedaling rate is 60 rpm, then

$$\text{power} = 2 \text{ kg} \times 6 \text{ m} \times 60 \text{ rpm} = 720 \text{ kgm·min}^{-1},$$
$$\text{or } 120 \text{ W}$$

To calculate the distance traveled by the flywheel of cycle ergometers with varying-sized flywheels, measure the circumference (in meters) of the resistance track on the flywheel and multiply the circumference by the number of flywheel revolutions during one complete revolution (360°) of the pedal (Gledhill and Jamnik 1995).

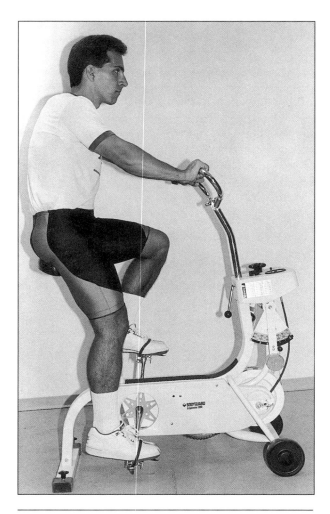

Figure 4.5 Bicycle ergometer (mechanically braked).

When you are standardizing the work performed on a friction-type bicycle ergometer, the client should maintain a constant pedaling rate. Some cycle ergometers have a speedometer that displays the individual's pedaling rate. Check this dial frequently to make certain that your client is maintaining a constant pedaling frequency throughout the test. If a speedometer is not available, use a metronome to establish your client's pedaling cadence. Controlling the pedaling rate on an electrically braked bicycle ergometer (figure 4.6) is unnecessary. An electromagnetic braking force adjusts the resistance for slower or faster pedaling rates, thereby keeping the power output constant. This type of bicycle ergometer, however, is difficult to calibrate.

Most cycle ergometer test protocols for untrained cyclists use a pedaling rate of 50 or 60 rpm, and power outputs are increased by 150 to 300 $kgm \cdot min^{-1}$ (25 to 50 W) in each stage of the test. However, you can use higher pedaling rates (≥ 80 rpm) for trained cyclists. A pedaling rate of 60 rpm produces the highest $\dot{V}O_2max$ when compared with rates of 50, 70, or 80 rpm (Hermansen and Saltin 1969). Figure 4.7 illustrates some widely used discontinuous and continuous maximal exercise test protocols for the bicycle ergometer.

To calculate the energy expenditure for bicycle ergometer exercise, use the ACSM equations provided in table 4.3. The total energy expenditure or

TESTING WITH BICYCLE ERGOMETERS

The following guidelines are suggested for the use of bicycle ergometers (Sinning 1975):

1. Calibrate the bicycle often by hanging known weights from the belt of the flywheel and reading the dial on the handwheel.

2. Always release the tension on the belt between tests.

3. Establish pedaling frequency before setting the workload.

4. Check the load setting frequently during the test because it may change as the belt warms up.

5. Set the metronome so that one revolution is completed for every two beats (e.g., set the metronome at 120 for a test requiring a pedaling frequency of 60 rpm).

6. Adjust the height of the seat so the knee is slightly flexed (about 5°) at maximal leg extension with the ball of the foot on the pedal.

7. Have the client assume an upright, seated posture with hands properly positioned on the handlebars.

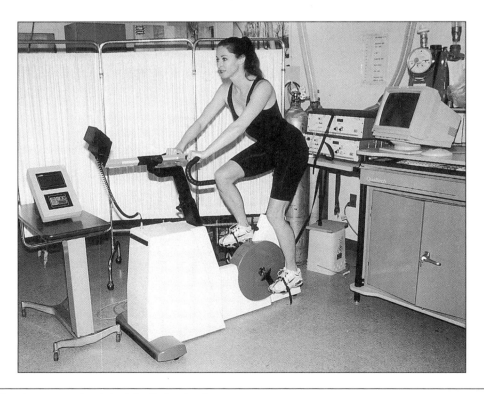

Figure 4.6 Bicycle ergometer (electrically braked).

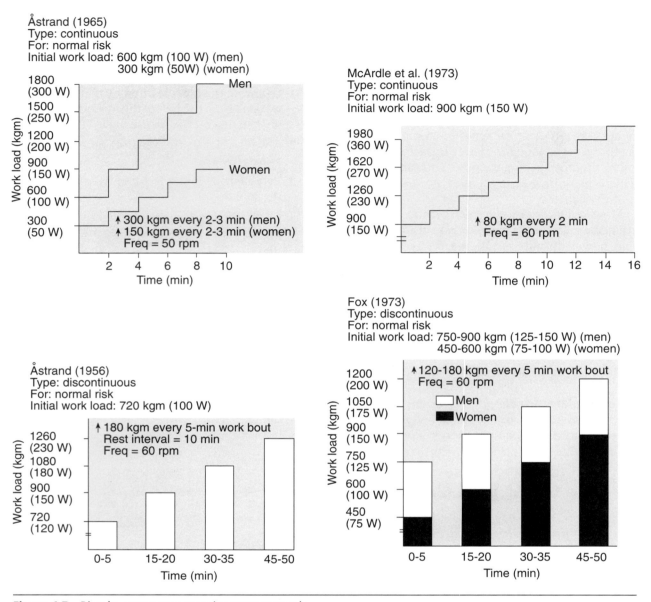

Figure 4.7 Bicycle ergometer exercise test protocols.

gross $\dot{V}O_2$, in ml·kg^{-1}·min^{-1}, is a function of the oxygen cost of pedaling against resistance (power output in watts), the oxygen cost of unloaded cycling (approximately 3.5 ml·kg^{-1}·min^{-1} at 50 to 60 rpm with zero resistance), and the resting oxygen consumption. The cost of cycling against an external load or resistance is approximately 1.8 ml·kg^{-1}·m^{-1} or 10.8 ml·kg^{-1}·W^{-1} (1 W = 6 kgm·min^{-1}; thus, 1.8 × 6 = 10.8 ml·kg^{-1}·W^{-1}). For an example calculation, see "ACSM Leg Ergometry Equation" on page 65.

Keep in mind that the leg and arm ergometry equations are accurate in estimating $\dot{V}O_2$ only if the client attains a steady state during the maxi-

mal GXT. If, for example, the client is able to complete only 1 min of exercise during the last stage of the maximal test protocol, the power output from the previous stage (in which the client reached steady state) should be used to estimate $\dot{V}O_2$max rather than the power output corresponding to the last stage.

Åstrand Bicycle Ergometer Maximal Test Protocol

For the Åstrand (1965) continuous test protocol (see figure 4.7), the initial power output is 300 kgm·min^{-1} (50 W) for women and 600 kgm·min^{-1}

ACSM LEG ERGOMETRY EQUATION

To calculate the energy expenditure of a 62-kg (136 lb) woman cycling at a work rate or power output of 60 W, follow these steps:

1. Calculate the energy cost of cycling at the specified power output.

$\dot{V}O_2$ = power output (W)/body mass (M) $\times$ 10.8
= 60 W/62 kg $\times$ 10.8
= 10.45 ml·kg^{-1}·min^{-1}

2. Add the estimated cost of cycling at zero load (i.e., 3.5 ml·kg^{-1}·min^{-1}).

$\dot{V}O_2$ = 10.45 ml·kg^{-1}·min^{-1} + 3.5 ml·kg^{-1}·min^{-1}
= 13.95 ml·kg^{-1}·min^{-1}

3. Add the estimated resting energy expenditure (3.5 ml·kg^{-1}·min^{-1}).

$\dot{V}O_2$ = 13.95 ml·kg^{-1}·min^{-1} + 3.5 ml·kg^{-1}·min^{-1}
= 17.45 ml·kg^{-1}·min^{-1}

(100 W) for men. Because the pedaling rate is 50 rpm, the resistance is 1 kg for women (1 kg $\times$ 6 m $\times$ 50 rpm = 300 kgm·min^{-1}) and 2 kg for men (2 kg $\times$ 6 m $\times$ 50 rpm = 600 kgm·min^{-1}). Have your client exercise at this initial workload for 2 min. Then increase the power output every 2 to 3 min in increments of 150 kgm·min^{-1} (25 W) and 300 kgm·min^{-1} (50 W) for women and men, respectively. Continue the test until the client is exhausted or can no longer maintain the pedaling rate of 50 rpm. Use the ACSM metabolic equation for leg ergometry to estimate $\dot{V}O_2$ from your client's power output during the last steady-state stage of the GXT.

Fox Bicycle Ergometer Maximal Test Protocol

The Fox (1973) protocol is a discontinuous test consisting of a series of 5-min exercise bouts with 10-min rest intervals. The starting workload is between 750 (125 W) and 900 kgm·min^{-1} (150 W) for men and 450 (75 W) and 600 kgm·min^{-1} (100 W) for women. The progressive increments in work depend on the client's HR response and usually are between 120 and 180 kgm·min^{-1} (20 and 30 W). The client exercises until exhausted or until no longer able to pedal for at least 3 min at a power output that is 60 to 90 kgm·min^{-1} (10 to 15 W) higher than the previous workload. You can use the metabolic equations to convert the power output from the last steady-state stage of this protocol to $\dot{V}O_2$max.

Bench Stepping Maximal Exercise Tests

The least desirable mode of exercise for maximum exercise testing is bench stepping. During bench stepping, the individual is performing both positive (up phase) and negative (down phase) work. Approximately one-quarter to one-third less energy is expended during negative work (Morehouse 1972). This factor, coupled with adjusting the step height and stepping rate for differences in body weight, makes standardization of the work extremely difficult.

General Procedures

Most step test protocols increase the intensity of the work by gradually increasing the height of the bench or stepping rate. The work (W) performed can be calculated using the equation W = F $\times$ D, where F is body weight in kilograms and D is bench height times number of steps per minute. For example, a 50-kg woman stepping at a rate of 22 steps/min on a 30-cm (0.30 m) bench is performing 330 kgm·min^{-1} of work (50 kg $\times$ 0.30 m $\times$ 22 steps·min^{-1}).

The following equations can be used to adjust the step height and stepping rate for differences in body weight to achieve a given work rate (Morehouse 1972):

step height (cm) = work (kg·cm·min^{-1})/body weight (kg) $\times$ stepping rate

stepping rate = work (kg·cm·min^{-1})
(steps·min^{-1}) $\div$ body weight (kg)
$\times$ step height (cm)

For example, if you devise a graded step test protocol that requires a client weighing 60 kg to exercise at a work rate of 300 kgm·min^{-1}, and the stepping rate is set at 18 steps/min, you need to determine the step height that corresponds to the work rate:

step height = 300 kgm·min^{-1}/60 kg $\times$ 18 steps·min^{-1}
= 0.28 m, or 28 cm

Alternatively, you may choose to keep the step height constant and vary the stepping cadence for each stage of the GXT. For example, if the step height is set at 30 cm (0.30 m), and the protocol requires that a client weighing 60 kg exercise at a work rate of 450 kgm·min^{-1}, you need to calculate the corresponding stepping rate for this client:

stepping rate = 450 kgm·min^{-1}/60 kg $\times$ 0.30 m
= 25 steps·min^{-1}

You can calculate the energy expenditure in METs using the ACSM metabolic equation for stepping exercise (see table 4.3). The total gross $\dot{V}O_2$ is a function of step frequency, step height, and the resting energy expenditure. The oxygen cost of the horizontal movement is approximately 0.2 $ml\cdot kg^{-1}$ for each four-count stepping cycle. The oxygen demand for stepping up is 1.8 $ml\cdot kg^{-1}\cdot m^{-1}$; approximately one-third more must be added (i.e., constant of 1.33 in equation) to account for the oxygen cost of stepping down. For an example of such calculations, see "ACSM Stepping Equation."

ACSM STEPPING EQUATION

To calculate the energy expenditure for bench stepping using a 16-in. step height at a cadence of 24 $steps\cdot min^{-1}$, use the following procedure:

$\dot{V}O_2$ in $ml\cdot kg^{-1}\cdot min^{-1}$ = [frequency (F) in $steps\cdot min^{-1}$ $\times$ 0.2] + (step height in m/step $\times$ F in $steps\cdot min^{-1}$ $\times$ 1.33 $\times$ 1.8) + resting $\dot{V}O_2$

1. Calculate the $\dot{V}O_2$ for the stepping frequency (F).

   $\dot{V}O_2$ = stepping frequency (F) $\times$ 0.20
   = 24 $steps\cdot min^{-1} \times 0.20$
   = 4.8 $ml\cdot kg^{-1}\cdot min^{-1}$

2. Convert the bench height to meters (1 in. = 2.54 cm or 0.0254 m).

   ht = 16 in. $\times$ 0.0254 m
   = 0.4064 m

3. Calculate the $\dot{V}O_2$ for the vertical work performed during stepping.

   $\dot{V}O_2$ = bench ht $\times$ stepping rate $\times$ 1.33 $\times$ 1.8
   = 0.4064 m $\times$ 24 $steps\cdot min^{-1} \times 1.33 \times 1.8$
   = 23.35 $ml\cdot kg^{-1}\cdot min^{-1}$

4. Add resting $\dot{V}O_2$ to the calculated $\dot{V}O_2$ from steps 1 and 3.

   $\dot{V}O_2$ = 4.8 $ml\cdot kg^{-1}\cdot min^{-1}$ + 23.35 $ml\cdot kg^{-1}\cdot min^{-1}$
   + 3.5 $ml\cdot kg^{-1}\cdot min^{-1}$
   = 31.65 $ml\cdot kg^{-1}\cdot min^{-1}$

Nagle, Balke, and Naughton Maximal Step Test Protocol

Nagle, Balke, and Naughton (1965) devised a graded step test for assessing work capacity. Have your client step at a rate of 30 steps/min on an automatically adjustable bench (2 to 50 cm). Set the initial bench height at 2 cm and increase the height 2 cm every minute of exercise. Use a metronome to establish the stepping cadence (4 beats per stepping cycle). To establish a cadence of 30 steps/min, set the metronome at 120 (30 $\times$ 4). Terminate the test when the subject is fatigued or can no longer maintain the stepping cadence. Use the ACSM metabolic equation for stepping exercise to calculate the energy expenditure ($\dot{V}O_2$max) corresponding to the step height and stepping cadence during the last work stage of this protocol.

SUBMAXIMAL EXERCISE TEST PROTOCOLS

It is desirable to directly determine the functional aerobic capacity of the individual for diagnosing CHD, classifying the cardiorespiratory fitness level, and prescribing an aerobic exercise program. However, it is not always practical to do so. The actual measurement of $\dot{V}O_2$max requires expensive laboratory equipment, a considerable amount of time to administer, and a high level of motivation on the part of the client.

Alternatively, you can use submaximal exercise tests to predict or estimate the $\dot{V}O_2$max of the individual. Many of these tests are similar to the maximal exercise tests described previously but differ in that they are terminated at some predetermined HR intensity. You will monitor the HR, BP, and RPE during the submaximal exercise test. The treadmill, bicycle ergometer, and bench stepping exercises are commonly used for submaximal exercise testing.

Assumptions of Submaximal Exercise Tests

Submaximal exercise tests assume a steady-state HR at each exercise intensity, as well as a linear relationship between HR, oxygen uptake, and work intensity. Although these relationships hold for light-to-moderate workloads, the relationship between oxygen uptake and work becomes curvilinear at heavier workloads.

Another assumption of submaximal testing is that the mechanical efficiency during cycling or treadmill exercise is constant for all individuals. However, a client with poor mechanical efficiency while cycling has a higher submaximal HR at a given workload, and the actual $\dot{V}O_2$max is underestimated due to this inefficiency (McArdle, Katch, and Katch 1996). As a result, $\dot{V}O_2$max predicted by submaximal exercise tests tends to be overestimated for highly trained individuals and underestimated for untrained, sedentary individuals.

Submaximal tests also assume that the maximal heart rate (HRmax) for clients of a given age is similar. The HRmax, however, has been shown to vary as much as ±11 bpm, even after controlling for variability due to age and training status (Londeree and Moeschberger 1984). Also, for submaximal tests, the HRmax is estimated from age. The equation HRmax = 220 – age yields a low estimate of the maximal heart rate, while the equation HRmax = 210 – (0.5 × age) gives a high estimate of maximal heart rate. The HRmax of approximately 5% to 7% of men and women is more than 15 bpm less than their age-predicted HRmax. On the other hand, 9% to 13% have HRmax values that exceed their age-predicted HRmax by more than 15 bpm (Whaley, Kaminsky, Dwyer, Getchell, and Norton 1992). Because of interindividual variability in HRmax and the potential inaccuracy with use of age-predicted HRmax, there may be considerable error (±10% to 15%) in estimating your client's $\dot{V}O_2$max, especially when submaximal data are extrapolated to an age-predicted HRmax.

Treadmill Submaximal Exercise Tests

Treadmill submaximal tests provide an estimate of functional aerobic capacity ($\dot{V}O_2$max) and assume a linear increase in HR with successive increments in workload. Compared to clients with low cardiorespiratory fitness levels, the well-conditioned individual presumably is able to perform a greater quantity of work at a given submaximal HR.

You can use treadmill maximal test protocols (figure 4.2) to identify the slope of the individual's HR response to exercise. The $\dot{V}O_2$max can be predicted from either one (single-stage model) or two (multistage model) submaximal HRs. Mahar, Jackson, Ross, Pivarnik, and Pollock (1985) reported that the accuracy of the single-stage model is similar to that of the multistage model.

Multistage Model

To estimate $\dot{V}O_2$max with the multistage model, use the HR and workload data from two or more submaximal stages of the treadmill test. Be sure your client reaches steady-state HRs between 115 and 150 bpm (Golding, Meyers, and Sinning 1989). Determine the slope *(b)* by calculating the ratio of the difference between the two submaximal

(SM) workloads (expressed as $\dot{V}O_2$) and the corresponding change in submaximal HRs:

$$b = (SM_2 - SM_1)/(HR_2 - HR_1)$$

Calculate the $\dot{V}O_2$ for each workload using the ACSM metabolic equation (table 4.3), and use the following equation to predict $\dot{V}O_2$max:

$$\dot{V}O_2max = SM_2 + b(HRmax - HR_2)$$

If the actual maximal HR is not known, estimate it using the formula 220 – age. The following example illustrates the use of the multistage model for estimating $\dot{V}O_2$max for a submaximal treadmill test given to a 38-year-old male.

Protocol: Bruce

Submaximal data:

Stage 2[a]	Stage 1[a]
$\dot{V}O_2{}^b$ = 24.5 ml·kg⁻¹·min⁻¹ (SM₂)	16.1 ml·kg⁻¹·min⁻¹ (SM₁)
HR = 145 bpm (HR₂)	130 bpm (HR₁)

Maximal HR: 220 – age = 182 bpm

$$\text{Slope } (b) = \frac{(SM_2 - SM_1)}{(HR_2 - HR_1)}$$

$$b = \frac{(24.5 - 16.1)}{(145 - 130)}$$

$$b = \frac{8.4}{15}$$

$$b = 0.56$$

$\dot{V}O_2$max: SM₂ + b(HR max – HR₂)

$$= 24.5 + 0.56(182 - 145)$$
$$= 24.5 + 20.72$$
$$\dot{V}O_2max = 45.22 \text{ ml·kg}^{-1}\text{·min}^{-1}$$

---

[a]Stage 1 and 2 refer to the last two stages of the GXT completed by the client, and not the first and second stage of the test protocol. For example, if the client completes three stages of the submaximal exercise test protocol, data from stage 2 and stage 3 are used to estimate $\dot{V}O_2$.

[b]$\dot{V}O_2$ is calculated using ACSM metabolic equations (see table 4.3). $\dot{V}O_2$ can be expressed in L·min⁻¹, ml·kg⁻¹·min⁻¹, or METs.

Single-Stage Model

To estimate $\dot{V}O_2$max with the single-stage model, use one submaximal HR and one workload. The steady-state submaximal HR during a single-stage GXT should reach 130 to 150 bpm. "Formulas for Men and Women" have been developed (Shephard 1972).

Formulas for Men and Women

Men

$\dot{V}O_2max = SM_{\dot{V}O_2} \times [(HRmax - 61)/(HR_{SM} - 61)]$

Women

$\dot{V}O_2max = SM_{\dot{V}O_2} \times [(HRmax - 72)/(HR_{SM} - 72)]$

$SM_{\dot{V}O_2}$ is calculated using the ACSM metabolic equations (see table 4.3). Estimate HRmax (if not known) using the formula 220 − age; HR_{SM} is the submaximal HR.

The following example illustrates the use of the single-stage model for estimating $\dot{V}O_2max$ for a treadmill submaximal test given to a 45-year-old female.

Protocol: Balke

Submaximal data: Stage 3

$\dot{V}O_2 = 5.0$ METs $(SM_{\dot{V}O_2})$
HR = 148 bpm (HR_{SM})

Maximal HR: 220 − age = 175 bpm

$\dot{V}O_2max: = SM_{\dot{V}O_2} \times [(HRmax - 72)/(HR_{SM} - 72)]$
$\qquad = 5 \times [(175 - 72)/(148 - 72)]$
$\qquad = 5 \times (103/76)$
$\qquad = 6.8$ METs

Single-Stage Treadmill Walking Test

Ebbeling, Ward, Puleo, Widrick, and Rippe (1991) developed a single-stage treadmill walking test suitable for estimating $\dot{V}O_2max$ of low-risk, healthy adults 20 to 59 years of age. For this protocol, walking speed is individualized and ranges from 2.0 to 4.5 mph (53.6 to 120.6 m·min⁻¹) depending on your client's age, gender, and fitness level. Establish a walking pace during a 4-min warm-up at 0% grade. The warm-up work bout should produce a heart rate within 50% to 70% of the individual's age-predicted HRmax. The test consists of brisk walking at the selected pace for an additional 4 min at 5% grade. Record the steady-state HR at this workload, and use it in the following equation to estimate $\dot{V}O_2max$:

$\dot{V}O_2max = 15.1 + 21.8(\text{speed in mph})$
(ml·kg⁻¹·min⁻¹) $- 0.327(\text{HR in bpm})$
$\qquad - 0.263(\text{speed} \times \text{age in years})$
$\qquad + 0.00504(\text{HR} \times \text{age})$
$\qquad + 5.48(\text{gender: female} = 0; \text{male} = 1)$

Single-Stage Treadmill Walking or Jogging Test

You can also estimate your client's $\dot{V}O_2max$ from one 6-min treadmill walk (50% $\dot{V}O_2max$) or run (70% $\dot{V}O_2max$) and steady-state HR from the last 2 min of exercise (Latin and Elias 1993). For the walking protocol, set the treadmill speed at 3.0 mph (80.4 m·min⁻¹) for women and 3.5 mph (93.8 m·min⁻¹) for men, and raise the grade to a level requiring 50% or 60% $\dot{V}O_2max$. For the running protocol, have the client run at a speed requiring about 70% to 80% $\dot{V}O_2max$ at 0% grade. Estimate the energy expenditure ($\dot{V}O_2$) of the exercise workload using the ACSM walking or running equation (see table 4.3). Plot the client's energy expenditure in L·min⁻¹ and the steady-state exercise HR in the corresponding columns of the Åstrand-Ryhming nomogram (see figure 4.8). Connect these points with a ruler and read the estimated $\dot{V}O_2max$ at the point where the line intersects the $\dot{V}O_2max$ column.

Single-Stage Treadmill Jogging Test

You can estimate the $\dot{V}O_2max$ of younger adults (18 to 28 years) using a single-stage treadmill jogging test (George, Vehrs, Allsen, Fellingham, and Fisher 1993). For this test, select a comfortable jogging pace ranging from 4.3 to 7.5 mph (115.2 to 201 m·min⁻¹), but not more than 6.5 mph (174.2 m·min⁻¹) for women and 7.5 mph (201 m·min⁻¹) for men. Have the client jog at a constant speed for about 3 min. The steady-state exercise HR should not exceed 180 bpm. Estimate $\dot{V}O_2max$ using the following equation:

$\dot{V}O_2max = 54.07 - 0.1938(\text{BW in kg})$
(ml·kg⁻¹·min⁻¹) $+ 4.47(\text{speed in mph})$
$\qquad - 0.1453(\text{HR in bpm})$
$\qquad + 7.062(\text{gender: female} = 0; \text{male} = 1)$

Bicycle Ergometer Submaximal Exercise Tests

Bicycle ergometer multistage submaximal tests can be used to predict $\dot{V}O_2max$. These tests are

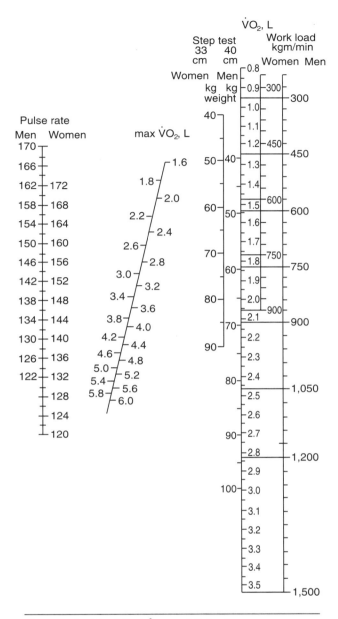

Figure 4.8 Modified Åstrand-Ryhming nomogram.
From "Aerobic Capacity in Men and Women with Special Reference to Age" by I. Åstrand, 1960, *Acta Physiologica Scandinavica* 49 (Suppl. 169), p. 51. Copyright 1960 by *Acta Physiologica Scandinavica*. Reprinted by permission.

either continuous or discontinuous and are based on the assumption that HR and oxygen uptake are linear functions of work rate. The HR response to submaximal workloads is used to predict $\dot{V}O_2$max.

YMCA Bicycle Ergometer Submaximal Exercise Test Protocol

Golding, Meyers, and Sinning (1989) developed a bicycle ergometer submaximal protocol for

women and men. This protocol uses three or four consecutive 3-min workloads on the bicycle ergometer designed to raise the HR to between 110 bpm and 85% of the age-predicted HRmax for at least two consecutive workloads. The pedal rate is 50 rpm, and the initial workload is 150 kgm·min⁻¹ (25 W). Use the HR during the last minute of the initial workload to determine subsequent workloads (see figure 4.9). If the HR is less than 80 bpm, set the second workload at 750 kgm·min⁻¹. If HR is 80 to 89 bpm or 90 to 100 bpm, the respective workloads are 600 or 450 kgm·min⁻¹ for the second stage of the protocol. If the HR at the end of the first workload exceeds 100 bpm, set the second workload at 300 kgm·min⁻¹.

Set the third and fourth workloads accordingly (see figure 4.9). Measure the HR during the last 30 sec of minutes 2 and 3 at each workload. If these HRs differ by more than 5 to 6 bpm, extend the workload an additional minute until the HR stabilizes. If the client's steady-state HR reaches or exceeds 85% of the age-predicted HRmax during the third workload, terminate the test.

Calculate the energy expenditure ($\dot{V}O_2$) for the last two workloads using the ACSM metabolic equations (see table 4.3). To estimate $\dot{V}O_2$max from these data, use the equations for the multistage model to calculate the slope of the line depicting the HR response to the last two workloads. Alternatively, you can graph these data to estimate $\dot{V}O_2$max (see figure 4.10). To do this, plot the $\dot{V}O_2$ for each workload and corresponding HRs. Connect these two data points with a straight edge, extending the line so that it intersects the predicted maximal HR line. To extrapolate $\dot{V}O_2$max, drop a perpendicular line from the point of intersection to the x-axis of the graph. If this is done carefully, the graphing method and multistage method will yield similar estimates of $\dot{V}O_2$max.

ACSM Bicycle Ergometer Submaximal Exercise Test Protocol

The ACSM (1999) developed a cycle ergometer submaximal exercise test protocol based on the individual's body weight and activity status (see table 4.6). To select the most appropriate protocol (A, B, or C), determine the client's body weight classification and activity status. Very active individuals are defined as those who have regularly participated in vigorous activities at least 20 min, three times per week, during the past three months.

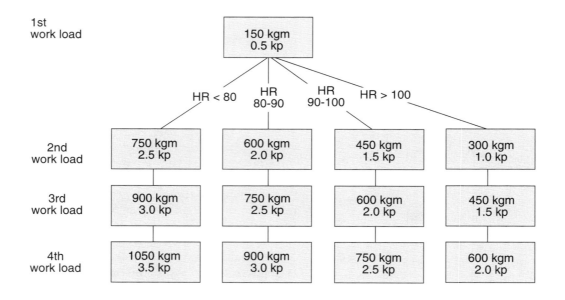

Directions:

1. Set the first work load at 150 kgm/min (0.5 kp)
2. If the HR in the third min is
   - less than (<) 80, set the second load at 750 kgm (2.5 kp);
   - 80-89, set the second load at at 600 kgm (2.0 kp);
   - 90-100, set the second load at 450 kgm (1.5 kp);
   - greater than (>) 100, set the second load at 300 kgm (1.0 kp)
3. Set the third and fourth (if required) loads according to the loads in the columns below the second loads.

Figure 4.9 YMCA bicycle ergometer protocol.

Data from Golding (2000). *YMCA Fitness Testing and Assessment Manual* (4th ed.), p. 140, Champaign, IL: Human Kinetics. Reprinted with permission of the YMCA of the USA, 101 N. Wacker Drive, Chicago, IL 60606.

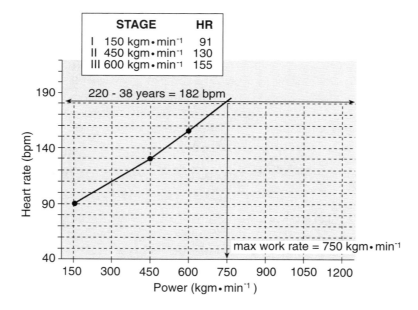

Figure 4.10 Plotting heart rate versus submaximal work rates to estimate maximal work capacity and VO$_2$max.

Each protocol consists of four 2-min workloads. Measure the HR during the last 15 sec of each workload, and stop the test when the client's HR reaches 65% to 70% of the HR range (Karvonen method) or 85% of the age-predicted maximal HR (ACSM 2000). Using the graphing method, estimate the $\dot{V}O_2$max by plotting the HR response to last two workloads and extending the line to the age-predicted HRmax (see figure 4.10). Alternatively, you can use the multistage model equations to estimate $\dot{V}O_2$max.

In the ACSM (1991) *Guidelines for Exercise Testing and Prescription* (4th edition), the termination point for this protocol was only 65% to 70% of the age-predicted HRmax, compared to the current recommendation of 85% HRmax (ACSM 2000). Greiwe, Kaminsky, Whaley, and Dwyer (1995) tested the reliability and validity of the ACSM protocol in estimating $\dot{V}O_2$max using the 65% to 70% HRmax termination criterion. They reported that this protocol significantly overestimated $\dot{V}O_2$max by 25% for women and men 21 to 54 years of age. Also, there were large intra-individual differences in the $\dot{V}O_2$max estimated from submaximal HR data

from two separate submaximal trials, indicating poor reliability for this protocol and termination criterion. Because of the low termination criterion and the short, 2-min stages for this protocol, the authors noted that subjects were unable to reach exercise intensities that would tend to decrease intra-individual variability in submaximal HR. Thus, there were large errors in estimating $\dot{V}O_2$max from the submaximal HR data. Using the revised termination criterion (85% age-predicted HRmax or 65% to 70% heart rate range) may overcome this problem. However, more validation studies are needed to test this hypothesis.

Åstrand-Ryhming Bicycle Ergometer Submaximal Exercise Test Protocol

The Åstrand-Ryhming protocol (1954) is a single-stage test that uses a nomogram to predict $\dot{V}O_2$max from HR response to one 6-min submaximal workload. A power output is selected that produces a heart rate between 125 and 170 bpm. The initial workload is usually 450 to 600 kgm·min⁻¹ (75 to 100 W) for trained, physically active women and

---

Table 4.6 ACSM Bicycle Ergometer Submaximal Test Protocols (ACSM 1999)

Stages (2 min each)	Test protocols[a]		
	A	B	C
1	25[b] (150)	25 (150)	50 (300)
2	50 (300)	50 (300)	100 (600)
3	75 (450)	100 (600)	150 (900)
4	100 (600)	150 (900)	200 (1200)

Selection criteria		

	Very active[c]	
Body weight in kg (lb)	No	Yes
≤73 (≤160)	A	A
74-90 (161-199)	A	B
≥91 (≥200)	B	C

[a]Terminate test protocol when heart rate reaches 70% heart rate reserve or 85% maximal heart rate.

[b]Workload in watts (kgm·min⁻¹).

[c]Very active = aerobic exercise 20 min, 3 days per week.

Reprinted, by permission, from American College of Sports Medicine, 1999, *ACSM health/fitness instructor certification study guide*. (Philadelphia: Lippincott, Williams, & Wilkins).

600 to 900 kgm·min⁻¹ (100 to 150 W) for trained, physically active men. An initial workload of 300 kgm·min⁻¹ (50 W) may be used for unconditioned or older individuals. Alternatively, you can use a nomogram (see figure 4.11) to estimate the initial workload for men by plotting the client's body weight and HR response after 1 min of cycling at 600 kgm·min⁻¹ (100 W) (Terry, Tolson, Johnson, and Jessup 1977). No such nomogram has been developed for women.

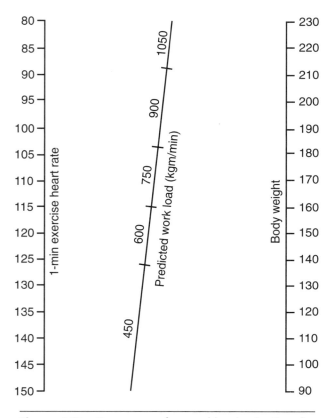

Figure 4.11 Nomogram for workload selection for Åstrand-Ryhming test.

Reprinted, by permission, from J.W. Terry et al., 1977, "A work load selection procedure for the Åstrand-Rhyming test," *Journal of Sports Medicine and Physical Fitness* 17:363.

During the test, measure the HR every minute and record the average HR during the fifth and sixth minutes. If the difference between these two HRs exceeds 5 to 6 bpm, extend the work bout until a steady-state HR is achieved. If the HR is less than 130 bpm at the end of the exercise bout, increase the workload by 300 kgm·min⁻¹ (50 W) and have the client exercise an additional 6 min.

To estimate $\dot{V}O_2$max for this protocol, use the modified Åstrand-Ryhming nomogram (see figure 4.8). This nomogram estimates $\dot{V}O_2$max (in L·min⁻¹) from submaximal treadmill, bicycle ergometer, and step test data. For each test mode, the sub-maximal HR is plotted with either oxygen cost of treadmill exercise ($\dot{V}O_2$ in L·min⁻¹), power output (kgm·min⁻¹) for bicycle ergometer exercise, or body weight (kg) for stepping exercise. The correlation between measured $\dot{V}O_2$max and the $\dot{V}O_2$max estimated from this nomogram is $r = 0.74$. The prediction error is ±10% and ±15%, respectively, for well-trained and untrained individuals (Åstrand and Rodahl 1977).

For clients younger or older than 25 years, you must use the following age-correction factors (table 4.7) to adjust the $\dot{V}O_2$max predicted from the nomogram for the effect of age. For example, if the estimated $\dot{V}O_2$max from the nomogram is 3.2 L·min⁻¹ for a 45-year-old client, the adjusted $\dot{V}O_2$max is 2.5 L·min⁻¹ (3.2 × 0.78 = 2.5 L·min⁻¹).

Table 4.7 Age-Correction Factors for Åstrand-Ryhming Nomogram

Age	Correction factor
15	1.10
25	1.00
35	0.87
40	0.83
45	0.78
50	0.75
55	0.71
60	0.68
65	0.65

Fox Single-Stage Bicycle Ergometer Test Protocol

You can modify the maximal exercise test protocol (see figure 4.7) designed by Fox (1973) to predict $\dot{V}O_2$max (ml·min⁻¹). Have your client perform a single workload (i.e., 900 kgm·min⁻¹ or 150 W) for 5 min. The standard error of estimate for this test is ±246 ml·min⁻¹, and the standard error of prediction is ±7.8%. The correlation between actual and predicted $\dot{V}O_2$max is $r = 0.76$. To estimate $\dot{V}O_2$max, measure the HR at the end of the fifth minute of exercise (HR_5) and use the following equation:

$$\dot{V}O_2max \ (ml \cdot min^{-1}) = 6300 - 19.26(HR_5)$$

Bench Stepping Submaximal Exercise Tests

Although there are many step tests available to evaluate cardiorespiratory fitness, few provide equations for predicting $\dot{V}O_2max$. Only step test protocols with prediction equations are included in this section.

Åstrand-Ryhming Step Test Protocol

As mentioned previously, you can use the Åstrand-Ryhming nomogram (see figure 4.8, p. 69) to predict $\dot{V}O_2max$ from postexercise HR and body weight during bench stepping. For this protocol, the client steps at a rate of 22.5 steps/min for 5 min. The bench height is 33 cm (13 in.) for women and 40 cm (15.75 in.) for men. Measure the postexercise HR by counting the number of beats between 15 and 30 sec immediately after exercise (convert this 15-sec count to beats per minute by multiplying by 4). Correct the predicted $\dot{V}O_2max$ from the nomogram if your client is older or younger than 25 years (see table 4.7).

Queens College Step Test Protocol

In a step test to predict $\dot{V}O_2max$ devised by McArdle, Katch, Pechar, Jacobson, and Ruck (1972), the client steps at a rate of 22 steps/min (females) or 24 steps/min (males) for 3 min. The bench height is 16.25 in. (41.3 cm). Have your client remain standing after the exercise. Wait 5 sec and then take a 15-sec HR count. Convert the count to beats per minute by multiplying by 4. If you are administering this test simultaneously to more than one client, you should teach your clients how to measure their own pulse rates (see p. 76). To estimate $\dot{V}O_2max$ in $ml \cdot kg^{-1} \cdot min^{-1}$, use the equations listed in table 4.8. The standard error of prediction for these equations is ±16%.

Table 4.8 Prediction Equations for Cardiorespiratory Field Tests

Field test	Equation[a]	Source
Distance run/walk		
1.0-mile steady-state jog	$\dot{V}O_2max = 100.5 - 0.1636(BW, kg) - 1.438(time, min) - 0.1928(HR, bpm) + 8.344(gender)^b$	George et al. 1993
1.0 mile run/walk (8-17 years)	$\dot{V}O_2max = 108.94 - 8.41(time, min) + 0.34(time, min)^2 + 0.21(age \times gender)^b - 0.84(BMI)^c$	Cureton et al. 1995
1.5-mile run/walk	$\dot{V}O_2max = 88.02 - 0.1656(BW, kg) - 2.76(time, min) + 3.716(gender)^b$	George et al. 1993
12-min run	$\dot{V}O_2max = 0.0268(distance, meters) - 11.3$	Cooper 1968
15-min run	$\dot{V}O_2max = 0.0178(distance, meters) + 9.6$	Balke 1963
1.0-mile walk	$\dot{V}O_2max = 132.853 - 0.0769(BW, lb) - 0.3877(age, years) + 6.315(gender)^b - 3.2649(time, min) - 0.1565(HR, bpm)$	Kline et al. 1987
Step tests		
Åstrand	Men: $\dot{V}O_2max \ (L \cdot min^{-1}) = 3.744[(BW + 5)/(HR - 62)]$ Women: $\dot{V}O_2max \ (L \cdot min^{-1}) = 3.750[(BW - 3)/(HR - 65)]$	Marley and Linnerud 1976
Queens College	Men: $\dot{V}O_2max = 111.33 - (0.42 \ HR, bpm)$ Women: $\dot{V}O_2max = 65.81 - (0.1847 \ HR, bpm)$	McArdle et al. 1972

[a]All equations estimate $\dot{V}O_2max$ in $ml \cdot kg^{-1} \cdot min^{-1}$ unless otherwise specified.

[b]For gender, substitute 1 for males and 0 for females.

[c]BMI = body mass index or body weight (body weight [BW] in kg)/ht^2 (in meters).

HR = heart rate.

Additional Modes for Submaximal Exercise Testing

If you are working in the context of a health or fitness club, you may have access to stair climbers and rowing ergometers. You can use some of these exercise machines for submaximal exercise testing of your clients.

Stair Climbing Submaximal Test Protocols

In light of the popularity of and continued interest in step aerobic training, you may choose to use a simulated stair climbing machine to estimate the aerobic capacity of some clients. The Stairmaster 4000 PT and 6000 PT are two step ergometers commonly used in health and fitness settings. The Stairmaster 4000 PT has step pedals that go up and down, whereas the 6000 PT model has a revolving staircase. Howley, Colacino, and Swensen (1992) reported that the HR response to increasing submaximal workloads (4.7 and 10 METs) on the Stairmaster 4000 PT step ergometer was linear. Also, compared to values with treadmill exercise, the HRs measured during stepping were systematically higher (7 to 11 bpm) at each submaximal intensity. However, the MET values read from the step ergometer were about 20% higher than the measured MET values. To obtain more accurate MET values for each submaximal intensity, use the following equation:

actual METs = 0.556 + 0.745(Stairmaster 4000 PT MET value)

To estimate $\dot{V}O_2$max, measure the steady-state HR and calculate the corrected MET value for each of two submaximal exercise intensities (e.g., 4 and 7 METs). Each stage of the test should last 3 to 6 min in order to produce steady state. Then use either the multistage model formulas (see p. 67) or the graphing method (see figure 4.10) to predict $\dot{V}O_2$max.

During the test, clients may hold the handrail lightly for balance but should not support their body weight. If they support their body weight, $\dot{V}O_2$max will be overestimated (Howley, Colacino, and Swenson 1992). Also, compared to the value with treadmill testing, your client's estimated $\dot{V}O_2$max may be lower because stair climbing produces systematically higher HRs at any given submaximal exercise intensity.

Rowing Ergometer Submaximal Test Protocols

Submaximal exercise protocols have been developed for the Concept II rowing ergometer and can be used to estimate your client's $\dot{V}O_2$max. The Hagerman (1993) protocol is designed for noncompetitive or unskilled rowers. Before beginning the test, set the fan blades in the fully closed position and select the small axle sprocket. For this test, select a submaximal exercise intensity (the HR should not exceed 170 bpm) that the client can sustain for 5 to 10 min. Measure the exercise HR at the end of each minute. Continue the rowing exercise until the client achieves a steady-state HR. Use the Hagerman nomogram (see figure 4.12)

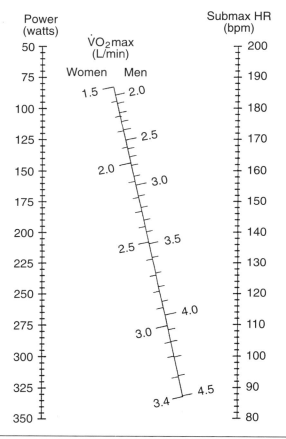

Figure 4.12 Concept II nomogram for estimating $\dot{V}O_2$max in noncompetitive and unskilled male and female rowers.

From "Concept II Rowing Ergometer Nomogram for Prediction of Maximal Oxygen Consumption" by Dr. Fritz Hagerman, Ohio University, Athens, OH. The nomogram is not appropriate for use with non-Concept II ergometers and is designed to be used by non-competitive or unskilled rowers participating in aerobic conditioning programs. Adapted by permission of CONCEPT II, INC. RR1, Box 1100, Morrisville, VT, (800) 245-5676.

to estimate $\dot{V}O_2$max from the submaximal power output (watts) and the steady-state HR during the last minute of exercise.

The Lakomy (1993) protocol is designed for both noncompetitive and skilled male rowers using the Concept II rowing ergometer. Prior to testing, set the fan blades in the fully closed position and select the large axle sprocket. The protocol begins with a 6-min warm-up that consists of rowing at an intensity of 50% to 60% HRmax. The warm-up is followed by a 2-min recovery period and a 6-min submaximal exercise bout, in which the client rows at an intensity of 80% to 90% HRmax while maintaining constant 500-m split times throughout. Measure your client's HR every 30 sec, and average the 5-, 5 1/2-, and 6-min HRs. Also, record the distance covered at the end of minutes 4 and 6.

Use the Lakomy nomogram (see figure 4.13) to estimate your client's $\dot{V}O_2$max from the distance covered during the last 2 min (subtract the 4-min distance from the 6-min distance) and the aver-

age exercise HR ([HR$_5$ + HR$_{5\,1/2}$ + HR$_6$]/3). This nomogram is based on an HRmax of 191 bpm. Therefore, you need to apply correction factors

Table 4.9 Maximal Heart Rate Correction Factors for the Lakomy Rowing Ergometer Protocol

HRmax	Factor
205	1.11
200	1.07
195	1.03
190	0.99
185	0.95
180	0.92
175	0.88
170	0.85

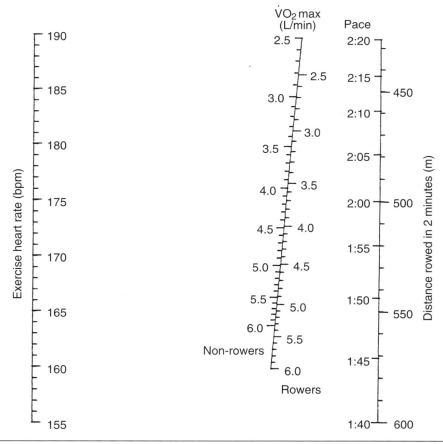

Figure 4.13 Concept II nomogram for estimating $\dot{V}O_2$max in noncompetitive and skilled male rowers.

From "Estimation of Maximum Oxygen Uptake from Submaximal Exercise on a Concept II Rowing Ergometer" by H.K.A. Lakomy and J. Lakomy, 1993, *Journal of Sports Sciences,* 11, p. 230. Adapted by permission of E. & F.N. Spon (an imprint of Chapman & Hall). © Taylor & Francis Ltd. (**http://www.tandf.co.uk/journals**).

for clients whose HRmax is greater or less than 191 bpm (table 4.9). Also, to estimate your client's HRmax for use with this nomogram, Lakomy and Lakomy (1993) recommend using the formula HRmax = 211 – age instead of the standard formula, HRmax = 220 – age. This adjustment accounts for the fact that the HRmax for rowing exercise is 8 to 10 bpm lower than the standard, age-predicted HRmax.

FIELD TESTS FOR ASSESSING AEROBIC FITNESS

The maximal and submaximal exercise tests using the treadmill or bicycle ergometer are not well suited for measuring the cardiorespiratory fitness of large groups in a field situation. Thus, a number of performance tests such as distance runs have been devised to predict $\dot{V}O_2$max (see table 4.8). These tests are practical, inexpensive, less time consuming than the treadmill or bicycle ergometer tests, and easy to administer to large groups; they can be used to classify the cardiorespiratory fitness level of healthy men (≤45 years) and women (≤55 years). You cannot use field tests to detect CHD because HR, ECG, and BP are usually not monitored during the performance. Most field tests used to assess cardiorespiratory endurance involve walking, running, swimming, cycling, or bench stepping; they require that clients be able to accurately measure their postexercise HR. Pollock, Broida, and Kendrick (1972) found that with practice, men could learn to measure their own pulse rates accurately. The correlation between manual and electronic measurements of pulse rate ranged between $r = 0.91$ and 0.94. Similar results ($r = 0.95$) were reported for college women for pulse rates measured manually and electronically (Witten 1973). Prior to administering field tests that require the measurement of HR, you should teach your clients how to measure their pulse rates using the palpation technique described in "How to Measure Your Pulse Rate."

Distance Run Tests

The most commonly used distance runs involve running distances of 1.0 or 1.5 miles (1600 to 2400 m) to evaluate aerobic capacity. Distance run tests are based on the assumption that the more fit individual will be able to run a given distance in less time or to run a greater distance in a given period of time. Using factor analysis, Disch, Frankiewicz,

---

HOW TO MEASURE YOUR PULSE RATE

1. Use your middle and index fingers to locate the radial pulse on the outside of your wrist just below the base of your thumb. Do not use your thumb to feel the pulse because it has a pulse of its own and may produce an inaccurate count.

2. If you cannot feel the radial pulse, try locating the carotid pulse by placing your fingers lightly on the front of your neck, just to the side of your voice box. Do not apply heavy pressure because this will cause your HR to slow down.

3. Use a stopwatch or the second hand of your wristwatch and count the number of pulse beats for a 6-, 10-, or 15-sec period.

4. Convert the pulse count to beats per minute using the following multipliers: 6-sec count times 10, 10-sec count times 6, and 15-sec count times 4.

5. Remember this value and record it on your scorecard.

---

and Jackson (1975) noted that runs greater than 1.0 mile tended to load exclusively on the endurance factor rather than the speed factor.

You should be aware that the relationship between distance runs and $\dot{V}O_2$max has not been firmly established. Although performance on a distance run can be accurately measured, it may not be an accurate index of $\dot{V}O_2$max or a substitute for the direct measurement of $\dot{V}O_2$max. Endurance running performance may be influenced by other factors such as motivation, percent fat (Cureton et al. 1978; Katch, McArdle, Czula, and Pechar 1973), running efficiency (pacing ability), and lactate threshold (Costill and Fox 1969; Costill, Thomason, and Roberts 1973).

The correlations between distance run tests and $\dot{V}O_2$max tend to vary considerably ($r = 0.27$ to 0.90) depending on the subjects, sample size, and testing procedures (George et al. 1993; Rikli, Petray, and Baumgartner 1992; Zwiren, Freedson, Ward, Wilke, and Rippe 1991). Generally, the longer the run, the higher the correlation with $\dot{V}O_2$max. On the basis of this observation, it is recommended that you select a test with a distance of at least 1.0 mile (1600 m) or a duration of at least 9 min.

The most widely used distance run tests are the 9- and 12-min runs and the 1.0- and 1.5-mile runs.

Some physical fitness test batteries for children and adolescents recommend using either the 9-min or 1.0-mile run tests.

Nine- or Twelve-Minute Run Tests

To administer the 9- or 12-min run test, use a 400-m track or flat course with measured distances so that the number of laps completed can be easily counted and multiplied by the course distance. Place markers to divide the course into quarters or eighths of a mile so that you can quickly determine the exact distance covered in 9 or 12 min. Instruct your clients to run as far as possible. Walking is allowed, but the objective of these tests is to cover as much distance as possible in either 9 or 12 min. At the end of the test, calculate the total distance covered in meters and use the appropriate equation in table 4.8 to estimate the client's $\dot{V}O_2$max.

1.5-Mile Run/Walk Test

The 1.5-mile run/walk test is conducted on a 400-m track or flat measured area. To measure the course, use an odometer or measuring wheel. For the 1.5-mile run, instruct your clients to cover the specified distance in the fastest possible time. Walking is allowed, but the objective is to cover the distance in the shortest possible time. Call out the elapsed time (in minutes and seconds) as the client crosses the finish line.

To use the $\dot{V}O_2$max prediction equation for the 1.5-mile run/walk test (see table 4.8), convert the seconds to minutes by dividing the seconds by 60. For example, if a client's time for the test is 12:30, the run time is converted to 12.5 min (30/60 sec = 0.5 min). This prediction equation estimates your client's $\dot{V}O_2$max from run time (in minutes), body weight (in kilograms), and gender.

1.0-Mile Jogging Test

One limitation of distance run tests is that individuals are encouraged to run as fast as possible and give a maximal effort, thereby increasing the risk of cardiovascular and orthopedic injuries. The potential risk is even greater for untrained individuals who do not run or jog regularly and have difficulty selecting a proper jogging pace. To address this problem, George et al. (1993) developed a submaximal 1-mile track jogging test for 18- to 29-year-old women and men that requires only moderate, steady-state exertion.

For this test, instruct your clients to select a comfortable, moderate jogging pace and to mea-sure their postexercise HR immediately following the test. The elapsed time for 1 mile should be at least 8 min for males and 9 min for females, and the postexercise HR (15-sec count $\times$ 4) should not exceed 180 bpm. To help establish a suitable pace, precede the timed 1-mile test with a 2- to 3-min warm-up. Use either an indoor or outdoor track for this test. Record the time required to jog 1 mile in minutes, and have your clients measure their postexercise HRs using the palpation technique (radial or carotid sites). Estimate the client's $\dot{V}O_2$max using the prediction equation for the 1.0-mile steady-state jog test (see table 4.8).

Walking Test

The Rockport Walking Institute (1986) has developed a walking test to assess cardiorespiratory fitness for men and women ages 20 to 69 years. Because this test requires only fast walking, it is useful for testing older or sedentary individuals (Fenstermaker, Plowman, and Looney 1992). The test was developed and validated for a large, heterogeneous sample of 86 women and 83 men (Kline et al. 1987). The cross-validation analysis resulted in a high validity coefficient and small standard error of estimate (*SEE*), indicating that the 1.0-mile walking test yields a valid submaximal assessment of estimated $\dot{V}O_2$max. Other researchers have substantiated the predictive accuracy of this equation for women 65 years of age and older (Fenstermaker et al. 1992).

To administer this test, instruct your clients to walk 1.0 mile as quickly as possible and to take their HR immediately at the end of the test by counting the pulse for 15 sec. It is important that clients know how to take their pulse accurately. The walking course should be a measured mile that is flat and uninterrupted, preferably a 400-m track. Clients should stretch for 5 to 10 min before the test and wear good walking shoes and loose-fitting clothes.

To estimate your client's $\dot{V}O_2$max, use the generalized equation for the 1.0-mile walking test (see table 4.8). Alternatively, you can use the Rockport relative fitness charts (appendix B.2, p. 292) to classify your client's cardiorespiratory fitness level. Locate the walking time and corresponding postexercise HR (bpm) on the appropriate chart for the individual's age and gender. These charts are based on body weights of 125 lb for women and 170 lb for men. If the client weighs substantially more than this, the cardiorespiratory fitness level will be overestimated.

Step Tests

The major advantage of using step tests to assess cardiorespiratory fitness is that they can be administered to large groups in a field situation without requiring expensive equipment or highly trained personnel. Most of these step tests use postexercise and recovery HRs to evaluate aerobic fitness, but they do not provide an estimate of the individual's $\dot{V}O_2$max. Step test protocols and scoring procedures are described in appendix B.3, "Step Test Protocols," page 294.

The validity of step tests is highly dependent on the accurate measurement of pulse rate. Step tests that use recovery HR tend to possess lower validity than those using the time required for the HR to reach a specified level during performance of a standardized workload (Baumgartner and Jackson 1975). The correlation coefficients between step test performance and $\dot{V}O_2$max range between $r = 0.32$ and 0.77 (Cureton and Sterling 1964; deVries and Klafs 1965; McArdle et al. 1972).

Additional Field Tests

In addition to running, walking, and step tests, cycling and swimming tests have been devised for use in field situations (Cooper 1977). The 12-min cycling test, using a bike with no more than three speeds, is conducted on a hard, flat surface when the wind velocity is less than 10 mph (268 m· min^{-1}). These conditions limit the effect of outside influences on the rider's performance. Five- and ten-speed bikes are not employed unless use of the lower gears can be restricted. Use an odometer to measure the distance traveled in 12 min. In the 12-min swimming test, the client may use any stroke and rest as needed. Norms for the 12-min cycling test and 12-min swimming test are available (Cooper 1977).

Of these two tests, the swimming test is the less preferred because the outcome is highly skill dependent. For example, a skilled swimmer with an average cardiorespiratory fitness level will probably be able to swim farther in 12 min than a poorly skilled swimmer with an above-average cardiorespiratory fitness level. In fact, Conley and colleagues (1991, 1992) reported that the 12-min swim has low validity ($r = 0.34$ to 0.42) as a cardiorespiratory field test for male and female recreational swimmers. Whenever possible, select an alternative field test and avoid using the 12-min swim test.

EXERCISE TESTING FOR CHILDREN AND OLDER ADULTS

You may need to modify the generic guidelines for exercise testing (see "General Principles of Exercise Testing," p. 55) of low-risk adults when you are assessing cardiorespiratory fitness of children and older adults (ACSM 2000). You must take into account growth, maturation, and aging when selecting exercise testing modes and protocols for these groups.

Assessing Cardiorespiratory Fitness of Children

In the laboratory setting, you can assess the cardiorespiratory fitness of children using either the treadmill or bicycle ergometer. Treadmill testing is usually preferable, especially for younger children, because their shortened attention span may not allow them to maintain a constant pedaling rate during a cycle ergometer test. Also, children younger than 8 years may not be tall enough to use a standard bicycle ergometer.

For treadmill testing, you should use the modified Balke protocol (see table 4.10) because the speed is constant and the intensity is increased by changing the grade. For cycle ergometer testing, ACSM (2000) recommends the McMaster protocol (see table 4.10). For this protocol, the pedaling frequency is 50 rpm, and increments in work rate are based on the child's height.

Cardiorespiratory field tests, such as the 1.0-mile (1600 m) run/walk, are widely used to assess the cardiorespiratory fitness of children 5 to 17 years of age. These tests are part of the Physical Best Program (American Alliance for Health, Physical Education, Recreation and Dance 1988), Fitnessgram (Cooper Institute for Aerobics Research 1994), and the President's Challenge Test (President's Council on Physical Fitness and Sports 1997), as well as national physical fitness surveys of children and youth (Ross and Pate 1987). To estimate $\dot{V}O_2$peak of 8- to 17-year-olds for the 1.0-mile run/walk test, you can use a generalized prediction equation (see table 4.8) (Cureton, Sloniger, O'Bannon, Black, and McCormack 1995). For younger children (5 to 7 years of age), the 0.5-mile run/walk test is recommended (Rikli, Petray, and Baumgartner 1992). Criterion-referenced standards for the 1.0-mile test are available elsewhere (American Alliance for Health, Physical Education, Recreation and Dance 1988; Cooper Institute for Aerobics Research 1994).

Table 4.10   Graded Exercise Test Protocols for Children (Skinner 1993)

Modified Balke Treadmill Protocol

Activity classification	Speed (mph)	Initial grade (%)	Increment (%)	Duration (min)
Poorly fit	3.0	6	2	2
Sedentary	3.25	6	2	2
Active	5.0	0	2.5	2
Athletes	5.25	0	2.5	2

McMaster Bicycle Ergometer Protocol

Height (cm)	Initial work rate: kgm·min^{-1} (watts)	Increments: kgm·min^{-1} (watts)	Duration (min)
<120	75 (12.5)	75 (12.5)	2
120-139.9	75 (12.5)	150 (25)	2
140-159.9	150 (25)	150 (25)	2
≥160	150 (25) 150 (25) for girls	300 (50) for boys	2

In Canada and Europe, the multistage 20-meter shuttle run test, developed by Leger and colleagues (1982, 1988), is a popular alternative to distance running/walking field tests to estimate the aerobic fitness of children (8-19 yr) in educational settings. This test has been cross-validated using other samples of European and Canadian children (Anderson 1992; vanMechelen, Holbil, and Kemper 1986).

For this test, children run back and forth continuously on a 20-meter (indoor or outdoor) course. The running speed is set using a sound signal emitted from a pre-recorded tape. The starting pace is 8.5 km·hr^{-1} and the speed is increased 0.5 km·hr^{-1} each minute until they can no longer maintain the pace. The maximal aerobic speed at this stage is used, in combination with age, in the following equation to estimate $\dot{V}O_2$max:

$$\dot{V}O_2\text{max} = 31.025 + 3.238(\text{speed, km·hr}^{-1})$$
$$(\text{ml·kg}^{-1}\text{·min}^{-1}) \quad - 3.248(\text{age, yr})$$
$$+ 0.1536(\text{age} \times \text{speed})$$

Assessing Cardiorespiratory Fitness of Older Adults

To assess the cardiorespiratory of elderly clients, you can use modified treadmill and bicycle ergometer protocols. The following modifications for standard GXT protocols are recommended:

- Extend the warm-up to more than 3 min.
- Set an initial exercise intensity of 2 to 3 METs; work increments should be 0.5 to 1.0 MET (e.g., Naughton treadmill protocol; see table 4.4, p. 61).
- Adjust (reduce) the treadmill speed to the walking ability of your client when needed.
- Extend the duration of each work stage (at least 3 min), allowing enough time for the client to attain steady state.
- Select a protocol likely to produce a total test time of 8 to 12 min.

Select treadmill protocols that increase grade, instead of speed, especially for older clients with poor ambulation. You can modify the standard Balke protocol (see figure 4.2) by having the client walk at 0% grade and 3.0 mph or slower initially and by increasing the duration of each stage to at least 3 min. If elderly clients are more comfortable holding on to the handrails during a treadmill test, you can use the standard Bruce protocol and the McConnell and Clark (1987) prediction equation to estimate their $\dot{V}O_2$max (see table 4.5). Alternatively, you could use bicycle ergometer GXTs for older individuals with poor balance, poor neuromuscular coordination, or impaired vision.

SOURCES FOR EQUIPMENT

Product	Manufacturer's Address
Bicycle ergometer (Lode electronically braked)	Physio-Dyne 1095 Broadhollow Rd. Farmingdale, NY 11735 (516) 694-6550 www.pb.net/~physio-dyne
Bicycle ergometer (Monark)	Monark 948 Greenbay Rd. Winnetka, IL 60093 (800) 359-4610 www.monarkbikes.com
Bicycle ergometer (Bodyguard, Tunturi, Schwinn)	U.S. Fitness Products 3072 Wake Forest Rd. Raleigh, NC 27609 (919) 875-1900 www.usafitness.com
Elliptical trainers	Life Fitness 10601 W. Belmont Ave. Franklin Park, IL 60131 (800) 735-3867 www.lifefitness.com Precor P.O. Box 3004 Bothell, WA 98041 (800) 786-8404 www.precor.com
Nordic ski machine	Nordic Track 104 Peavey Rd. Chaska, MN 55138 (800) 220-1256 www.nordictrack.com
Rowing ergometer	Concept II, Inc. 105 Industrial Park Dr. Morrisville, VT 05661 (800) 245-5676 www.concept2.com
Stair climbing machines	StairMaster Sports/Medical Products, Inc. 12421 Willows Rd. N.E., Ste. 100 Kirkland, WA 98034 (800) 635-2936 www.stairmaster.com
Treadmill (Quinton)	Quinton Instrument Co. 3303 Monte Villa Pkwy. Bothell, WA 98021 (800) 426-0347 www.quinton.com

KEY POINTS

- The best way to assess aerobic capacity (cardiorespiratory fitness) is through a GXT in which the functional $\dot{V}O_2$max is measured.

- Unless contraindications to exercise are observed, you should administer a maximal exercise test to moderate-risk men ($\geq$45 years) and women ($\geq$55 years) before they begin a vigorous exercise program.

- Before, during, and after a maximal or submaximal exercise test, closely monitor the HR, BP, and RPE.

- Treadmill, bicycle ergometer, and bench stepping are the most commonly used modes of exercise for exercise testing.

- The choice of exercise mode and exercise test protocol depends on the age, gender, purpose of the test, and the health and fitness status of the individual.

- Submaximal exercise tests are used to estimate the functional aerobic capacity by predicting the $\dot{V}O_2$max of the individual. Failure to meet the assumptions underlying submaximal exercise tests produces a $\pm$10% to 20% error in the prediction of $\dot{V}O_2$max from submaximal HR data.

- Field tests are the least desirable way of assessing aerobic capacity and should not be used for diagnostic purposes. However, field tests are useful for assessing the cardiorespiratory fitness of large groups.

- Commonly used field tests include distance runs, walking tests, and step tests.

- Distance runs should last at least 9 min to assess aerobic function. Distance runs usually range between 1 and 2 miles (1600 to 3200 m) or 9 to 12 min.

- The validity of step tests for assessing cardiorespiratory fitness is highly dependent on the accurate measurement of HR and is usually somewhat lower than the validity of distance run tests.

KEY TERMS

Learn the definition for each of the following key terms. Definitions of key terms can be found in "Glossary of Terms," page 349.

absolute $\dot{V}O_2$
cardiorespiratory endurance
graded exercise test
gross $\dot{V}O_2$
maximal exercise test
maximum oxygen uptake
net $\dot{V}O_2$

peak $\dot{V}O_2$
ratings of perceived exertion
relative $\dot{V}O_2$
respiratory exchange ratio
submaximal exercise test
$\dot{V}O_2$max

REVIEW QUESTIONS

In addition to being able to define each of the key terms listed, test your knowledge and understanding of the material by answering the following review questions.

1. What is the most valid and direct measure of functional aerobic capacity?

2. What is the difference between absolute and relative $\dot{V}O_2$?

3. What is the difference between gross and net $\dot{V}O_2$?

4. What is the difference between $\dot{V}O_2$max and $\dot{V}O_2$peak?

5. What factors should you consider when choosing a maximal or submaximal exercise test protocol for your client?

6. Identify the ACSM criteria for attainment of $\dot{V}O_2$max during a GXT.

7. During a GXT, what three variables are monitored at regular intervals?

8. List three reasons for stopping a GXT.

9. What is active recovery, and why is it recommended for graded exercise testing?

10. What is the difference between continuous, discontinuous, and ramp exercise testing protocols?

11. Calculate the gross $\dot{V}O_2$ for a 60-kg woman running on a treadmill at a speed of 6.0 mph and a grade of 10%.

12. Calculate the gross $\dot{V}O_2$ for an 80-kg man cycling on Monark bicycle ergometer at a pedaling frequency of 70 rpm and a resistance of 3.5 kg.

13. Calculate the energy expenditure for bench stepping using an 8-in. step and a cadence of 30 steps/min.

14. Name three types of field tests for estimating aerobic capacity.

15. Which type of testing, treadmill or bicycle ergometer, should be used for assessing the cardiorespiratory fitness of children?

16. How should standard GXT protocols be modified for testing of older adults?

REFERENCES

American Alliance for Health, Physical Education, Recreation and Dance. 1988. *The AAHPERD physical best program*. Reston, VA: Author.

American College of Sports Medicine (ACSM). 1991. *Guidelines for exercise testing and prescription,* 4th ed. Philadelphia: Lea & Febiger.

American College of Sports Medicine. 1999. *ACSM health/fitness instructor certification study guide.* Philadelphia: Lippincott, Williams & Wilkins.

American College of Sports Medicine. 2000. *ACSM's guidelines for exercise testing and prescription,* 6th ed. Philadelphia: Lippincott Williams & Wilkins.

Anderson, G.S. 1992. The 1600-m and multistage 20-m shuttle run as predictive tests of aerobic capacity in children. *Pediatric Exercise Science* 4: 312–318.

Åstrand, I. 1960. Aerobic capacity in men and women with special reference to age. *Acta Physiologica Scandinavica* 49(Suppl. 169): 1–92.

Åstrand, P.O. 1956. Human physical fitness with special reference to age and sex. *Physiological Reviews* 36: 307–335.

Åstrand, P.O. 1965. *Work tests with the bicycle ergometer.* Varberg, Sweden: AB Cykelfabriken Monark.

Åstrand, P.O., and Rodahl, K. 1977. *Textbook of work physiology.* New York: McGraw-Hill.

Åstrand, P.O., and Ryhming, I. 1954. A nomogram for calculation of aerobic capacity (physical fitness) from pulse rate during submaximal work. *Journal of Applied Physiology* 7: 218–221.

Atterhog, J.H., Jonsson, B., and Samuelsson, R. 1979. Exercise testing: A prospective study of complication rates. *American Heart Journal* 98: 572-580.

Balke, B. 1963. A simple field test for the assessment of physical fitness. *Civil Aeromedical Research Institute Report,* 63–18. Oklahoma City: Federal Aviation Agency.

Balke, B., and Ware, R. 1959. An experimental study of physical fitness of Air Force personnel. *US Armed Forces Medical Journal* 10: 675–688.

Baumgartner, T.A., and Jackson, A.S. 1975. *Measurement for evaluation in physical education.* Boston: Houghton Mifflin.

Borg, G. 1982. Psychophysical bases of perceived exertion. *Medicine & Science in Sports & Exercise* 14: 377–381.

Bruce, R.A., Kusumi, F., and Hosmer, D. 1973. Maximal oxygen intake and nomographic assessment of functional aerobic impairment in cardiovascular disease. *American Heart Journal* 85: 546–562.

Conley, D., Cureton, K., Dengel, D., and Weyand, P. 1991. Validation of the 12-min swim as a field test of peak aerobic power in young men. *Medicine & Science in Sports & Exercise* 23: 766–773.

Conley, D., Cureton, K., Hinson, B., Higbie, E., and Weyand, P. 1992. Validation of the 12-minute swim as a field test of peak aerobic power in young women. *Research Quarterly for Exercise and Sport* 63: 153–161.

Cooper, K.H. 1968. A means of assessing maximal oxygen intake. *Journal of the American Medical Association* 203: 201–204.

Cooper, K.H. 1977. *The aerobics way.* New York: Evans.

Cooper Institute for Aerobics Research. 1994. *Fitnessgram user's manual.* Dallas: Author.

Cooper Institute for Aerobics Research. 1997. *The fitness specialist certification manual.* Dallas: Author.

Costill, D.L., and Fox, E.L. 1969. Energetics of marathon running. *Medicine and Science in Sports* 1: 81–86.

Costill, D.L., Thomason, H., and Roberts, E. 1973. Fractional utilization of the aerobic capacity during distance running. *Medicine and Science in Sports* 5: 248–252.

Cureton, K., Sloniger, M., O'Bannon, J., Black, D., and McCormack, W. 1995. A generalized equation for prediction of $\dot{V}O_2$peak from 1-mile run/walk performance. *Medicine & Science in Sports & Exercise* 27: 445–451.

Cureton, K.J., Sparling, P.B., Evans, B.W., Johnson, S.M., Kong, U.D., and Purvis, J.W. 1978. Effect of experimental alterations in excess weight on aerobic capacity and distance running performance. *Medicine and Science in Sports* 10: 194–199.

Cureton, T.K., and Sterling, L.F. 1964. Interpretation of the cardiovascular component resulting from the factor analysis of 104 test variables measured in 100 normal young men. *Journal of Sports Medicine and Physical Fitness* 4: 1–24.

deVries, H.A., and Klafs, C.E. 1965. Prediction of maximal oxygen intake from submaximal tests. *Journal of Sports Medicine and Physical Fitness* 5: 207–214.

Disch, J., Frankiewicz, R., and Jackson, A. 1975. Construct validation of distance run tests. *Research Quarterly* 46: 169–176.

Ebbeling, C., Ward, A., Puleo, E., Widrick, J., and Rippe, J. 1991. Development of a single-stage submaximal treadmill walking test. *Medicine & Science in Sports & Exercise* 23: 966–973.

Fenstermaker, K., Plowman, S., and Looney, M. 1992. Validation of the Rockport walking test in females 65 years and older. *Research Quarterly for Exercise and Sport* 63: 322–327.

Foster, C., Jackson, A.S., Pollock, M.L., Taylor, M.M., Hare, J., Sennett, S.M., Rod, J.L., Sarwar, M., and Schmidt, D.H. 1984. Generalized equations for predicting functional capacity from treadmill performance. *American Heart Journal* 107: 1229–1234.

Foster, C., Pollock, M.L., Rod, J.L., Dymond, D.S., Wible, G., and Schmidt, D.H. 1983. Evaluation of functional capacity during exercise radionuclide angiography. *Cardiology* 70: 85–93.

Fox, E.L. 1973. A simple, accurate technique for predicting maximal aerobic power. *Journal of Applied Physiology* 35: 914–916.

George, J., Vehrs, P., Allsen, P., Fellingham, G., and Fisher, G. 1993. $\dot{V}O_2$max estimation from a submaximal 1-mile track jog for fit college-age individuals. *Medicine & Science in Sports & Exercise* 25: 401–406.

Gibbons, R.A., Balady, G.J., Beasely, J.W., Bricker, J.T., Duvemoy, W.F., Froelicher, V.F., Mark, D.B., Marwick, T.H., McCallister, B.D., Thompson, P.D. Jr., Winters, W.L., Yanowitz, F.G., Ritchie, J.L., Gibbons, R.J., Cheitlin, M.D., Eagle, K.A., Gardner, T.J., Garson, A. Jr., Lewis, R.P., O'Rourke, R.A., and Ryan, T.J. 1997. ACC/AHA guidelines for exercise testing. A report of the American College of Cardiology/ American Heart Association Task Force on Prac-

tice Guidelines. *Journal of the American College of Cardiology* 30: 260–311.

Gledhill, N., and Jamnik, R. 1995. Determining power outputs for cycle ergometers with different sized flywheels. *Medicine & Science in Sports & Exercise* 27: 134–135.

Golding, L., Meyers, C., and Sinning, W., eds. 1989. *The Y's way to physical fitness.* Champaign, IL: Human Kinetics.

Greiwe, J., Kaminsky, L., Whaley, M., and Dwyer, G. 1995. Evaluation of the ACSM submaximal ergometer test for estimating $\dot{V}O_2$max. *Medicine & Science in Sports & Exercise* 27: 1315–1320.

Hagerman, F. 1993. *Concept II rowing ergometer nomogram for prediction of maximal oxygen consumption* [abstract]. Morrisville, VT: Concept II.

Hanson, P. 1988. Clinical exercise testing. In *Resource manual for guidelines for exercise testing and prescription,* ed. S.N. Blair, P. Painter, R. Pate, L.K. Smith, and C.B. Taylor, 248–255. Philadelphia: Lea & Febiger.

Hermansen, L., and Saltin, B. 1969. Oxygen uptake during maximal treadmill and bicycle exercise. *Journal of Applied Physiology* 26: 31–37.

Howley, E., Colacino, D., and Swensen, T. 1992. Factors affecting the oxygen cost of stepping on an electronic stepping ergometer. *Medicine & Science in Sports & Exercise* 24: 1055–1058.

Katch, F.I., McArdle, W.D., Czula, R., and Pechar, G.S. 1973. Maximal oxygen intake, endurance running performance, and body composition in college women. *Research Quarterly* 44: 301–312.

Kattus, A.A., Hanafee, W.N., Longmire, W.P., MacAlpin, R.N., and Rivin, A.U. 1968. Diagnosis, medical and surgical management of coronary insufficiency. *Annals of Internal Medicine* 69: 115–136.

Kline, G.M., Porcari, J.P., Hintermeister, R., Freedson, P.S., Ward, A., McCarron, R.F., Ross, J., and Rippe, J.M. 1987. Estimation of $\dot{V}O_2$max from a one-mile track walk, gender, age, and body weight. *Medicine & Science in Sports & Exercise* 19: 253–259.

Lakomy, H., and Lakomy, J. 1993. Estimation of maximum oxygen uptake from submaximal exercise on a Concept II rowing ergometer. *Journal of Sports Sciences* 11: 227–232.

Latin, R., and Elias, B. 1993. Predictions of maximum oxygen uptake from treadmill walking and running. *Journal of Sports Medicine and Physical Fitness* 33: 34–39.

Leger, L.A., and Lambert, J. 1982. A maximal multistage 20-m shuttle run test to predict $\dot{V}O_2$max. *European Journal of Applied Physiology and Occupational Physiology* 49: 1–12.

Leger, L.A., Mercier, D., Gadoury, C., and Lambert, J. 1988. The multistage 20-metre shuttle run test for aerobic fitness. *Journal of Sports Sciences* 6: 93–101.

Levine, B., Zuckerman, J., and Cole, C. 1998. Medical complications of exercise. In *ACSM's resource manual for guidelines for exercise testing and prescription*, ed. J.L. Roitman, 488–498. Philadelphia: Lippincott Williams & Wilkins.

Londeree, B., and Moeschberger, M. 1984. Influence of age and other factors on maximal heart rate. *Journal of Cardiac Rehabilitation* 4: 44–49.

Mahar, M.T., Jackson, A.S., Ross, R.M., Pivarnik, J.M., and Pollock, M.L. 1985. Predictive accuracy of single and double stage submax treadmill work for estimating aerobic capacity. *Medicine & Science in Sports & Exercise* 17: 206–207.

Maksud, M.G., and Coutts, K.D. 1971. Comparison of a continuous and discontinuous graded treadmill test for maximal oxygen uptake. *Medicine and Science in Sports* 3: 63–65.

Marley, W., and Linnerud, A. 1976. A three-year study of the Åstrand-Ryhming step test. *Research Quarterly* 47: 211–217.

McArdle, W.D., Katch, F.I., and Katch, V.L. 1996. *Exercise physiology: Energy, nutrition and human performance*, 4th ed. Baltimore: Williams & Wilkins.

McArdle, W.D., Katch, F.I., and Pechar, G.S. 1973. Comparison of continuous and discontinuous treadmill and bicycle tests for $\dot{V}O_2$max. *Medicine and Science in Sports* 5: 156–160.

McArdle, W.D., Katch, F.I., Pechar, G.S., Jacobson, L., and Ruck, S. 1972. Reliability and interrelationships between maximal oxygen intake, physical working capacity and step-test scores in college women. *Medicine and Science in Sports* 4: 182–186.

McConnell, T., and Clark, B. 1987. Prediction of maximal oxygen consumption during handrail-supported treadmill exercise. *Journal of Cardiopulmonary Rehabilitation* 7: 324–331.

McInnis, K., and Balady, G. 1994. Comparison of submaximal exercise responses using the Bruce vs modified Bruce protocols. *Medicine & Science in Sports & Exercise* 26: 103–107.

Morehouse, L.E. 1972. *Laboratory manual for physiology of exercise*. St. Louis: Mosby.

Nagle, F.S., Balke, B., and Naughton, J.P. 1965. Gradational step tests for assessing work capacity. *Journal of Applied Physiology* 20: 745–748.

Naughton, J., Balke, B., and Nagle, F. 1964. Refinement in methods of evaluation and physical conditioning before and after myocardial infarction. *American Journal of Cardiology* 14: 837.

Pollock, M.L., Bohannon, R.L., Cooper, K.H., Ayres, J.J., Ward, A., White, S.R., and Linnerud, A.C. 1976. A comparative analysis of four protocols for maximal treadmill stress testing. *American Heart Journal* 92: 39–46.

Pollock, M.L., Broida, J., and Kendrick, Z. 1972. Validity of the palpation technique of heart rate determination and its estimation of training heart rate. *Research Quarterly* 43: 77–81.

Pollock, M.L., Foster, C., Schmidt, D., Hellman, C., Linnerud, A.C., and Ward, A. 1982. Comparative analysis of physiologic responses to three different maximal graded exercise test protocols in healthy women. *American Heart Journal* 103: 363–373.

Pollock, M.L., Wilmore, J.H., and Fox, S.M. III. 1978. *Health and fitness through physical activity*. New York: Wiley.

President's Council on Physical Fitness and Sports. 1997. *The presidential physical fitness award program*. Washington, D.C.: author.

Rikli, R., Petray, C., and Baumgartner, T. 1992. The reliability of distance run tests for children in grades K-4. *Research Quarterly for Exercise and Sport* 63: 270–276.

Rochmis, P., and Blackburn, H. 1971. Exercise tests. A survey of procedures, safety and litigation experience in approximately 170,000 tests. *Journal of the American Medical Association* 217: 1061–1066.

Rockport Walking Institute. 1986. *Rockport fitness walking test*. Marlboro, MA: Author.

Ross, J., and Pate, R. 1987. The national children and youth fitness study II: A summary of findings. *Journal of Physical Education, Recreation and Dance* 58: 51–56.

Shephard, R.J. 1972. *Alive man: The physiology of physical activity*. Springfield, IL: Charles C Thomas.

Shephard, R.J. 1977. Do risks of exercise justify costly caution? *The Physician and Sportsmedicine* 5: 58–65.

Sinning, W. 1975. *Experiments and demonstrations in exercise physiology*. Philadelphia: Saunders.

Skinner, J. 1993. *Exercise testing and exercise prescription for special cases*. Philadelphia: Lea & Febiger.

Terry, J.W., Tolson, H., Johnson, D.J., and Jessup, G.T. 1977. A work load selection procedure for the Åstrand-Ryhming test. *Journal of Sports Medicine and Physical Fitness* 17: 361–366.

Thompson, P.D. 1993. The safety of exercise testing and participation. In *ACSM's resource manual for guidelines for exercise testing and prescription*, ed. S.N. Blair, P. Painter, R. Pate, L.K. Smith, and C.B. Taylor, 361–370. Philadelphia: Lea & Febiger.

VanMechelen, W., Hibil, H., and Kemcer, H.C. 1986. Validation of two running tests as estimates of maximal erobic power in children. *European Journal of Applied Physiology and Occupational Physiology* 55: 503–506.

Whaley, M., Kaminsky, L., Dwyer, G., Getchell, L., and Norton, J. 1992. Predictors of over- and under-achievement of age-predicted maximal heart rate. *Medicine & Science in Sports & Exercise* 24: 1173–1179.

Wilson, P.K., Winga, E.R., Edgett, J.W., and Gushiken, T.J. 1978. *Policies and procedures of a cardiac rehabilitation program—immediate to long term care.* Philadelphia: Lea & Febiger.

Witten, C. 1973. Construction of a submaximal cardiovascular step test for college females. *Research Quarterly* 44: 46–50.

Zwiren, L., Freedson, P., Ward, A., Wilke, S., and Rippe, J. 1991. Estimation of $\dot{V}O_2$max: A comparative analysis of five exercise tests. *Research Quarterly for Exercise and Sport* 62: 73–78.

chapter 5

Designing Cardiorespiratory Exercise Programs

- What are the basic components of an aerobic exercise prescription?
- How is the aerobic exercise prescription individualized to meet each client's goals and interests?
- What methods are used to prescribe and monitor exercise intensity?
- Which exercise modes are best suited for an aerobic exercise prescription?

- How often does a client need to exercise to improve and maintain aerobic fitness?
- How long does a client need to exercise to improve aerobic fitness?
- Is discontinuous aerobic training as effective as continuous training?
- How effective are multimodal, cross-training programs?
- What are the physiological benefits of aerobic exercise training?

Once you have assessed an individual's cardiorespiratory fitness status, you are responsible for planning an aerobic exercise program to develop and maintain the cardiorespiratory endurance of that program participant—a program designed to meet the individual's needs and interests, taking into account age, gender, physical fitness level, and exercise habits. Appendix A.5, "Lifestyle Evaluation," page 270, provides forms that will help you determine your clients' exercise patterns and preferences.

In designing the exercise prescription, keep in mind that some people engage in aerobic exercise to improve their health status or reduce their disease risk, while others are primarily interested in enhancing their physical fitness ($\dot{V}O_2max$) levels. Given that the quantity of exercise needed to promote health is less than that needed to develop and maintain higher levels of physical fitness, you must adjust the exercise prescription according to your client's primary goal.

This chapter provides guidelines for writing individualized exercise prescriptions that promote health status as well as develop and maintain cardiorespiratory fitness. The chapter compares various training methods and aerobic exercise modes, and presents examples of individualized exercise programs.

THE EXERCISE PRESCRIPTION

It is important to consider your client's goals and purposes for engaging in an exercise program. The primary goal for exercising may affect the mode, intensity, frequency, duration, and progression of the exercise prescription. For example, the quantity of physical activity needed to achieve health benefits or reduce one's risk of illness and death is less than the amount of activity typically prescribed when the client's goal is to make substantial improvements in cardiorespiratory fitness.

When the primary goal for the exercise prescription is improved health, refer to "Guidelines for Exercise Prescription for Improved Health," below.

On the other hand, when the primary goal for the exercise prescription is to improve cardiorespiratory fitness, refer to "ACSM Guidelines for Exercise Prescription for Cardiorespiratory Fitness," below.

Elements of a Cardiorespiratory Exercise Workout

Each exercise workout of the aerobic exercise prescription and program should include the following phases:

- Warm-up
- Endurance
- Cool-down

The purpose of the warm-up is to increase blood flow to the working cardiac and skeletal muscles, increase body temperature, decrease the chance of muscle and joint injury, and lessen the chance of abnormal cardiac rhythms. During the warm-up, the tempo of the exercise is gradually increased to prepare the body for a higher intensity of exercise performed during the conditioning phase. The warm-up period usually includes 5 to 10 min of stretching exercises and light calisthenics for the legs, lower back, abdomen, hips, groin, and shoulders (for specific exercises, see appendix F.1, "Selected Flexibility Exercises," p. 336), as well as 5 to 10 min of low-intensity aerobic activity (e.g., brisk walking during warm-up for clients who jog during their endurance phase).

During the endurance phase of the workout, the aerobic exercise is performed according to the exercise prescription. This phase usually lasts 20

GUIDELINES FOR EXERCISE PRESCRIPTION FOR IMPROVED HEALTH

The following guidelines are from the U.S. Department of Health and Human Services (1996).

1. Mode: Select endurance-type physical activities, including formal aerobic exercise training, housework and yard work, and physically active recreational pursuits.

2. Intensity: Prescribe at least moderate-intensity physical activities ($\geq$45% $\dot{V}O_2$max).

3. Frequency: Schedule physical activity for most, preferably all, days of the week.

4. Duration: Accumulate at least 30 min of moderate activity each day. Duration varies according to the type and intensity of activity (see "Examples of Moderate Amounts of Physical Activity," chapter 1, p. 4).

ACSM GUIDELINES FOR EXERCISE PRESCRIPTION FOR CARDIORESPIRATORY FITNESS

These are the ACSM 2000 guidelines:

1. Mode: Select rhythmical aerobic activities that can be maintained continuously and that involve large muscle groups (see "Classification of Aerobic Exercise Modalities," p. 89).

2. Intensity: Prescribe intensities between 55/60% and 90% of maximal heart rate or between 40/50% and 85% of the oxygen uptake reserve ($\dot{V}O_2R$) or heart rate reserve (HRR). For individuals with very low initial cardiorespiratory fitness, use intensities between 40% and 50% $\dot{V}O_2R$.

3. Frequency: Schedule exercise three to five days a week.

4. Duration: Schedule 20 to 60 min of continuous aerobic activity, depending on the exercise intensity.

5. Rate of progression: Adjust the exercise prescription for each client in accordance with the conditioning effect, participant characteristics, new exercise test results, or performance during the exercise sessions. The rate of progression depends on the individual's age, functional capacity, health status, and goals. For apparently healthy adults, the aerobic exercise prescription consists of three stages: initial conditioning, improvement, and maintenance.

to 60 min, depending on the exercise intensity, and is followed immediately by the cool-down phase.

A cool-down phase immediately after endurance exercise is needed to reduce the risk of cardiovascular complications caused by stopping exercise suddenly. During cool-down, the individual continues exercising (e.g., walking, jogging, or cycling) at a low intensity for about 5 to 10 min. This light activity allows the heart rate (HR) and blood pressure (BP) to return to near baseline levels, prevents the pooling of blood in the extremities, and reduces the possibility of dizziness and fainting. The continued pumping action of the muscles increases the venous return and speeds up the recovery process. Stretching exercises may be repeated during the cool-down phase to reduce the chance of muscle cramps or muscle soreness.

Modes of Exercise

If the primary goal of the exercise program is to develop and maintain cardiorespiratory fitness, prescribe aerobic activities using large muscle groups in a continuous, rhythmical fashion. In the initial and improvement stages of the exercise program, it is important to closely monitor the exercise intensity. Therefore, you should select modes of exercise that allow the individual to maintain a constant exercise intensity and are not highly dependent on the participant's skill. **Group I activities,** such as walking, cycling, and simulated stair climbing (see below), are best suited for this purpose.

For **Group II activities** such as aerobic dance, step aerobics, and swimming, the rate of energy expenditure is highly dependent on the participant's skill level. You may prescribe Group II activities in the initial and improvement stages only for skilled individuals who are able to maintain constant exercise intensity while performing the activity. However, you should consider using Group II activities to add variety in the later stages (maintenance stage) of your client's exercise program.

Group III activities such as racquetball, basketball, and volleyball are highly variable in terms of exercise intensity and skill. Incorporate these activities only on a limited basis in the maintenance stage to add variety and fun to the exercise program. It is best that you do not emphasize competitive aspects of these activities, especially for high-risk and symptomatic participants.

In addition to walking, jogging, and cycling, there are other exercise modalities that provide a sufficient cardiorespiratory demand for improving aerobic fitness. Exercise modalities such as bench

Classification of Aerobic Exercise Modalities[a]

Group I activities	Group II activities	Group III activities
Cycling (indoors)	Aerobic dancing	Basketball
Jogging	Bench step aerobics	Country and western dancing
Running	Cycling (outdoors)	Handball
Walking	Hiking	Racquet sports
Rowing[b]	In-line skating	Volleyball
Stair climbing[b]	Nordic skiing (outdoors)	Super circuit weight training
Simulated climbing[b]	Rope skipping	
Nordic skiing[b]	Swimming	
Elliptical training[b]	Water aerobics	
Aerobic riding[bc]		

[a]Group I activities provide constant intensity and are not skill dependent; Group II activities may provide constant or variable intensity, depending on skill. Group III activities provide variable intensity and are highly skill dependent.

[b]Machine-based activities.

[c]May not provide adequate training intensity for above-average fitness levels.

step aerobics, machine-based stair climbing, elliptical training, and rowing offer your exercise program participants a variety of options for their exercise prescription. Many individuals prefer to cross-train to add variety and enjoyment to their aerobic workouts. But are these exercise modes just as effective as traditional Group I activities (walking, jogging, and cycling)? The answer to this question is not simple and depends on the method (%$\dot{V}O_2$max or perceived exertion) used to equate different exercise modalities.

During exercise at a prescribed percentage of $\dot{V}O_2$max, Thomas, Ziogas, Smith, Zhang, and Londeree (1995) noted that six different aerobic exercise modes (treadmill jogging, Nordic skiing, shuffle skiing, stepping, cycling, and rowing) produced relatively similar cardiovascular responses (see figure 5.1), but that cycling resulted in a significantly higher perceived exertion (RPE) compared to the other modes. Likewise, other researchers have reported that compared to the value for treadmill jogging, the relationship between HR and $\dot{V}O_2$ at constant, submaximal intensities was similar for in-line skating (Wallick et al. 1995) and aerobic dancing with arms used extensively above the head or kept below the shoulders (Berry, Cline, Berry, and Davis 1992). In

contrast, Parker, Hurley, Hanlon, and Vaccaro (1989) reported that the average steady-state HR during 20 min of aerobic dancing was significantly higher than that for treadmill jogging when the subjects exercised at the same relative intensity (60% $\dot{V}O_2$max). Likewise, Howley, Colacino, and Swensen (1992) noted that HR response during electronic stepping ergometer exercise was systematically higher than that with treadmill exercise at the same submaximal $\dot{V}O_2$. Also, supporting the body weight during step ergometer exercise significantly reduced the HR and oxygen consumption compared to lightly holding on to the handrails for balance.

When exercise modes are equated using subjective ratings of perceived exertion (RPEs), research suggests that treadmill jogging may be superior to other aerobic exercise modes in terms of total oxygen consumption and rate of energy expenditure (Kravitz, Robergs, and Heyward 1996; Kravitz, Robergs, Heyward, Wagner, and Powers 1997; Zeni, Hoffman, and Clifford 1996). Subjects exercising on seven different modalities at a somewhat hard (RPE = 13 to 14) intensity for 15 to 20 min experienced a greater total oxygen consumption for treadmill jogging compared to stepping, rowing, Nordic skiing, cycling, shuffle skiing, and

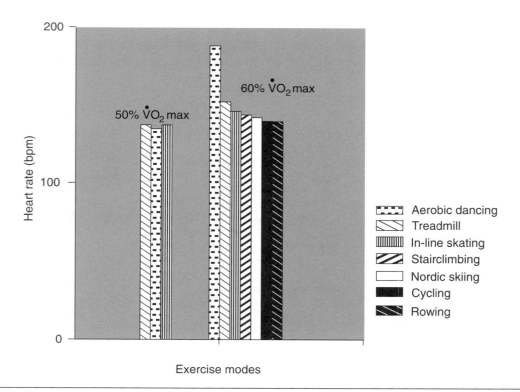

Figure 5.1 Comparison of steady-state heart rate response at submaximal exercise intensities for various aerobic exercise modes.

aerobic riding (Kravtiz, Robergs, et al. 1997; Thomas et al. 1995). Also, the rate of energy expenditure during treadmill exercise was 20% to 40% greater than during stationary cycling (Kravitz, Robergs, et al. 1997; Zeni et al. 1996) and 57% greater than during aerobic riding (Kravitz et al. 1996, Kravitz, Robergs, et al. 1997). In addition, steady-state exercise HRs were higher (see figure 5.2) for treadmill jogging compared to cycling and aerobic riding (Kravitz et al. 1996; Kravitz, Robergs, et al. 1997; Zeni et al. 1996).

When selecting aerobic exercise modes for your client's exercise prescription, you should consider how easily the exercise intensity can be graded and adjusted in order to overload the cardiorespiratory system throughout the improvement stage. For aerobic dance and bench step aerobic exercise, work rates can be progressively increased by means of quicker cadences, different bench heights (Olson, Williford, Blessing, and Greathouse 1991), and upper-body exercise using light (1 to 4 lb) handheld weights (Kravitz, Heyward, Stolarczyk, and Wilmerding 1997). The intensity of in-line skating can be effectively graded by increasing the skating velocity (Wallick et al. 1995). The intensity of rowing, stair climbing, and simulated whole-body climbing exercise can be incremented progressively using a variety of exercise machines (Brahler and Blank 1995; Howley et al. 1992).

Prescribe rope-skipping activities with caution; the exercise intensity for skipping 60 to 80 skips/min is approximately 9 METs. This value exceeds the maximum MET capacity of most sedentary individuals. Also, the exercise intensity is not easily graded because doubling the rate of skipping increases the energy requirement by only 2 to 3 METs. Town, Sol, and Sinning (1980) reported an average energy expenditure of 11.7 to 12.5 METs for skipping at rates of 125, 135, and 145 skips/min. They concluded that rope skipping is a strenuous exercise that may not be well suited as a form of graded, aerobic exercise.

When selecting exercise modes for your older clients, you need to consider their functional aerobic capacity, musculoskeletal problems, and neuromuscular coordination (impaired vision or balance). Select activities that are enjoyable and convenient. For many older adults, walking is an excellent mode. Stationary cycling and aquatic exercise can be used for individuals with impaired vision or balance. Research suggests that tai chi increases balance, muscular strength, and flexibility, as well as cardiorespiratory fitness ($\dot{V}O_2$peak)

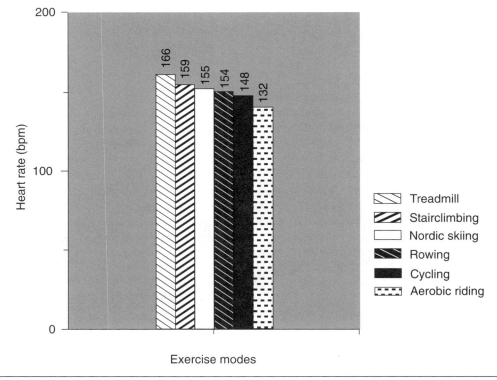

Figure 5.2 Comparison of steady-state heart rate response at somewhat hard intensity (rating of perceived exertion = 13 to 14) for various aerobic exercise modes.

of older adults (Chewning, Yu, and Johnson 2000; Lan, Lai, Chen, and Wong 1998).

Intensity of Exercise

Traditionally, exercise intensity has been expressed as a straight percentage of either the individual's maximal aerobic capacity ($\dot{V}O_2$max), peak oxygen consumption ($\dot{V}O_2$peak), or HRR. However, research has suggested that the %$\dot{V}O_2$max is not equivalent (1:1 ratio) to the %HRR for cycling and treadmill exercise (Swain and Leutholtz 1997; Swain, Leutholtz, King, Haas, and Branch 1998). Therefore, ACSM (2000) recently changed its recommendation regarding the method used to calculate exercise intensity for aerobic exercise prescriptions. Instead of expressing relative intensity as a straight percentage of $\dot{V}O_2$max (%$\dot{V}O_2$max), ACSM now recommends using the **percent $\dot{V}O_2$ reserve (%$\dot{V}O_2$R)**. The $\dot{V}O_2$R is the difference between the $\dot{V}O_2$max and resting oxygen consumption ($\dot{V}O_2$ rest). With this modification, percent values for the %$\dot{V}O_2$R and %HRR methods for prescribing exercise intensity are approximately equal, thereby improving the accuracy of calculating a target $\dot{V}O_2$, particularly for clients who are engaging in low-intensity aerobic exercise (Swain 1999).

Regardless of the method used, intensity and duration of exercise are indirectly related. In other words, the higher the exercise intensity, the shorter the duration of exercise required and vice versa. Before prescribing the exercise intensity for aerobic exercise, carefully evaluate the individual's initial cardiorespiratory fitness classification, goals for the program, exercise preferences, and injury risks. Your client can improve cardiorespiratory fitness with either lower-intensity, longer-duration exercise or higher-intensity, shorter-duration exercise. For most individuals, low-to-moderate intensities of longer duration are recommended; higher-intensity exercise increases the risk of orthopedic injury and discourages continued participation in the exercise program.

Part of the art of exercise prescription is being able to select an exercise intensity that is adequate to stress the cardiovascular system without overtaxing it. According to ACSM (2000), the initial exercise intensity for apparently healthy adults is 40/50% to 85% $\dot{V}O_2$R. Lower-intensity exercise (40% to 50% $\dot{V}O_2$R) may be sufficient to provide important health benefits for sedentary clients and/or older individuals with low initial cardiorespiratory fitness levels. For most individuals, intensities of 60% to 80% $\dot{V}O_2$R are sufficient to improve cardiorespiratory fitness. As a general rule, the more fit the individual, the higher the exercise intensity needs to be to produce further improvement in cardiorespiratory fitness. Exercise intensity can be prescribed using the $\dot{V}O_2$reserve, HR, or RPE method.

$\dot{V}O_2$ reserve (MET) Method

First, measure the client's functional aerobic capacity ($\dot{V}O_2$max or $\dot{V}O_2$peak) using a graded exercise test (see chapter 4). Express the client's $\dot{V}O_2$max in relative terms, that is, $ml \cdot kg^{-1} \cdot min^{-1}$ or METs (metabolic equivalents). Given that 1 MET approximately equals $3.5 \ ml \cdot kg^{-1} \cdot min^{-1}$, a $\dot{V}O_2$max of $35 \ ml \cdot kg^{-1} \cdot min^{-1}$, for example, would be equivalent to 10 METs (35/3.5 = 10 METs).

Next determine the $\dot{V}O_2$reserve ($\dot{V}O_2$R). As mentioned previously, the $\dot{V}O_2$R is the difference between $\dot{V}O_2$max and $\dot{V}O_2$rest ($\dot{V}O_2$R = $\dot{V}O_2$max – $\dot{V}O_2$rest). The percent of $\dot{V}O_2$R depends on the initial cardiorespiratory fitness level of the client. To calculate the target $\dot{V}O_2$ (in METs) based on the $\dot{V}O_2$R, use the following equation:

$$\text{target } \dot{V}O_2 = [\text{relative exercise intensity (\%)} \times \dot{V}O_2\text{R}] + \dot{V}O_2\text{rest}$$

For example, the target $\dot{V}O_2$ corresponding to 50% $\dot{V}O_2$R for a client with a $\dot{V}O_2$max of 10 METs is calculated as follows:

$$\text{target } \dot{V}O_2 = [0.50 \times (10 - 1 \text{ MET})] + 1 \text{ MET}$$
$$= (0.50 \times 9 \text{ METs}) + 1 \text{ MET}$$
$$= 4.5 + 1.0 \text{ METs, or } 5.5 \text{ METs}$$

The exercise intensity (METs) for walking, jogging, running, cycling, and bench stepping activities is directly related to the speed of movement, power output, or mass lifted. Use the ACSM equations (table 4.3, p. 57) to calculate the speed or work rates corresponding to a specific MET intensity for the exercise prescription. For example, to estimate how fast a woman should jog on a level course to be exercising at an intensity of 8 METs, follow these steps:

1. Convert the METs to $ml \cdot kg^{-1} \cdot min^{-1}$.
$$\dot{V}O_2 = 8 \text{ METs} \times 3.5 \ ml \cdot kg^{-1} \cdot min^{-1}$$
$$= 28 \ ml \cdot kg^{-1} \cdot min^{-1}$$

2. Substitute known values into the ACSM running equation and solve for speed.
$$28 \ ml \cdot kg^{-1} \cdot min^{-1} = [\text{speed } (m \cdot min^{-1}) \times 0.2] + 3.5 \ ml \cdot kg^{-1} \cdot min^{-1}$$

$$28.0 \ \mathrm{ml \cdot kg^{-1} \cdot min^{-1}} - 3.5 = \text{speed (m \cdot min^{-1})} \times 0.2$$
$$122.5 \ \mathrm{m \cdot min^{-1}} = \text{speed}$$

3. Convert speed to mph.

$$1 \ \mathrm{mph} = 26.8 \ \mathrm{m \cdot min^{-1}}$$

$$122.5 \ \mathrm{m \cdot min^{-1}} / 26.8 \ \mathrm{m \cdot min^{-1}} = 4.57 \ \mathrm{mph}$$

4. Convert mph to minute per mile pace.

$$\text{pace} = 60 \ \mathrm{min \cdot hr^{-1}} / \mathrm{mph}$$

$$= 60 \ \mathrm{min \cdot hr^{-1}} / 4.57 \ \mathrm{mph}$$

$$= 13.1 \ \mathrm{min \cdot mile^{-1}} \ (\text{or } 8.1 \ \mathrm{min \cdot km^{-1}})$$

Average MET values for selected conditioning exercises, sports, and recreational activities are presented in appendix E.4, "Gross Energy Expenditure (METs) for Conditioning Exercises, Sports, and Recreational Activities," page 330. When prescribing the exercise intensity, be sure to consider factors such as altitude, humidity, temperature, terrain, running surface, and additional equipment. Because these factors may alter the actual exercise intensity, you may want to use the HR or the RPE method along with the MET method to ensure that the exercise intensity does not exceed safe limits.

Heart Rate Method

There are three ways to prescribe exercise intensity for your clients using HR data. Each of these approaches is based on the assumption that HR is a linear function of exercise intensity (i.e., the higher the exercise intensity, the higher the HR).

Heart Rate Versus MET Graphing Method

When a submaximal or maximal graded exercise test (GXT) is administered, the client's steady-state HR response to each stage of the exercise test can be plotted (see figure 5.3). The HRmax is the HR observed at the highest exercise intensity during a maximal GXT. For submaximal GXTs, you can estimate your client's HRmax using 220 – age. From this graph, you can obtain HRs corresponding to given percentages of the estimated functional capacity or $\dot{V}O_2$max. In our example, the functional capacity of the individual is 7.4 METs, and the HRmax is 195 bpm. The HRs corresponding to exercise intensities of 4.8 and 6.4 METs (60% to 85% $\dot{V}O_2$R) are 139 and 175 bpm, respectively. During exercise workouts, the individual should

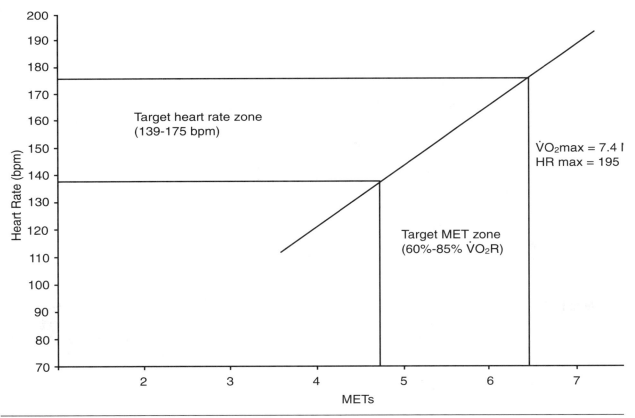

Figure 5.3 Plotting target heart rate zone using graded exercise test data (heart rate vs. METs). HRmax = maximal heart rate; $\dot{V}O_2$R = oxygen reserve.

measure the HR using a heart rate monitor or palpation to verify that the appropriate exercise intensity is reached.

It is important to note that the HR response to graded exercise is dependent to some extent on the mode of exercise testing. For example, compared to treadmill testing, exercising on an electronic step ergometer elicits higher HRs, and stationary cycling typically results in somewhat lower HRs at the same relative exercise intensities. When using this method to obtain HRs for an exercise prescription, be sure to match the exercise testing and training modes by selecting a testing mode that elicits HR responses that are similar to those obtained for the training mode (see figure 5.1). For example, if your client chooses in-line skating as a training mode, you should administer a treadmill GXT, given that the relationship between HR and $\dot{V}O_2$ at submaximal exercise intensities is similar for these two exercise modes (Berry et al. 1992).

Heart Rate Reserve Method

When HR data from a GXT are not available, you can use the **Karvonen,** or **percent heart rate reserve (%HRR), method** to determine target HRs for your client's exercise prescription. The **heart rate reserve (HRR)** method takes into account the resting heart rate and maximal HR. The HRR is the difference between the maximal HR and resting HR. A percentage of HRR is added to the client's resting HR to determine the target exercise HR:

$$\text{target HR} = [\% \text{ exercise intensity} \times (\text{HRmax} - \text{HRrest})] + \text{HRrest}$$

As previously mentioned, the percent values for the HRR method are approximately equal to the percent values for the $\dot{V}O_2R$ method. The ACSM (2000) recommends using 40/50% to 85% HRR. For example, if

$$\text{maximal HR} = 178 \text{ bpm},$$

$$\text{resting HR} = 68 \text{ bpm, and}$$

$$\text{exercise intensity} = 60\% \text{ HRR, then}$$

$$\text{target exercise HR} = 0.60 \,(178 - 68) + 68$$
$$\text{or } 134 \text{ bpm}$$

Table 5.1 presents alternative guidelines for determining minimal, average, and maximal training HRs using this method based on your client's initial fitness level (deVries 1980).

Percentage of Maximal Heart Rate Method

You also can use a straight percentage of maximal HR (**percent heart rate maximum; %HRmax**) to estimate exercise intensity and determine target exercise HR. This method is based on the fact that the %HRmax is related to % $\dot{V}O_2R$ and %HRR. In table 5.2, we can see that 55% and 90% HRmax correspond to exercise intensities of 40% and 85% $\dot{V}O_2R$ or HRR. The ACSM (2000) recommends prescribing target HRs between 55/60% and 90% HRmax depending on the fitness level of your client.

With use of this technique, the actual maximal HR must be known or must be predicted either from the HR response to submaximal workloads or from the formula 220 – age in years. For example, if the age-predicted maximal HR is 180 bpm and the exercise intensity is set at 70% HRmax, the target exercise HR is equal to 126 bpm.

$$\%\text{HRmax} \times \text{HRmax} = \text{target HR}$$
$$0.70 \times 180 \text{ bpm} = 126 \text{ bpm}$$

Compared to the Karvonen (%HRR) method, the %HRmax method tends to give a lower value when the same relative intensity is used. If in our example the client's resting HR is 80 bpm, the target HR using the Karvonen method is 150 bpm [0.70 × (180 – 80) + 80 bpm] compared to 126 bpm for the %HRmax method.

The ACSM (2000) recommends using the %HRmax method to prescribe exercise intensity for your older clients. The %HRmax provides a

Table 5.1 Prescription of Exercise Intensity Using %HRR[a] Method for Various Fitness Levels			
	High (%)	**Low (%)**	**Average (%)**
Minimum HR	40	60	70
Average HR	50-60	70-75	80-85
Maximum HR	75	85	90
[a]Target HR = %HRR (HRmax – HRrest) + HRrest. HRR = heart rate reserve.			

Table 5.2 Comparison of Methods for Prescribing Exercise Intensity for Healthy Adults[a]

Classification	Relative intensity		
	% $\dot{V}O_2R$ or %HRR	%HRmax	RPE (6-20 scale)
Very light	<20	<35	<10
Light	20-39	35-54	10-11
Moderate	40-59	55-69	12-13
Hard	60-84	70-89	14-16
Very hard	≥85	≥90	17-19
Maximal	100	100	20

[a]Based on data from Pollock et al. 1998.

HRR = heart rate reserve; RPE = rating of perceived exertion.

more accurate estimate of % $\dot{V}O_2$peak of older adults than the %HRR method; using the %HRR method results in a higher-than-expected percentage of $\dot{V}O_2$max (Kohrt, Spina, Holloszy, and Ehsani 1998). However, you should measure, not predict (220 – age), the client's HRmax, for two reasons. Older individuals (>65 years of age) have large variability in HRmax, and they are more likely to be taking medications that affect peak HR.

Limitations of Heart Rate Methods

Exclusive use of HR to develop intensity recommendations for your client's exercise prescription may lead to large errors in estimating relative exercise intensities (% $\dot{V}O_2R$) for some individuals. This is especially true when HRmax is predicted from age (220 – age) instead of being directly measured. In about 30% of the population, an age-predicted prescription of 60% HRR may be as low as 70% and as high as 80% of the actual HRmax (Dishman 1994). Also, medications, emotional states, and environmental factors (such as temperature, humidity, and air pollution) can affect your client's exercise training HRs. Thus, you should consider alternative methods for monitoring exercise intensity.

Ratings of Perceived Exertion Method

In light of the limitations associated with using HR for setting exercise intensity, consider using a combination of HR and RPE in developing prescriptions for your clients. You can use RPEs to pre-scribe and monitor exercise intensity (Birk and Birk 1987). The RPE scales (see table 4.2) are valid and reliable tools for assessing the level of physical exertion during continuous, aerobic exercise (Birk and Birk 1987; Borg and Linderholm 1967; Dunbar et al. 1992).

During the GXT, the client rates the intensity of each stage of the test using the RPE scale. You can use the intensities (METs) corresponding to ratings of 12 (somewhat hard) and 16 (hard) to set the minimum and maximum training intensities for the exercise prescription. Compared to the %HRR method, RPEs between 12 and 16 closely approximate 40% and 84% HRR, respectively (Pollock et al. 1998). With practice an individual can learn to associate RPE with a specific target exercise HR, especially at higher exercise intensities (Smutok, Skrinar, and Pandolf 1980). Thus, the RPE can be used instead of HR, or in combination with HR, to monitor training intensity and to adjust the exercise prescription for conditioning effects.

One advantage of RPE as a method of monitoring exercise intensity is that your clients do not need to stop exercising in order to check their HRs. For an extensive review of research pertaining to the use of perceived exertion for prescribing exercise intensity, see Dishman 1994.

Frequency of Exercise

The frequency of the exercise sessions depends on your client's caloric goals, health and fitness level, preferences, and time constraints. For health benefits, individuals should exercise at a moderate intensity most, if not all, days of the week. Individuals with functional capacities > 5 METs should exercise at a moderate to vigorous intensity a minimum of three times per week to produce significant changes in cardiorespiratory endurance (ACSM 2000). As the fitness level increases, however, the frequency should be increased to five times per week for continued improvement (Pollock 1973). For individuals with functional capacities < 3 METs, multiple daily exercise sessions are advisable.

In terms of improving $\dot{V}O_2max$, the sequence of exercise sessions seems to be less important than the total work performed during the training. Similar improvements were noted for individuals who trained every other day (M-W-F) and three consecutive days (M-T-W) (Moffatt, Stamford, and Neill 1977). The ACSM (2000) recommends exercising on alternate days during the initial stages of training to lessen the chance of bone or joint injury. Also, older adults who can tolerate vigorous exercise should work out at least three times per week, with a day of rest between each exercise session (ACSM 2000).

Once people reach the desired level of cardiorespiratory fitness, they may maintain it by exercising two to four days per week, provided that the intensity and duration of the workouts are similar to those used to achieve the current fitness level (Brynteson and Sinning 1973; Hickson and Rosenkoetter 1981).

Duration of Exercise

As an exercise specialist, you must prescribe an appropriate combination of exercise intensity and duration so that the individual adequately stresses the cardiorespiratory system without overexertion. As mentioned earlier, the intensity and duration of exercise are inversely related (the lower the exercise intensity, the longer the duration of the exercise). The ACSM (2000) recommends 20 to 60 min of continuous, aerobic activity. Apparently healthy individuals usually can sustain exercise intensities of 60% to 85% $\dot{V}O_2R$ for 20 to 30 min. During the improvement stage, duration can be increased every two to three weeks until participants can exercise continuously for 30 min at a moderate to vigorous intensity (ACSM 2000). Poorly conditioned and older individuals may be able to exercise continuously at a low intensity (40% $\dot{V}O_2R$) for only 5 to 10 min. They may need to perform multiple sessions (e.g., four to six 5-min exercise bouts or two to three 10-min exercise bouts) in a given day to accumulate 20 to 30 min of aerobic exercise.

An alternative way of estimating the duration of exercise is to use the caloric cost of the exercise. To achieve health benefits, ACSM (2000) recommends target **caloric thresholds** of 150 to 400 kcal per exercise session, and a minimal weekly caloric threshold of 1000 kcal from physical activity or exercise.

During the initial stage of the exercise program, however, weekly exercise caloric expenditure may be considerably lower (200 to 600 kcal per week). Throughout the improvement stage, the goal is to increase your client's caloric expenditure from 1000 to 2000 kcal per week by gradually increasing the frequency, intensity, and duration of the exercise. For example, in order for a 60-kg woman who is exercising at an intensity of 7 METs, five times per week, to reach a weekly net caloric threshold of 1500 kcal per week, she needs to expend 300 kcal per exercise session (1500 kcal/5 = 300 kcal). You can estimate the net caloric cost of her exercise ($kcal \cdot min^{-1}$) using the following formula:

$$net\ cal\ cost\ (kcal \cdot min^{-1}) = METs \times 3.5 \\ \times body\ mass\ in\ kg/200$$

To calculate the net caloric expenditure from her activity, subtract the resting oxygen consumption (1 MET) from the gross $\dot{V}O_2$ ($\dot{V}O_2$ cost of exercise + $\dot{V}O_2rest$) and substitute this value (7 – 1 = 6 METs) into the equation:

$$net\ cal\ cost = 6\ METs \times 3.5 \times 60\ kg/200 \\ = 7.35\ kcal \cdot min^{-1}$$

Therefore, she needs to exercise approximately 41 min (300 kcal/7.35 $kcal \cdot min^{-1}$), five times per week, in order to achieve her weekly caloric expenditure goal of 1500 kcal.

Rate of Progression

Physiological changes associated with aerobic endurance training (see "Physiological Changes Induced by Cardiorespiratory Endurance Training," p. 97) enable the individual to increase the total work performed. The greatest conditioning effects occur during the first six to eight weeks of the exercise program. Aerobic endurance may improve as much as 3% per week during the first month, 2% per week for the second month, and 1% per week or less thereafter (Sharkey 1979). For continued improvements, the cardiorespiratory system must be overloaded through adjustments in the intensity and duration of the exercise to the new level of fitness. The degree of improvement is dependent on the age, health status, and initial fitness level of the participant. For the average person, aerobic training programs generally produce a 5% to 20% increase in $\dot{V}O_2$max (Pollock 1973). Sedentary, inactive persons may improve as much as 40% in aerobic fitness, while elite athletes may improve only 5% because they begin at a level much closer to their genetic limits. We do not expect older individuals entering the exercise program to improve as quickly as younger individuals even when the initial fitness levels are the same.

Stages of Progression

As discussed in chapter 3, the three stages of progression for cardiorespiratory exercise programs are the **initial conditioning, improvement,** and **maintenance stages** (ACSM 2000).

Initial Conditioning

The initial conditioning stage typically lasts up to four weeks and consists of stretching exercises, light calisthenics, and moderate-level aerobic activity. The ACSM (2000) suggests that the initial exercise intensity be set at 40% to 60% HRR. The duration of the aerobic exercise during this stage should be at least 15 to 20 min, increasing to 30 min in four weeks. Individuals starting a moderate-intensity conditioning program should exercise a minimum of three to four days per week. Active individuals with good-to-excellent initial cardiorespiratory fitness levels may skip the initial conditioning stage of the program.

Improvement

The improvement stage usually lasts 16 to 20 weeks. During this stage, the rate of progression is more rapid. Intensity, duration, and frequency

Physiological Changes Induced by Cardiorespiratory Endurance Training

Increases	Decreases
Cardiorespiratory system	
Heart size and volume	Resting heart rate
Blood volume and total hemoglobin	Submaximal exercise heart rate
Stroke volume—rest and exercise	Blood pressure (if high)
Cardiac output—maximum	
$\dot{V}O_2$max	
Oxygen extraction from blood	
Lung volumes	
Musculoskeletal system	
Mitochondria—number and size	
Myoglobin stores	
Triglyceride stores	
Oxidative phosphorylation	
Other systems	
Strength of connective tissues	Body weight (if overweight)
Heat acclimatization	Body fat
High-density lipoprotein cholesterol	Total cholesterol
	Low-density lipoprotein cholesterol

of exercise should always be increased independently. Increase the duration of exercise every two to three weeks when the client is able to sustain moderate to vigorous exercise intensities for 20 to 30 min. The exercise intensity is increased gradually within the upper half of the target range (e.g., 50% to 85% HRR). Increase the frequency of exercise from three to five times per week. Rate of progression during this stage depends on a number of factors. Cardiac patients, older adults, and less fit individuals may need more time for the body to adapt to a higher conditioning intensity. In such cases, the exercise duration should be at least 20 to 30 min before the exercise intensity increases (ACSM 2000).

Maintenance

After achieving the desired level of cardiorespiratory fitness, an individual enters the maintenance stage of the exercise program. This stage usually begins six months after the start of training and continues on a regular, long-term basis if the individual has made a lifetime commitment to exercise.

During this stage, a variety of enjoyable activities from Group II and III (see "Classification of Aerobic Exercise Modalities," p. 89) can be included in the exercise program to counteract boredom and to maintain the interest level of the participant. For example, an individual who was running five days per week at the end of the improvement stage may choose to run only three days per week and substitute in-line skating and racquetball on the other two days.

AEROBIC TRAINING METHODS AND MODES

Either continuous or discontinuous training methods can improve cardiovascular endurance. **Continuous training** involves one continuous, aerobic exercise bout performed at low-to-moderate intensities without rest intervals. **Discontinuous training** consists of several intermittent low- to high-intensity aerobic exercise bouts interspersed with rest periods. Research indicates that continuous training and discontinuous training are equally effective in improving cardiorespiratory fitness. However, Pollock et al. (1977) reported that the dropout rate of adults in a high-intensity interval (discontinuous) training program was twice that of those in a continuous jogging program.

Continuous Training

All of the exercise modes listed as Group I and II activities (see p. 89) are suitable for continuous training. One advantage of continuous training is that a prescribed exercise intensity (e.g., 75% HRR) is maintained fairly consistently throughout the duration of the steady-paced exercise. Generally, continuous exercise at low-to-moderate intensities is safer, more comfortable, and better suited for individuals initiating an aerobic exercise program.

Walking, Jogging, and Cycling

The most popular modes of continuous training are walking, jogging or running, and cycling. Exercise programs using walking, jogging, and cycling provide similar cardiovascular benefits (Magel et al. 1974; Pollock, Cureton, and Greninger 1969; Pollock et al. 1971; Pollock, Dimmick, Miller, Kendrick, and Linnerud 1975; Wilmore et al. 1980). Improvements in $\dot{V}O_2$max are comparable for most commonly used exercise modes. Pollock et al. (1975) compared running, walking, and cycling exercise programs of middle-aged men who trained at 85% to 90% HRmax. All three groups showed significant improvements in $\dot{V}O_2$max. These results indicate that improvement in $\dot{V}O_2$max is independent of the mode of training when frequency, intensity, and duration of exercise are held constant and are prescribed in accordance with sound, scientific principles.

Aerobic Dance

Aerobic dance is a popular mode of exercise for improving and maintaining cardiorespiratory fitness. A number of excellent books provide detailed information about aerobic dance methods and techniques (Kuntzelman 1979; Wilmoth 1986). A typical aerobic dance workout consists of 8 to 10 min of stretching, calisthenics, and low-intensity exercise. This is followed by 15 to 45 min of either high- or low-impact aerobic dancing at the target training intensity. Handheld weights (1 to 4 lb) can be used to increase exercise intensity. Heart rates should be monitored at least six times during the exercise to ensure that the HR stays within the target zone (Russell 1983). The 10-min cool-down period usually includes more stretching and calisthenic-type exercises.

Several studies conducted to assess the cardiorespiratory effect of aerobic dance training have documented average increases in $\dot{V}O_2$max of 10% or greater (Blessing, Wilson, Puckett, and Ford

1987; Milburn and Butts 1983; Parker et al. 1989; Williford, Blessing, Barksdale, and Smith 1988). Milburn and Butts (1983) reported that aerobic dance was as effective as jogging for improving cardiorespiratory endurance when performed at similar intensity, frequency, and duration. The subjects trained 30 min, four days a week for seven weeks, at 83% to 84% HRmax.

Bench Step Aerobics

Health and fitness clubs throughout the United States are promoting bench step training as an effective high-intensity, low-impact aerobic exercise mode. Step training uses whole-body movements on steps or benches, ranging in height from 4 to 12 in. (10.2 to 30.5 cm). Choreographed movement routines are performed to music. A typical bench step aerobic workout consists of 5 to 10 min of warm-up and 20 to 30 min of step training. This is followed by a short (3 to 5 min) cool-down. Exercise training intensity can be graded through use of variations in stepping cadence or bench height and the use of 1- to 4-lb hand weights (Kravitz, Heyward, et al. 1997).

Studies confirm that continuous step training at bench heights ranging from 6 to 12 in. (15.2 to 30.5 cm) provides an adequate training stimulus that meets ACSM (2000) guidelines for intensity and duration (Olson, Williford, Blessing, and Greathouse 1991; Petersen, Verstraete, Schultz, and Stray-Gundersen 1993; Woodby-Brown, Berg, and Latin 1993). Following 8 to 12 weeks of step aerobic training, $\dot{V}O_2$max improves as much as 8% to 16% (Kravitz, Cizar, Christensen, and Setterlund 1993; Kravitz, Heyward, et al. 1997; Velasquez and Wilmore 1992). In a study comparing bench step exercise with and without hand weights, use of 2- to 4-lb hand weights did not result in a greater improvement in $\dot{V}O_2$max than to step training without hand weights (Kravitz, Heyward, et al. 1997).

Step Ergometry and Stair Climbing

Step ergometry (machine-based stair climbing) is a popular exercise mode in health and fitness clubs. Research shows a linear HR response to graded submaximal exercise performed on stair climbing ergometers. However, the MET levels displayed on the Stairmaster 4000 PT overestimate the actual MET intensity of the exercise (Howley, Colacino, and Swensen 1992). When prescribing exercise intensity using this type of stair climber, be certain to adjust the machine's estimates for each MET level using the following equation:

$$\text{actual METs} = 0.556 + 0.745(\text{Stairmaster MET setting})$$

Although machine-based stair climbing provides a training stimulus that meets guidelines for exercise intensity, presently there is no research comparing the effectiveness of stair climbing training to other aerobic training modes.

Elliptical Training

Elliptical training machines have recently become popular in the fitness industry. Elliptical trainers are designed for either upper-body or combined upper- and lower-body exercise. The lower-body motion during exercise on an elliptical trainer is a cross between the actions performed with machine-based stair climbing and upright stationary cycling. With elliptical trainers, the feet move in an egg-shaped or elliptical pattern, and the feet stay in contact with the footpads of the device throughout the exercise. Unlike running or jogging, this form of exercise may provide a high-intensity workout with low-impact forces comparable to walking (Porcari, Foster, and Schneider 2000). Although there is no research documenting the long-term effects of this type of training on cardiovascular fitness, preliminary data suggest that this exercise modality meets ACSM (2000) guidelines for developing and maintaining cardiorespiratory fitness (Kravitz, Wax, Mayo, Daniels, and Charette 1998; Porcari et al. 2000). Kravitz et al. (1998) reported that the average energy expenditure during forward/backward exercise with no resistance and against resistance for 5 min (125 strides/min) was, respectively, 8.1 and 10.7 kcal·min⁻¹. Exercise intensities ranged between 72.5% and 83.5% HRmax (age-predicted). Compared to treadmill exercise, upper-body elliptical training at self-selected intensities produced similar $\dot{V}O_2$, HR, and RPE responses (Crommett, Kravitz, Wongsathikun, and Kemerly 1999; Porcari et al. 2000). Although there was no difference in $\dot{V}O_2$ between combined upper-/lower-body elliptical training and treadmill exercise, upper-/lower-body elliptical training produced a significantly higher HR and RPE (Crommett et al. 1999).

Aerobic Riding

Aerobic riding involves both upper- and lower-body muscle groups. For this reason, some manufacturers claim that this mode of exercise will automatically burn more calories than lower-body-only exercise modes such as jogging, cycling, and stair climbing. One study, however, noted that the energy expenditure during 10 min of steady-state exercise at a somewhat hard intensity (RPE = 13) on an aerobic rider was significantly lower than the caloric expenditure for treadmill jogging, stationary cycling, and Nordic skiing (Kravitz, Robergs et al. 1997). Subjects reported that they felt a similar workout intensity, in terms of RPE, during aerobic riding. Aerobic riding appears to challenge the muscular system (subjects complained of muscular discomfort) more than the cardiovascular system. In fact, the relative submaximal $\dot{V}O_2$ (47% $\dot{V}O_2$max) for aerobic riding was significantly less than that for treadmill jogging (74% $\dot{V}O_2$max), Nordic skiing (68% $\dot{V}O_2$max), and stationary cycling (64% $\dot{V}O_2$max). Thus, aerobic riding may not be suitable for aerobic exercise prescriptions, particularly for individuals with above-average cardiorespiratory fitness.

Discontinuous Training

As mentioned previously, discontinuous training involves a series of low- to high-intensity exercise bouts interspersed with rest or relief periods. All of the exercise modes listed as Group I and II activities (see p. 89) are suitable for discontinuous training. Because of the intermittent nature of this form of training, the exercise intensity and total amount of work performed can be greater than with continuous training, making discontinuous training a versatile method that is widely used by athletes, as well as individuals with low cardiorespiratory fitness. In fact, ACSM (2000) recommends the use of discontinuous (intermittent) training for symptomatic individuals who are able to tolerate only low-intensity exercise for short periods of time (3 to 5 min). Interval training, Treading, and circuit resistance training are examples of intermittent or discontinuous training.

Interval Training

Interval training involves a repeated series of exercise work bouts interspersed with rest or relief periods. This method is popular among athletes because it allows the athlete to exercise at higher relative intensities during the work interval than are possible with longer-duration, continuous training. Interval training programs also can be designed to improve speed and anaerobic endurance, as well as aerobic endurance, simply by means of modifications in the exercise intensity and length of the work and relief intervals.

AN INTERVAL TRAINING PRESCRIPTION TO DEVELOP AEROBIC ENDURANCE

Sets: 1

Repetitions: 3

Distance: 1100 yd

Time: 3 to 4 min

Rest-relief interval: 1.5 to 2 min

Each work interval consists of running at a pace such that a distance of 1100 yd is covered in 3 to 4 min. The work interval is followed by a rest-relief interval of 1.5 to 2 min. This sequence is repeated three times. During the rest-relief interval, the individual usually walks or jogs while recovering from the work bout. For aerobic interval training, the ratio of work to rest-relief is usually 1:1 or 1:0.5. Each work interval is 3 to 5 min and is repeated three to seven times. The exercise intensity usually ranges between 70% and 85% $\dot{V}O_2$max. Apply the overload principle by increasing the exercise intensity or length of the work interval, decreasing the length of the rest-relief interval, or increasing the number of work intervals per exercise session. For a discussion of interval training and sample programs, including programs for developing speed and anaerobic endurance, refer to Fox and Mathews 1974.

Treading

Treading is a type of interval training that has recently gained popularity in fitness clubs because of the variety and enjoyment it offers. Treading is a group-led exercise that involves walking, jogging, and/or running at various speeds and grades on the treadmill. A typical Treading workout consists of 1:1 or 1.5:1 work-recovery intervals or stages that are repeated for a specified duration. For example, a 30-min workout may consist of six stages. Each stage lasts 5 min (i.e., 3-min work interval and 2-min recovery interval). One can advance the intensity of the work interval by increasing the treadmill speed or grade. During the recovery interval, both the speed and grade of the treadmill are decreased (e.g., 2.5 mph and 0% grade). Instructors individualize and adapt the workouts for their clients by adjusting the duration of the work-recovery intervals and varying the speed and grade.

In one study researchers designed 30-min Treading workouts for walkers and runners (Nichols, Sherman, and Abbott 2000). They reported that the average intensity of the walking protocol was 40% to 49% $\dot{V}O_2$max for male and female walkers, respectively. For the running protocol, the average intensity of the work intervals was 76% to 80% $\dot{V}O_2$max for male and female runners, respectively. The researchers suggested that these average intensities, as well as the duration of the workout (30 min), are sufficient to meet ACSM (2000) standards for an aerobic exercise prescription. More research is needed to determine the long-term training effects of Treading on cardiorespiratory fitness.

Circuit Resistance Training

Use of circuit resistance training for the development of aerobic fitness, as well as muscular strength and tone, has received much attention. An example of a circuit resistance training program is presented in chapter 7, page 141 (see figure 7.1). Circuit resistance training usually consists of several circuits of resistance training with a minimal amount of rest between the exercise stations (15 to 20 sec). Alternatively, instead of rest, you can have your clients perform 1 to 3 min of aerobic exercise between each station. The aerobic stations may include activities such as stationary cycling, jogging in place, rope skipping, stair climbing, bench stepping, and rowing. This modification of the circuit is known as **super circuit resistance training.**

Gettman and Pollock (1981) reviewed the research dealing with the physiological benefits of circuit resistance training. Because it produces only a 5% increase in aerobic capacity as compared to a 15% to 25% increase with other forms of aerobic training, the authors concluded that circuit resistance training should not be used to develop aerobic fitness. Rather, it may be used during the maintenance stage of an aerobic exercise program.

PERSONALIZED EXERCISE PROGRAMS

The aerobic exercise prescription should be individualized to meet each client's training goals and interests. To do this, you need to consider your client's age, gender, physical fitness level, and exercise preferences. This section presents a sample case study and examples of individualized exercise prescriptions to illustrate how the exercise prescription may be personalized for each client.

Case Study

Like any preventive or therapeutic intervention, exercise should be prescribed carefully. You must be able to evaluate your client's medical history, medical condition, physical fitness status, lifestyle characteristics, and interests before designing the exercise program. In addition, to test your ability to extract, analyze, and evaluate all pertinent information needed to design a safe exercise program for your client, many professional certification examinations require that you be able to analyze a case study. For these reasons this section includes a sample case study.

A case study is a written narrative that summarizes client information that you will need to develop an accurate and safe individualized exercise prescription (Porter 1988). Important elements to focus on when reading and analyzing a case study are listed in "Essential Elements of a Case Study" (see next page). First, identify the client's coronary heart disease (CHD) risk factors by focusing on information provided about family history of CHD, blood lipid profile (total cholesterol, high- and low-density lipoprotein cholesterol [HDL-C and LDL-C]), blood glucose levels, resting BP, physical activity, body fat level, and smoking. Become familiar with ideal or typical values for various blood chemistry tests so that you will be able to recognize normal or abnormal test results. Remember that each of the following factors place individuals at greater risk for CHD:

- Triglycerides ≥ 150 mg·dl^{-1}
- Total cholesterol ≥ 200 mg·dl^{-1}
- LDL-cholesterol ≥ 130 mg·dl^{-1}
- HDL-cholesterol <40 mg·dl^{-1}
- Total cholesterol/HDL ratio >5.0
- Blood glucose ≥ 110 mg·dl^{-1}
- Systolic BP ≥ 140 or diastolic BP ≥ 90 mmHg

Use the demographic data (age and gender) and CHD risk factors to determine the client's CHD risk classification (low, moderate, or high risk). The CHD risk classification dictates how closely the client's exercise program needs to be monitored.

Pay close attention to information about the client's *medical history* and *physical examination* results. These may reveal signs or symptoms of

Essential Elements of a Case Study

Demographic Factors

Age

Gender

Ethnicity

Occupation

Height

Body weight

Family history of coronary heart disease

Medical History

Present symptoms

Dyspnea or shortness of breath

Angina or chest pain

Leg cramps or claudication

Musculoskeletal problems or limitations

Medications

Past history

Diseases

Injuries

Surgeries

Lab tests

Lifestyle Assessment

Alcohol and caffeine intake

Smoking

Nutritional intake/eating patterns

Physical activity patterns and interests

Sleeping habits

Occupational stress level

Mental status/family lifestyle

Physical Examination

Blood pressure

Heart/lung sounds

Orthopedic problems/limitations

Laboratory Tests (Ideal or Typical Values)

Triglycerides (<150 mg·dl^{-1})

Total cholesterol (<200 mg·dl^{-1})

LDL-cholesterol (<130 mg·dl^{-1})

HDL-cholesterol (>40 mg·dl^{-1})

Total cholesterol/HDL-cholesterol (<3.5)

Blood glucose (60-110 mg·dl^{-1})

Hemoglobin: 13.5-17.5 g·dl^{-1} (men)

11.5-15.5 g·dl^{-1} (women)

Hematocrit: 40-52% (men)

36-48% (women)

Potassium (3.5-5.5 meq·dl^{-1})

Blood urea nitrogen (4-24 mg·dl^{-1})

Creatinine (0.3-1.4 mg·dl^{-1})

Iron: 40-190 μg·dl^{-1} (men)

35-180 μg·dl^{-1} (women)

Calcium (8.5-10.5 mg·dl^{-1})

Physical Fitness Evaluation

Cardiorespiratory fitness (HR, BP, $\dot{V}O_2$max)

Body composition (% body fat)

Musculoskeletal fitness (muscle and bone strength)

Flexibility

Neuromuscular tension/stress

CHD, particularly if shortness of breath, chest pains, or leg cramps are reported or high BP is detected. It is also important to note the types of medication the client is using. Drugs such as digitalis, beta-blockers, diuretics, vasodilators, bronchodilators, and insulin may alter the body's physiological responses during exercise and could affect the HR and BP responses reported for the GXT. Keep in mind that exercise programs need to be modified for individuals with musculoskeletal disorders such as arthritis, low back pain, osteoporosis, and chondromalacia. Next, be certain to key in on information regarding the client's lifestyle. Factors such as smoking, lack of physical activity, or diets high in saturated fats or cholesterol increase the risk of CHD, atherosclerosis, and hypertension. You often can target these factors for modification; they also help you assess the likelihood of the client's adherence to the exercise program. (See "Factors Related to Exercise Program Adherence," p. 43.)

Examine the BP, HR, and RPE data for the *graded exercise test* used to assess the client's functional aerobic capacity and cardiorespiratory fitness level. You need to be acutely aware of the normal and abnormal physiological responses to graded exercise. After assessing the client's CHD risk and cardiorespiratory fitness level, you can design an aerobic exercise program using a personalized exercise prescription of intensity, frequency, duration, mode, and progression. To write the exercise prescription, use the results from the GXT (HR, RPE, functional MET capacity).

The sample case study on page 104 is provided to test your ability to evaluate risk factors and GXT results and to prescribe an accurate and safe aerobic exercise program for this individual. See the results of the analysis in appendix A.8, "Analysis of Sample Case Study," page 285.

Sample Cycling Program

The sample cycling program on page 105 shows a personalized cycling program for a 27-year-old female who was given a maximal GXT on a stationary bicycle ergometer. Her measured $\dot{V}O_2$max is 7.4 METs. The exercise intensity is based on a percentage of her $\dot{V}O_2$ reserve (%$\dot{V}O_2$R), and the target exercise HRs corresponding to 50% (4.2 METs) and 80% $\dot{V}O_2$R (6.1 METs) are 126 bpm and 168 bpm, respectively (see figure 5.3). Thus, the training exercise HR should fall within this HR range. During the initial stage of the exercise program, the woman will cycle at a work rate corresponding to 50% $\dot{V}O_2$R (4.2 METs) for three weeks. The work rates (power output) corresponding to each exercise intensity are calculated using the ACSM formulas for leg ergometry (see table 4.3). During the fourth week, relative exercise intensity will be increased by 10%.

To calculate the net energy cost (kcal·min^{-1}) of cycling, subtract the resting $\dot{V}O_2$ (1 MET) from the gross $\dot{V}O_2$ for each intensity. Convert this net MET value to kcal·min^{-1} using the following formula:

kcal·min^{-1} = METs × 3.5 × body mass (kg)/200
(e.g., 3.2 × 3.5 × 65 kg/200 = 3.6 kcal·min^{-1})

In the initial stages of the program, the weekly net energy expenditure is between 218 and 387 kcal. In the improvement stage, the exercise intensity, duration, and frequency are progressively increased, and the weekly net caloric expenditure ranges between 387 and 1160 kcal. During the last 12 weeks of the improvement stage, this client's net caloric expenditure due to exercise meets the caloric threshold (>1000 kcal per week from physical activity) recommended by ACSM (2000). In the maintenance phase, tennis and aerobic dancing are added to give variety and to supplement the cycling program. The ACSM (2000) guidelines were followed to calculate each component of this exercise prescription.

Sample Jogging Program

The sample jogging program on page 106 is designed for a 29-year-old male who has an excellent cardiorespiratory fitness level. Since a GXT could not be administered, the $\dot{V}O_2$max was predicted from performance on the 12-min distance run test. The maximal HR was predicted using the formula 220 − age. Because this client is accustomed to jogging and his cardiorespiratory fitness level is classified as excellent, he is exempted from the initial stage and enters the improvement stage of the program immediately. During this time (20 weeks), the exercise intensity is increased from 70% to 85% of the estimated $\dot{V}O_2$R. The speed corresponding to each MET intensity is calculated using the ACSM formulas for running on a level course (see table 4.3). The intensity, duration, and frequency of the exercise sessions provide a weekly *net* caloric expenditure between 673 and 1984 kcal. During the first four weeks of the program, this client's *net* rate of energy expenditure due to exercise is 10.2 kcal·min^{-1} (8.3 METs × 3.5 × 70 kg/200 = 10.2 kcal·min^{-1}); thus, he will expend approximately 673 kcal, jogging 22 min at an 11:06 min per mile pace three times per week (22 min × 10.2 kcal·min^{-1} × 3). The distance covered is figured by dividing the exercise duration by the running pace: 22 min/11.1 min·mile^{-1} = 2 miles. During the improvement stage, the frequency of exercise sessions gradually progresses from three to five days a week. During the maintenance stage, the running is reduced to three days per week, and handball and basketball are added to the aerobic exercise program. The ACSM (2000) guidelines were followed to calculate each component of this exercise prescription.

A 28-year-old female police officer (5 ft 5 in. or 165.1 cm; 140 lb or 63.6 kg, and 28% body fat) has enrolled in the adult fitness program. Her job demands a fairly high level of physical fitness—a level she was able to achieve six years ago when she passed the physical fitness test battery used by the police department. Before becoming a police officer, she jogged 20 min, usually three times a week. Since starting her job, she has had little or no time for exercise and has gained 15 lb (6.8 kg). She works 8 hr a day, is divorced, and takes care of two children, ages 7 and 9. At least three times a week, she and the children dine out, usually at fast-food restaurants like Burger King and Taco Bell. She reports that her job, along with the sole responsibility for raising her two children, is quite stressful. Occasionally she experiences headaches and a tightness in the back of her neck. Usually in the evening she has one glass of wine to relax.

Her medical history reveals that she smoked one pack of cigarettes a day for four years while she was in college. She quit smoking three years ago. The past two years she has tried some quick weight loss diets, with little success. She was hospitalized on two occasions to give birth to her children. She reports that her father died of heart disease when he was 52 and that her older brother has high blood pressure. Recently she had her blood chemistry analyzed because she was feeling light-headed and dizzy after eating. In an attempt to lose weight, she eats only one large meal a day, at dinnertime. Results of the blood analysis were total cholesterol = 220 mg·dl^{-1}; triglycerides = 98 mg·dl^{-1}; glucose = 82 mg·dl^{-1}; high-density lipoprotein cholesterol = 37 mg·dl^{-1}; and total cholesterol/high-density lipoprotein cholesterol ratio = 5.9.

The exercise evaluation yielded the following data:

- Mode/protocol: Treadmill/modified Bruce
- Resting data: HR = 75 bpm; BP = 140/82 mm Hg
- End point: Stage 4 (2.5 mph, 12% grade). Test terminated because of fatigue.

Stage	METs	Duration (min)	HR (bpm)	BP (mm Hg)	RPE
1	2.3	3	126	145/78	8
2	3.5	3	142	160/78	11
3	4.6	3	165	172/80	14
4	7.0	3	190	189/82	18

Analysis

- Evaluate the client's CHD risk profile. Be certain to address each of the positive and negative risk factors.
- Describe any special problems or limitations that need to be considered in designing an exercise program for this client.
- Were the HR, BP, and RPE responses to the graded exercise test normal? Explain.
- What is the client's functional aerobic capacity in METs? Categorize her cardiorespiratory fitness level (see table 4.1)
- Plot the HR versus METs on graph paper.
- From the graph, determine the client's target heart rate zone for the aerobic exercise program. What HRs and RPEs correspond to 60%, 70%, and 75% of the client's $\dot{V}O_2$reserve?
- The client expressed an interest in walking outside on a level track to develop aerobic fitness. Calculate her walking speed for each of the following training intensities: 60%, 70%, and 75% $\dot{V}O_2$reserve. Use the ACSM equations presented in table 4.3.
- In addition to starting an aerobic exercise program, what suggestions do you have for this client for modifying her lifestyle?

Sample Cycling Program

Client data

Age	27 years
Gender	Female
Body weight	65 kg (143 lb)
Resting heart rate	67 bpm
Maximal heart rate	195 bpm (measured)
$\dot{V}O_2$max	26 ml·kg^{-1}·min^{-1} (measured) 7.4 METs
Graded exercise test	Bicycle ergometer
Initial cardiorespiratory fitness level	Poor

Exercise prescription

Mode	Stationary cycling
Intensity	50-80% $\dot{V}O_2$ reserve 14.7-21.4 ml·kg^{-1}·min^{-1} 4.2-6.1 METs
Exercise heart rates (from figure 5.3)	126 bpm minimum 168 bpm maximum
RPE	10-16
Duration	20-40 min
Frequency	3-5 times/week

Cycling program

Phase (weeks)	Intensity % $\dot{V}O_2$ reserve	METs	HR (bpm)	RPE	Power output (watts)	Resistance (kg)	Pedal rate (rpm)	Net kcal/min	Time (min)	Frequency	Weekly net expenditure (kcal)
Initial											
1	50	4.2	126	10	46	0.9	50	3.6	20	3	218
2	50	4.2	126	10	46	0.9	50	3.6	25	3	270
3	50	4.2	126	10	46	0.9	50	3.6	30	3	324
4	60	4.8	138	11	59	1.2	50	4.3	30	3	387
Improvement											
5-8	60-70	4.8-5.5	138-152	11-12	59-74	1.2-1.5	50	4.3-5.1	30	3-4	387-612
9-12	60-70	4.8-5.5	138-152	11-12	59-74	1.2-1.5	50	4.3-5.1	35	3-4	452-714
13-16	70-75	5.5-5.9	152-162	12-14	74-82	1.5-1.6	50	5.1-5.6	35	3-4	535-784
17-20	70-75	5.5-5.9	152-162	12-14	74-82	1.5-1.6	50	5.1-5.6	40	4-5	816-1120
21-24	75-80	5.9-6.1	162-168	14-16	82-86	1.6-1.7	50	5.6-5.8	40	4-5	896-1160
25-28	75-80	5.9-6.1	162-168	14-16	82-86	1.6-1.7	50	5.6-5.8	40	5	1120-1160
Maintenance											
24+											
Cycling	75-80	5.9-6.1	162-168	14-16	82-86	1.6-1.7	50	5.6-5.8	40	3	672-696
Low-impact aerobics	65% HRR	5.0	150	13-14				4.5	30	1	136
Tennis		7.0		16-18				6.8	60	1	408

Sample Multimodal Exercise Program

Some clients may prefer to engage in a variety of exercise modes (cross training) to develop their cardiorespiratory fitness (see "Multimodal Exercise Program" on p. 107). For these cases, it is difficult to systematically prescribe increments in exercise intensity using METs or target HRs. Although MET equivalents for various activities are available (ACSM 2000), typically a range of values is given, making it difficult for you to

Sample Jogging Program

Client data

Age	29 years
Gender	Male
Body weight	70 kg (154 lb)
Resting heart rate	50 bpm
Maximal heart rate	191 bpm (age-predicted)
$\dot{V}O_2max$	45 ml·kg^{-1}·min^{-1} (predicted) 12.9 METs
Graded exercise test	None
Initial cardiorespiratory fitness level	Excellent

Exercise prescription

Mode	Jogging and running
Intensity	70-85% $\dot{V}O_2$reserve 32.5-38.8 ml·kg^{-1}·min^{-1} 9.3-11.1 METs
Exercise heart rates	149 bpm minimum (70% HRR) 170 bpm maximum (85% HRR)
RPE	12-16
Duration	22-32 min
Frequency	3-5 times/week

Jogging program

Phase (weeks)	Intensity % $\dot{V}O_2$ reserve	METs	HR (bpm)	RPE	Pace: mph (min/mile)	Distance (miles)	Net kcal/min	Time (min)	Frequency	Weekly net expenditure (kcal)
Improvement										
1-4	70	9.3	149	12	5.4 (11:06)	2.0	10.2	22	3	673
5-8	70-80	9.3-10.5	149-163	12-13	5.4-6.2 (9:40)	2.0-2.5	10.2-11.6	22-24	3	673-835
9-12	70-80	9.3-10.5	149-163	12-13	5.4-6.2 (9:40)	2.3-2.6	10.2-11.6	25	4	1020-1160
13-16	80-85	10.5-11.1	163-170	14-16	6.2-6.6 (9:05)	2.6-3.3	11.6-12.4	25-30	4	1160-1488
17-20	80-85	10.5-11.1	163-170	14-16	6.2-6.6 (9:05)	3.1-3.6	11.6-12.4	30-32	5	1740-1984
Maintenance										
21+										
Jogging	85	11.2	170	14-16	6.6 (9:05)	3.6	12.4	32	3	1190
Handball	60	8.0		12-13			9.2	60	1	552
Basketball	60	8.0		12-13			9.2	60	1	552

accurately prescribe work rates corresponding to specific intensity recommendations in an exercise prescription. Also, the HR response to a given MET level is highly dependent on the exercise mode.

The degree of muscle mass involved in the activity, as well as whether the body weight is supported during exercise, can affect the HR response to a prescribed exercise intensity. For example, whole-body exercise modes, such as Nordic skiing and aerobic dancing, involve both upper- and lower-body musculature. These produce higher submaximal HRs than lower-body exercise modes (e.g., cycling and jogging). Also, at any given exercise intensity, the HR response during weight-bearing exercise, such as jogging, is greater than that for non-weight-bearing exercise (e.g., cycling).

Therefore, you should use RPEs to progressively increase exercise intensity throughout the improvement stage of a multimodal aerobic exercise program (see table 4.2). To use the RPE safely and effectively, you will need to teach your clients to focus on and learn to monitor important exertional cues such as breathing effort (rate and depth of breathing) and muscular sensations (e.g., pain, warmth, and fatigue).

Guidelines for developing multimodal exercise prescriptions are presented on page 108. For **multimodal exercise programs,** you should set exercise frequency and weekly *net* caloric

Sample Multimodal Exercise Program

Client data

Age	44 years
Sex	Female
Weight	68 kg (150 lb)
Resting heart rate	70 bpm
Maximal heart rate	170 bpm
$\dot{V}O_2max$ (measured)	30 ml·kg^{-1}·min^{-1} 8.6 METs
Graded exercise test	Treadmill maximal GXT (Bruce protocol)
Initial cardio-respiratory fitness level	Fair

Exercise prescription

Modes and estimates of gross caloric expenditure (METs) and net caloric expenditure (kcal·min^{-1})^a	Stationary cycling (100 W): 5.5 METs; 5.4 kcal·min^{-1} Step aerobics (6-8 in. step): 8.5 METs; 8.9 kcal·min^{-1} Rowing (100 W): 7.0 METs; 7.1 kcal·min^{-1} Swimming (moderate effort): 7.0 METs; 9.5 kcal·min^{-1} Stair climbing (machine): 9.0 METs; 7.1 kcal·min^{-1} Hiking: 6.0 METs; 5.9 kcal·min^{-1} Resistance training (free weights/machines): 3.0 METs; 2.4 kcal·min^{-1}
Intensity	RPE: 10 to 16
Duration	20 to 60 min
Frequency	3 to 5 days per week
Weekly caloric expenditure	500 to 1250 kcal per week

Multimodal exercise program

Phase (weeks)	Intensity (RPE)	Minimal duration (min)	Minimal frequency	Average kcal/workout	Weekly caloric goal
Initial					
1-2	10	20	3	133	500
3-4	10	25	3	200	600
Improvement					
5-8	12	25	3	200	700
9-12	12	30	3	233	800
13-16	12-13	30	4	225	900
17-20	14-15	30	4	250	1000
21-24	15-16	30	5	250	1250
Maintenance					
24+	15-16	30	5	250	1250

Examples

Week 1	Activity	Net kcal·min^{-1} estimates	Time (min)	Frequency	Kcal/workout (net)	Activity group^b
Monday	Stationary cycling	5.4	20	1	108	I
Wednesday	Step aerobics	8.9	20	1	178	II
Friday	Stair climbing	9.5	30	1	285	I
	Totals*		70	3	571	3
	Goals		60	3	500	3

Week 21	Activity	Net kcal·min^{-1} estimates	Time (min)	Frequency	Kcal/workout (net)	Activity group^b
Monday	Swimming	7.1	35	1	248	II
Tuesday	Rowing	7.1	35	1	248	I
Wednesday	Stair climbing	9.5	30	1	285	I
Friday	Resistance training	2.4	40	1	96	III
Sunday	Hiking	5.9	60	1	354	II
	Totals*		200	5	1231	4
	Goals		150	5	1250	4

^{a}Gross MET levels for activities from Ainsworth et al. (2000); net energy expenditure in kcal·min^{-1} = net MET level × 3.5 × body mass (kg)/200.

^{b}Check all Group I and II activities.

*Compare weekly totals to weekly goals.

expenditure goals for each client (see "Sample Multimodal Exercise Program"). Provide your clients with estimates of *net* energy expenditure (kcal·min⁻¹) for each of the aerobic activities they select for their exercise prescriptions. The exercise duration to achieve a specified weekly *net* caloric expenditure goal will vary depending on the activity mode chosen for each exercise session. Any combination of Group I and II activities can be used, provided that the client is able to maintain the prescribed RPE intensity for at least 20 min.

Flexibility is the key to successful multimodal exercise prescriptions. Clients should be free not only to select exercise modes of interest but also to decide on various combinations of frequency and duration as long as they meet the caloric thresholds specified in their exercise prescriptions for each week.

The primary advantages of multimodal exercise programs over single-mode (e.g., jogging or cycling) programs for many of your clients are

- greater likelihood of engaging in a safe and effective exercise program,

- overall greater enjoyment of physical activity and exercise,

- better understanding of how their bodies respond to exercise,

- more direct involvement and sense of control in developing and monitoring their exercise programs, and

- increased likelihood of incorporating physical activity and exercise into their lifestyles.

GUIDELINES FOR MULTIMODAL EXERCISE PRESCRIPTIONS

- Modes: Select at least three per week from Group I and II activities.

- Frequency: Three to seven sessions a week. Engage in either Group I or II activities at least three times per week.

- Intensity: Rating of perceived exertion between 10 and 16.

- Duration: At least 15 min, preferably 20 to 30 min. Duration depends on energy cost (kcal·min⁻¹) of exercise mode.

- Caloric expenditure: 1000 to 2000 kcal·week⁻¹. Group III activities can be used to reach weekly caloric expenditure goal but cannot be counted as one of the required aerobic activities.

KEY POINTS

- Always personalize cardiorespiratory exercise programs to meet the needs, interests, and abilities of each participant.

- The exercise prescription includes mode, frequency, intensity, duration, and progression of exercise.

- Aerobic endurance activities involving large muscle groups are well suited for developing cardiorespiratory fitness. Group I activities such as walking, jogging, and cycling allow the individual to maintain steady-state exercise intensities and are not highly dependent on skill.

- Exercise intensity can be prescribed using the HR, $\dot{V}O_2$reserve, or RPE methods, or a combination of these methods.

- For the average healthy person, the cardiorespiratory exercise program should be at an intensity of 60% to 85% $\dot{V}O_2R$, a duration of 20 to 60 min, and a frequency of three to five days per week.

- The cardiorespiratory exercise program includes three stages of progression: initial conditioning, improvement, and maintenance.

- Each exercise session includes warm-up, aerobic conditioning exercise, and cool-down.

- Continuous and discontinuous training methods are equally effective for improving cardiorespiratory fitness.

- Multimodal exercise prescriptions use a variety of Group I and II aerobic activities to improve cardiorespiratory endurance.

KEY TERMS

Learn the definition for each of the following key terms. Definitions of key terms can be found in "Glossary of Terms," page 349.

caloric threshold

continuous training

cross training

discontinuous training

Group I aerobic activities

Group II aerobic activities

Group III aerobic activities

heart rate reserve (HRR)

improvement stage

initial conditioning stage

interval training

Karvonen method

maintenance stage

percent heart rate maximum (%HRmax)

percent heart rate reserve (%HRR)

percent $\dot{V}O_2$ reserve (%$\dot{V}O_2$R)

super circuit resistance training

Treading

$\dot{V}O_2$ reserve ($\dot{V}O_2$R)

multimodal exercise program

REVIEW QUESTIONS

In addition to being able to define each of the key terms, test your knowledge and understanding of the material by answering the following review questions.

1. Name the four components of any aerobic exercise prescription.

2. What are the guidelines for an exercise prescription for improved health?

3. What are the guidelines for an exercise prescription for cardiorespiratory fitness?

4. Identify the three parts of an aerobic exercise workout and state the purpose of each part.

5. To classify an aerobic exercise mode as either a Group I, II, or III activity, what criteria are used?

6. Give three examples each for Group I, II, and III aerobic activities.

7. Describe three methods used to prescribe intensity for an aerobic exercise prescription.

8. Using the $\dot{V}O_2$ reserve method, calculate the target $\dot{V}O_2$ for a client whose $\dot{V}O_2$max is 12 METs and relative exercise intensity is 70% $\dot{V}O_2$R.

9. Which method of prescribing intensity (%HRR or %HRmax), corresponds 1:1 with the %$\dot{V}O_2$R method?

10. What are the limitations of using HR methods to monitor intensity of aerobic exercise?

11. Describe how RPEs can be used to prescribe and monitor the intensity of aerobic exercise.

12. What target caloric thresholds are recommended by ACSM for aerobic exercise workouts and weekly caloric expenditure from physical activity and exercise?

13. What is the recommended frequency of activity and exercise for improved health benefits? For improved cardiorespiratory fitness?

14. Name the three stages of a cardiorespiratory exercise program. For the average individual, what is the typical length (in weeks) of each stage?

15. What is the difference between continuous and discontinuous aerobic exercise training? Give examples of continuous and discontinuous training methods.

16. What are the essential elements of a client case study?

REFERENCES

Ainsworth, B.E., Haskell, W.L., Whitt, M.C., Irwin, M.L., Swartz, A.M., Strath, S.J., O'Brien, W.L., Bassett, D.R. Jr., Schmitz, K.H., Emplaincourt, P.O., Jacobs, D.R., and Leon, A.S. 2000. Compendium of physical activities: An update of activity codes and MET intensities. *Medicine & Science in Sports & Exercise* 32(Suppl.): S498–S516.

American College of Sports Medicine (ACSM). 2000. *ACSM's guidelines for exercise testing and prescription.* Philadelphia: Lippincott Williams & Wilkins.

Berry, M.J., Cline, C.C., Berry, C.B., and Davis, M. 1992. A comparison between two forms of aerobic dance and treadmill running. *Medicine & Science in Sports & Exercise* 24: 946–951.

Birk, T.J., and Birk, C.A. 1987. Use of ratings of perceived exertion for exercise prescription. *Sports Medicine* 4: 1–8.

Blessing, D.L., Wilson, D.G., Puckett, J.R., and Ford, H.T. 1987. The physiological effects of 8 weeks of aerobic dance with and without hand-held weights. *American Journal of Sports Medicine* 15: 508–510.

Borg, G.V., and Linderholm, H. 1967. Perceived exertion and pulse rate during graded exercise in various age groups. *Acta Medica Scandinavica* 472(Suppl.): 194–206.

Brahler, C.J., and Blank, S.E. 1995. VersaClimbing elicits higher $\dot{V}O_2$max than does treadmill running or rowing ergometry. *Medicine & Science in Sports & Exercise* 27: 2499–254.

Brynteson, P., and Sinning, W.E. 1973. The effects of training frequencies on the retention of cardiovascular fitness. *Medicine and Science in Sports* 5: 29–33.

Chewning, B., Yu, T., and Johnson, J. 2000. T'ai chi (part 2): Effects on health. *ACSM's Health & Fitness Journal* 4(3): 17–19, 28, 30.

Crommett, A., Kravitz, L., Wongsathikun, J., and Kemerly, T. 1999. Comparison of metabolic and subjective response of three modalities in college-age subjects. *Medicine & Science in Sports & Exercise* 31(Suppl.): S158 [abstract].

deVries, H.A. 1980. *Physiology of exercise for physical education and athletics.* Dubuque, IA: Brown.

Dishman, R.K. 1994. Prescribing exercise intensity for healthy adults using perceived exertion. *Medicine & Science in Sports & Exercise* 26: 1087–1094.

Dunbar, C.C., Robertson, R.J., Baun, R., Blandin, M.F., Metz, K., Burdett, R., and Goss, F.L. 1992. The validity of regulating exercise intensity by ratings of perceived exertion. *Medicine & Science in Sports & Exercise* 24: 94–99.

Fox, E.L., and Mathews, D.K. 1974. *Interval training: Conditioning for sports and general fitness.* Philadelphia: Saunders.

Gettman, L.R., and Pollock, M.L. 1981. Circuit weight training: A critical review of its physiological benefits. *The Physician and Sportsmedicine* 9: 44–60.

Hickson, R.C., and Rosenkoetter, M.A. 1981. Reduced training frequencies and maintenance of increased aerobic power. *Medicine & Science in Sports & Exercise* 13: 13–16.

Howley, E.T., Colacino, D.L., and Swensen, T.C. 1992. Factors affecting the oxygen cost of stepping on an electronic stepping ergometer. *Medicine & Science in Sports & Exercise* 24: 1055–1058.

Kohrt, W.M., Spina, R.J., Holloszy, J.O., and Ehsani, A.A. 1998. Prescribing exercise intensity for older women. *Journal of the American Geriatric Society* 46: 129–133.

Kravitz, L., Cizar, C., Christensen, C., and Setterlund, S. 1993. The physiological effects of step training with and without handweights. *Journal of Sports Medicine and Physical Fitness* 33: 348–358.

Kravitz, L., Heyward, V., Stolarczyk, L., and Wilmerding, V. 1997. Effects of step training with and without handweights on physiological profiles of women. *Journal of Strength and Conditioning Research* 11: 194–199.

Kravitz, L., Robergs, R., and Heyward, V. 1996. Are all aerobic exercise modes equal? *Idea Today* 14: 51–58.

Kravitz, L., Robergs, R.A., Heyward, V.H., Wagner, D.R., and Powers, K. 1997. Exercise mode and gender comparisons of energy expenditure at self-selected intensities. *Medicine & Science in Sports & Exercise* 29: 1028–1035.

Kravitz, L., Wax, B., Mayo, J.J., Daniels, R., and Charette, K. 1998. Metabolic response of elliptical exercise training. *Medicine & Science in Sports & Exercise* 30(Suppl.): S169 [abstract].

Kuntzelman, B.A. 1979. *The complete guide to aerobic dancing.* Skokie, IL: Publications International.

Lan, C., Lai, J., Chen, S., and Wong, M. 1998. 12-month tai chi training in the elderly: Its effects on health fitness. *Medicine & Science in Sports & Exercise* 30: 345–351.

Magel, J.R., Foglia, G.F., McArdle, W.D., Gutin, B., Pechard, G.S., and Katch, F.I. 1974. Specificity of swim training on maximum oxygen uptake. *Journal of Applied Physiology* 38: 151–155.

Milburn, S., and Butts, N.K. 1983. A comparison of the training responses to aerobic dance and jogging in college females. *Medicine & Science in Sports & Exercise* 15: 510–513.

Moffatt, R.J., Stamford, B.A., and Neill, R.D. 1977. Placement of tri-weekly training sessions: Importance regarding enhancement of aerobic capacity. *Research Quarterly* 48: 583–591.

Nichols, J.F., Sherman, C.L., and Abbott, E. 2000. Treading is new and hot: 30 minutes meets the ACSM recommendations for cardiorespiratory fitness and caloric expenditure. *ACSM's Health & Fitness Journal* 4(2): 12–17.

Olson, M.S., Williford, H.N., Blessing, D.L., and Greathouse, R. 1991. The cardiovascular and metabolic effects of bench stepping exercise in females. *Medicine & Science in Sports & Exercise* 23: 1311–1318.

Parker, S.B., Hurley, B.F., Hanlon, D.P., and Vaccaro, P. 1989. Failure of target heart rate to accurately monitor intensity during aerobic dance. *Medicine & Science in Sports & Exercise* 21: 230–234.

Petersen, T., Verstraete, D., Schultz, W., and Stray-Gundersen, J. 1993. Metabolic demands of step aerobics. *Medicine & Science in Sports & Exercise* 25: S79 [abstract].

Pollock, M.L. 1973. The quantification of endurance training programs. In *Exercise and Sport Sciences Reviews,* ed. J.H. Wilmore, 1: 155–188. New York: Academic Press.

Pollock, M., Cureton, T.K., and Greninger, L. 1969. Effects of frequency of training on working capacity, cardiovascular function, and body composition of adult men. *Medicine and Science in Sports* 1: 70–74.

Pollock, M., Dimmick, J., Miller, H., Kendrick, Z., and Linnerud, A.C. 1975. Effects of mode of training on cardiovascular function and body composition of adult men. *Medicine and Science in Sports* 7: 139–145.

Pollock, M., Gaesser, G.A., Butcher, J.D., Despres, J.P., Dishman, R.K., Franklin, B.A., and Garber, C.E. 1998. The recommended quantity and quality of exercise for developing and maintaining cardiorespiratory and muscular fitness, and flexibility in healthy adults. *Medicine & Science in Sports & Exercise* 30: 975–991.

Pollock, M., Gettman, L., Milesis, C., Bah, M., Durstine, L., and Johnson, R. 1977. Effects of frequency and duration of training on attrition and incidence of injury. *Medicine and Science in Sports* 9: 31–36.

Pollock, M.L., Miller, H.S., Janeway, R., Linnerud, A.C., Robertson, B., and Valentino, R. 1971. Effects of walking on body composition and cardiovascular function of middle-aged men. *Journal of Applied Physiology* 30: 126–130.

Porcari, J., Foster, C., and Schneider, P. 2000. Exercise response to elliptical trainers. *Fitness Management* 16(9): 50–53.

Porter, G.H. 1988. Case study evaluation for exercise prescription. In *Resource manual for guidelines for exercise testing and prescription*, ed. S.N. Blair, P. Painter, R.R. Pate, L.K. Smith, and C.B. Taylor, 248–255. Philadelphia: Lea & Febiger.

Russell, P.J. 1983. Aerobic dance programs: Maintaining quality and effectiveness. *Physical Educator* 40: 114–120.

Sharkey, B.J. 1979. *Physiology of fitness*. Champaign, IL: Human Kinetics.

Smutok, M.A., Skrinar, G.S., and Pandolf, K.B. 1980. Exercise intensity: Subjective regulation by perceived exertion. *Archives of Physical Medicine and Rehabilitation* 61: 569–574.

Swain, D.P. 1999. $\dot{V}O_2$ reserve: A new method for exercise prescription. *ACSM's Health & Fitness Journal* 3(5): 10–14.

Swain, D.P., and Leutholtz, B.C. 1997. Heart rate reserve is equivalent to % $\dot{V}O_2$ reserve, not to $\dot{V}O_2$ max. *Medicine & Science in Sports & Exercise* 29: 410–414.

Swain, D.P., Leutholtz, B.C., King, M.E., Haas, L.A., and Branch, J.D. 1998. Relationship between % heart rate reserve and % $\dot{V}O_2$ reserve in treadmill exercise. *Medicine & Science in Sports & Exercise* 30: 318–321.

Thomas, T.R., Ziogas, G., Smith, T., Zhang, Q., and Londeree, B.R. 1995. Physiological and perceived exertion responses to six modes of submaximal exercise. *Research Quarterly for Exercise and Sport* 66: 239–246.

Town, G.P., Sol, N., and Sinning, W. 1980. The effect of rope skipping rate on energy expenditure of males and females. *Medicine & Science in Sports & Exercise* 12: 295–298.

U.S. Department of Health and Human Services. 1996. *Physical activity and health: A report of the Surgeon General—At a glance*. Atlanta: U.S. Department of Health and Human Services, Centers for Disease Control and Prevention, National Center for Chronic Disease Prevention and Health Promotion.

Velasquez, K.S., and Wilmore, J.H. 1992. Changes in cardiorespiratory fitness and body composition after a 12-week bench step training program. *Medicine & Science in Sports & Exercise* 24: S78 [abstract].

Wallick, M.E., Porcari, J.P., Wallick, S.B., Berg, K.M., Brice, G.A., and Arimond, G.R. 1995. Physiological responses to in-line skating compared to treadmill running. *Medicine & Science in Sports & Exercise* 27: 242–248.

Williford, H.N., Blessing, D.L., Barksdale, J.M., and Smith, F.H. 1988. The effects of aerobic dance training on serum lipids, lipoproteins, and cardiopulmonary function. *Journal of Sports Medicine and Physical Fitness* 28: 151–157.

Wilmore, J.H., Davis, J.A., O'Brien, R.S., Vodak, P.A., Walder, G.R., and Amsterdam, E.A. 1980. Physiological alterations consequent to 20-week conditioning programs of bicycling, tennis and jogging. *Medicine & Science in Sports & Exercise* 12: 1–9.

Wilmoth, S.K. 1986. *Leading aerobic dance-exercise.* Champaign, IL: Human Kinetics.

Woodby-Brown, S., Berg, K., and Latin, R.W. 1993. Oxygen cost of aerobic bench stepping at three heights. *Journal of Strength and Conditioning Research* 7: 163–167.

Zeni, A.I., Hoffman, M.D., and Clifford, P.S. 1996. Energy expenditure with indoor exercise machines. *Journal of the American Medical Association* 275: 1424–1427.

Assessing Strength and Muscular Endurance

Muscular strength and endurance are two important components of physical fitness. Minimal levels of muscular fitness are needed to perform activities of daily living, to maintain functional independence as one ages, and to partake in active leisure-time pursuits without undue stress or fatigue. Adequate levels of muscular fitness lessen the chance of developing low back problems, osteoporotic fractures, and musculoskeletal injuries.

This chapter describes a variety of laboratory and field tests for assessing all forms of muscular strength and endurance. In addition, this chapter compares types of exercise machines, addresses factors affecting muscular fitness tests, and discusses sources of measurement error.

DEFINITION OF TERMS

Muscular strength is defined as the ability of a muscle group to develop maximal contractile force against a resistance in a single contraction. The force generated by a muscle or muscle group, however, is highly dependent on the velocity of movement. Maximal force is produced when the limb is not rotating (i.e., zero velocity). As the speed of joint rotation increases, the muscular force decreases. Thus, *strength for dynamic movements* is defined as the maximal force generated in a single contraction at a specified velocity (Knuttgen and Kraemer 1987). **Muscular endurance** is the ability of a muscle group to exert submaximal force for extended periods.

Both strength and muscular endurance can be assessed for static and dynamic muscular contractions. If the resistance is immovable, the muscle contraction is **static** or **isometric** ("iso," same; "metric," length), and there is no visible movement of the joint. **Dynamic contractions,** in which there is visible joint movement, are either concentric, eccentric, or isokinetic (see figure 6.1, *a* and *b*).

If the resistance is less than the force produced by the muscle group, the contraction is **concentric,** allowing the muscle to shorten as it exerts

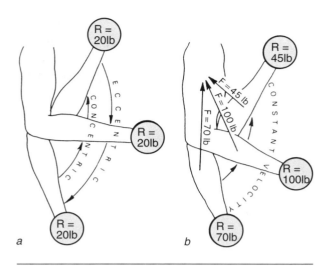

Figure 6.1 Types of muscle contraction.

tension to move the bony lever. The muscle is also capable of exerting tension while lengthening. This is known as **eccentric contraction** and typically occurs when the muscles produce a braking force to decelerate rapidly moving body segments or to resist gravity (e.g., slowly lowering a barbell). Both concentric and eccentric contractions are sometimes called **isotonic** ("iso," same; "tonic," tension). The term "isotonic contraction" is a misnomer because the tension produced by the muscle group fluctuates greatly even though the resistance is constant throughout the range of motion (ROM). This fluctuation in muscular force is due to the change in muscle length and angle of pull as the bony lever is moved, creating a strength curve that is unique for each muscle group (Kreighbaum and Barthels 1981). For example, the strength of the knee flexors is maximal at 160° to 170° (see figure 6.2).

In regular (concentric and eccentric), dynamic exercise, because of the change in mechanical and physiological advantage as the limb is moved, the muscle group is not contracting maximally throughout the ROM. Thus, the greatest resistance that can be used during regular, dynamic exercise is equal to the maximum weight that can be moved at the *weakest* point in the ROM.

Isokinetic contraction (see figure 6.1b) is a maximal contraction of a muscle group at a constant velocity throughout the entire range of joint motion ("iso," same; "kinetic," motion). The velocity of contraction is controlled mechanically so that the limb rotates at a set velocity (e.g., 120°·sec⁻¹). Electromechanical devices vary the resistance to match the muscular force produced at each point in the ROM. Thus, isokinetic exercise machines allow the muscle group to encounter variable but maximal resistances during the movement.

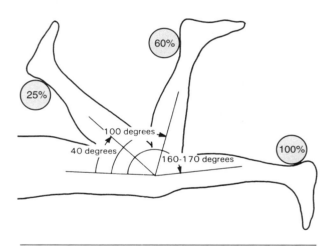

Figure 6.2 Strength variations in relation to knee joint angle.

Table 6.1	Strength Testing Modes	
Testing mode	**Equipment**	**Measure***
Static	Isometric dynamometers, cable tensiometers, and load cells	MVC (kg)
Dynamic		
Constant resistance	Free weights (barbells and dumbbells) and exercise machines	1-RM (lb or kg)
Variable resistance	Exercise machines	NA
Isokinetic and omnikinetic	Isokinetic and omnikinetic dynamometers	Peak torque (Nm or ft-lb)
*MVC = maximal voluntary contraction; 1-RM = one-repetition maximum; NA = not applicable; Nm = newton-meter; ft-lb = foot-pound.		

STRENGTH AND MUSCULAR ENDURANCE TESTING

Static strength and muscular endurance are measured using dynamometers, cable tensiometers, and load cells. Free weights (barbells and dumbbells), as well as constant-resistance, variable-resistance, and isokinetic exercise machines, are used to assess dynamic strength and endurance (see table 6.1.). The testing procedures vary depending on the type of test (i.e., strength or endurance) and equipment.

Isometric Muscle Testing Using Dynamometers

You can use isometric dynamometers to measure static strength and endurance of the grip squeezing muscles and leg and back muscles (see figure 6.3). The handgrip dynamometer has an adjustable handle to fit the size of the hand and measures forces between 0 and 100 kilograms (kg), in 1-kg increments. The back and leg dynamometer consists of a scale that measures forces ranging from 0 to 2500 lb in 10-lb increments. Both dynamometers are spring devices. As force is applied to the dynamometer, the spring is compressed and moves the indicator needle a corresponding amount.

Grip Strength Testing Procedures

Before using the handgrip dynamometer, adjust the handgrip size to a position that is comfortable for the individual. Alternatively, you can measure the hand width with a caliper and use this value to set the optimum grip size (Montoye and Faulkner 1964). The individual stands erect, with the arm and forearm positioned as follows (Fess 1992): shoulder adducted and neutrally rotated, elbow flexed at 90°, forearm in the neutral position, and

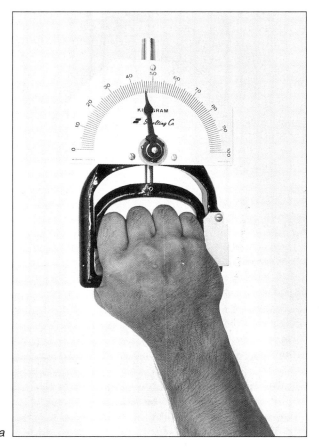

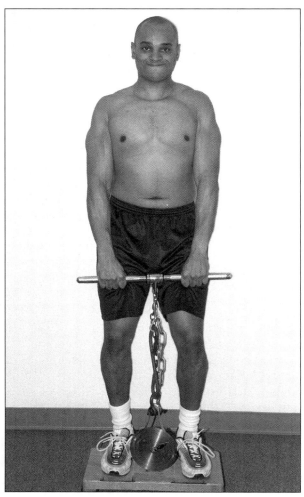

Figure 6.3 Dynamometers for measuring static strength and endurance: *(a)* handgrip dynamometer and *(b)* back and leg dynamometer.

wrist in slight extension (0° to 30°). For some test protocols, however, the client must keep the arm straight and slightly abducted when measuring the grip strength of each hand (Canadian Society for Exercise Physiology 1998). The individual squeezes the dynamometer as hard as possible using one brief maximal contraction and no extraneous body movement. Administer three trials for each hand, allowing a 1-min rest between trials, and use the best score as the client's static strength.

Grip-Endurance Testing Procedures

Once the grip size is adjusted, instruct the client to squeeze the handle as hard as possible and to continue squeezing for 1 min. Record the initial force and the final force exerted at the end of 1 min. The greater the endurance, the less the rate and degree of decline in force. The relative endurance score is the final force divided by the initial force times 100.

Alternatively, you can assess static grip endurance by having your client exert a submaximal force, which is a given percentage of the individual's maximum voluntary contractile (MVC) strength (e.g., 50% MVC). The relative endurance score is the amount of time that this force level is maintained. During the test, the client must watch the dial of the dynamometer and adjust the amount of force exerted as necessary in order to maintain the appropriate submaximal force level.

Leg Strength Testing Procedures

Using the back and leg dynamometer, the individual stands on the platform with trunk erect and the knees flexed to an angle of 130° to 140°. The client holds the hand bar using a pronated grip and positions it across the thighs by adjusting the length of the chain (see figure 6.3b). If a belt is available, attach it to each end of the hand bar after positioning the belt around the client's hips. The belt helps to stabilize the bar and to reduce the stress placed on the hands during the leg lift. Without using the back, the client slowly exerts as much force as possible while extending the knees. The maximum indicator needle remains at the peak force achieved. Administer two or three trials with a 1-min rest interval. Divide the maximum score (in pounds) by 2.2 to convert it to kilograms.

Back Strength Testing Procedures

Using the back and leg dynamometer, the individual stands on the platform with the knees fully extended and the head and trunk erect. The client grasps the hand bar using a pronated grip with the right hand and a supinated grip with the left. Position the hand bar across the client's thighs. Without leaning backward, the client pulls the hand bar straight upward using the back muscles and is instructed to roll the shoulders backward during the pull. Clients should be reminded before lifting to flex the trunk minimally and to keep the head and trunk erect during the test. Administer two trials with a 1-min rest between the trials. Divide the maximum score (in pounds) by 2.2 to convert it to kilograms.

Static Strength Norms

Norms are available to assess the grip strength of each hand (right and left) separately (see table 6.2), as well as combined (right plus left hand) scores. The *Canadian Physical Activity, Fitness and Lifestyle Appraisal* provides age- and gender-based norms for combined grip strength scores of individuals between 15 and 69 years of age (Canadian Society for Exercise Physiology 1998).

You can also use norms developed for men and women to assess your client's static strength for each dynamometric test item (see table 6.2). Calculate your client's total strength score by adding the right grip, left grip, leg strength, and back strength scores. Before doing this, convert the leg and back strength scores (measured in pounds) to kilograms. To calculate the relative strength score, divide the total strength score by body mass (expressed in kilograms).

Isometric Muscle Testing Using Cable Tensiometers

You can use cable tensiometry to assess the static strength of 38 different muscle groups throughout the body. Standardized testing procedures have been described elsewhere in detail and should be followed closely to ensure the validity and reliability of the test results (Clarke 1966). The instrumentation includes a tensiometer, steel cables, testing table, wall hooks, straps, and goniometer. Attach one end of the cable to the wall or table hooks and, using a strap, attach the other end to the body part to be tested. Always position the cable at a right angle to the pulling bony lever. Use a goniometer to measure the appropriate joint angle. Place the tensiometer on a taut cable. As the individual exerts force on the cable, the riser of the tensiometer is depressed and a maximum indicator needle registers the static

Table 6.2 Static Strength Norms

Classification	Left grip (kg)	Right grip (kg)	Back strength (kg)	Leg strength (kg)	Total strength (kg)	Relative strength*
Men						
Excellent	>68	>70	>209	>241	>587	>7.50
Good	56-67	62-69	177-208	214-240	508-586	7.10-7.49
Average	43-55	48-61	126-176	160-213	375-507	5.21-7.09
Below average	39-42	41-47	91-125	137-159	307-374	4.81-5.20
Poor	<39	<41	<91	<137	<307	<4.81
Women						
Excellent	>37	>41	>111	>136	>324	>5.50
Good	34-36	38-40	98-110	114-135	282-323	4.80-5.49
Average	22-33	25-37	52-97	66-113	164-281	2.90-4.79
Below average	18-21	22-24	39-51	49-65	117-163	2.10-2.89
Poor	<18	<22	<39	<49	<117	<2.10

*Relative strength is determined by dividing total strength by body mass (kg).

For persons over age 50, reduce scores by 10% to adjust for muscle tissue loss due to aging. Data from Corbin et al. (1978).

strength score. Tensiometers measure forces ranging between 0 and 400 lb (0 to 181.8 kg). However, the larger tensiometers are less accurate in the lower range; therefore, you should use a small tensiometer, which measures forces between 0 and 100 lb (0 to 45.4 kg), to obtain greater accuracy in the lower range.

Cable tensiometry tests can be used to assess strength impairment at specific joint angles and to monitor progress during rehabilitation. As with all forms of static strength testing, you should be aware that strength is specific to the joint angle and muscle group being tested. Therefore, test at least three to four muscle groups to provide an adequate estimation of static strength.

Test batteries and norms have been developed for males and females 9 years old through college age (Clarke 1975; Clarke and Monroe 1970). The test battery for males of all ages includes the same three strength tests: shoulder extension, knee extension, and ankle plantar flexion. For elementary and junior high school girls, the test battery includes shoulder extension, hip extension, and trunk flexion. The three test items in the battery developed for senior high school and college women are shoulder flexion, hip flexion, and ankle plantar flexion.

Dynamic Muscle Testing Using Constant-Resistance and Variable-Resistance Modes

Although either a **constant-resistance** or a **variable-resistance exercise** mode can be used to assess dynamic (concentric and eccentric) muscle strength and endurance, you will be better served if you use either free weights or constant-resistance exercise machines.

A major disadvantage of free weights, dumbbells, and constant-resistance exercise machines, however, is that they measure dynamic strength only at the weakest point in the ROM. The reason is that the resistance cannot be varied to account for fluctuations in muscular force caused by the changing mechanical (angle of pull of muscle) and physiological (length of muscle) advantage of the musculoskeletal system during the movement.

In an attempt to overcome this deficiency, equipment manufacturers have designed variable-resistance machines that vary the resistance during the ROM. Variable-resistance machines have a moving connection (i.e., lever, cam, or pulley) between the resistance and the point of force application. As the weight is lifted, the mechanical advantage of the machine decreases. Therefore, more force must be applied to continue moving the resistance. The variable-resistance mode of exercise attempts to match the force capability of the musculoskeletal system throughout the ROM. However, many variable-resistance exercise machines fail to match the strength curves of different muscle groups. Also, with variable-resistance machines, it is difficult to assess the client's maximal force or strength because the resistance is modified by the levers, pulleys, and cams, causing the movement velocity to vary. Variable-resistance exercise machines, therefore, have limited usefulness for maximal testing. Still, these types of machines are well suited for resistance training.

Although free weights and constant-resistance exercise machines are generally recommended for muscular fitness testing, there are advantages and limitations to each of these modalities. Compared to exercise machines, free weights require more neuromuscular coordination in order to stabilize body parts and maintain balance during lifting of the barbell or dumbbell. While exercise machines reduce the need for spotting during the test, these machines limit the individual's range of joint motion and plane of movement. Also, some exercise machines have relatively large weight plate increments so that you must attach smaller weights to the weight stack in order to measure your client's strength accurately. Although most exercise machines have adjustable seats and lever arms, some cannot accommodate individuals with short limbs. Machines designed specifically for children and smaller adults must be used to standardize such clients' starting positions for testing. Body size and weight increments are less of a problem with free weights. The following dynamic strength and muscular endurance test protocols were specifically developed for constant-resistance exercise machines.

Dynamic Strength Tests

Dynamic strength is usually measured as the **one-repetition maximum** (**1-RM**), which is the maximum weight that can be lifted for one complete repetition of the movement. The 1-RM strength value is obtained through trial and error.

Although 1-RM strength tests can be safely administered to individuals of all ages, you should take precautions to decrease the risk of injury when clients attempt to lift maximal loads. Be certain that your client warms up before attempting the lift and starts with a weight that is below the

---

STEPS FOR 1-RM MAXIMUM TESTING

The following basic steps are recommended for 1-RM testing (Kraemer and Fry 1995).

1. Have your client warm up by completing 5 to 10 repetitions of the exercise at 40% to 60% of the estimated 1-RM.

2. During a 1-min rest, have the client stretch the muscle group. This is followed by three to five repetitions of the exercise at 60% to 80% of the estimated 1-RM.

3. Increase the weight conservatively, and have the client attempt the 1-RM lift. If the lift is successful, the client should rest 3 to 5 min before attempting the next weight increment. Follow this procedure until the client fails to complete the lift. The 1-RM typically is achieved within three to five trials.

4. Record the 1-RM value as the maximum weight lifted for the last successful trial.

---

individual's expected 1-RM. When you administer these tests, you should spot your clients and closely monitor their lifting technique and breathing.

The ACSM (2000) recommends the bench press and leg press (upper plate of constant-resistance exercise machine) for assessing strength of the upper and lower body, respectively. To determine **relative strength,** divide the 1-RM values by the client's body mass. Norms for men and women are provided in tables 6.3 and 6.4.

Another test of dynamic strength includes six test items: bench press, arm curl, latissimus pull, leg press, leg extension, and leg curl. For each exercise, express and evaluate the 1-RM as a percentage of body mass. For example, if a 120-lb (54.5 kg) woman bench presses 60 lb (27.2 kg), her strength-to-body mass ratio is 0.50 (60 divided by 120), and she scores 3 points for that exercise. Follow this procedure for each exercise; then add the total points to determine the overall strength and fitness category of the individual. Strength-to-body mass ratios with corresponding point values for college-age men and women are presented in table 6.5.

Dynamic Muscle Endurance Tests

You can assess your client's dynamic muscle endurance by having the individual perform as many repetitions as possible using a weight that is a set

Table 6.3	Age-Gender Norms for 1-RM Maximum Bench Press (1-RM/BM)				
Percentile rankings* for men	Age				
	20-29	30-39	40-49	50-59	60+
90	1.48	1.24	1.10	0.97	0.89
80	1.32	1.12	1.00	0.90	0.82
70	1.22	1.04	0.93	0.84	0.77
60	1.14	0.98	0.88	0.79	0.72
50	1.06	0.93	0.84	0.75	0.68
40	0.99	0.88	0.80	0.71	0.66
30	0.93	0.83	0.76	0.68	0.63
20	0.88	0.78	0.72	0.63	0.57
10	0.80	0.71	0.65	0.57	0.53

Percentile rankings* for women	Age					
	20-29	30-39	40-49	50-59	60-69	70+
90	0.54	0.49	0.46	0.40	0.41	0.44
80	0.49	0.45	0.40	0.37	0.38	0.39
70	0.42	0.42	0.38	0.35	0.36	0.33
60	0.41	0.41	0.37	0.33	0.32	0.31
50	0.40	0.38	0.34	0.31	0.30	0.27
40	0.37	0.37	0.32	0.28	0.29	0.25
30	0.35	0.34	0.30	0.26	0.28	0.24
20	0.33	0.32	0.27	0.23	0.26	0.21
10	0.30	0.27	0.23	0.19	0.25	0.02

*Descriptors for percentile rankings: 90 = well above average; 70 = above average; 50 = average; 30 = below average; 10 = well below average.

Data for men provided by The Cooper Institute for Aerobics Research, Dallas, TX, 1994. Data for women provided by the Women's Exercise Research Center, The George Washington University Medical Center, Washington, D.C., 1998. Published in *The Physical Fitness Specialist Certification Manual*, The Cooper Institute for Aerobics Research, Dallas, TX, revised 1997.

percentage of the body weight or maximum strength (1-RM). Pollock, Wilmore, and Fox (1978) recommend using a weight that is 70% of the 1-RM value for each exercise. Although norms for this test have not been established, these authors suggest, on the basis of their testing and research findings, that the average individual should be able to complete 12 to 15 repetitions.

The YMCA (2000) recommends using a bench press test to assess dynamic muscular endurance of the upper body. For this absolute endurance test, use a flat bench and barbell. The client per-

forms as many repetitions as possible at a set cadence of 30 repetitions per minute. Use a metronome to establish the exercise cadence. Male clients lift an 80-lb (36.4 kg) barbell, whereas female clients use a 35-lb (15.9 kg) barbell. Terminate the test when the client is unable to maintain the exercise cadence. Table 6.6 presents norms for this test.

Alternatively, you can use a test battery consisting of seven items to assess dynamic muscular endurance. Select the weight to be lifted using a set percentage of the individual's body mass. The

Table 6.4　Age-Gender Norms for 1-RM Leg Press (1-RM/BM)

Percentile rankings* for men	Age				
	20-29	30-39	40-49	50-59	60+
90	2.27	2.07	1.92	1.80	1.73
80	2.13	1.93	1.82	1.71	1.62
70	2.05	1.85	1.74	1.64	1.56
60	1.97	1.77	1.68	1.58	1.49
50	1.91	1.71	1.62	1.52	1.43
40	1.83	1.65	1.57	1.46	1.38
30	1.74	1.59	1.51	1.39	1.30
20	1.63	1.52	1.44	1.32	1.25
10	1.51	1.43	1.35	1.22	1.16

Percentile rankings* for women	Age					
	20-29	30-39	40-49	50-59	60-69	70+
90	2.05	1.73	1.63	1.51	1.40	1.27
80	1.66	1.50	1.46	1.30	1.25	1.12
70	1.42	1.47	1.35	1.24	1.18	1.10
60	1.36	1.32	1.26	1.18	1.15	0.95
50	1.32	1.26	1.19	1.09	1.08	0.89
40	1.25	1.21	1.12	1.03	1.04	0.83
30	1.23	1.16	1.03	0.95	0.98	0.82
20	1.13	1.09	0.94	0.86	0.94	0.79
10	1.02	0.94	0.76	0.75	0.84	0.75

*Descriptors for percentile rankings: 90 = well above average; 70 = above average; 50 = average; 30 = below average; 10 = well below average.

Data for men provided by The Cooper Institute for Aerobics Research, Dallas, TX, 1994. Data for women provided by the Women's Exercise Research Center, The George Washington University Medical Center, Washington, D.C., 1998. Published in *The Physical Fitness Specialist Certification Manual*, The Cooper Institute for Aerobics Research, Dallas, TX, revised 1997.

client lifts this weight up to a maximum of 15 repetitions. Table 6.7 provides percentages for each test item, as well as the scoring system and norms for college-age men and women.

Dynamic Muscle Testing Using Isokinetic and Omnikinetic Exercise Modes

Isokinetic dynamometers provide an accurate and reliable assessment of strength, endurance, and power of muscle groups (see figure 6.4). The speed of limb movement is kept at a constant preselected velocity. Any increase in muscular force produces an increased resistance rather than increased acceleration of the limb. Thus, fluctuations in muscular force throughout the ROM are matched by an equal counterforce or **accommodating resistance.**

Isokinetic dynamometers measure muscular torque production at speeds of $0°$ to $300°\cdot sec^{-1}$. From the recorded output, you can evaluate peak torque, total work, and power. Some less expen-

Table 6.5   Strength-to-Body Mass Ratios for Selected 1-RM Tests

Bench press	Arm curl	Lat pull-down	Leg press	Leg extension	Leg curl	Points
Men						
1.50	0.70	1.20	3.00	0.80	0.70	10
1.40	0.65	1.15	2.80	0.75	0.65	9
1.30	0.60	1.10	2.60	0.70	0.60	8
1.20	0.55	1.05	2.40	0.65	0.55	7
1.10	0.50	1.00	2.20	0.60	0.50	6
1.00	0.45	0.95	2.00	0.55	0.45	5
0.90	0.40	0.90	1.80	0.50	0.40	4
0.80	0.35	0.85	1.60	0.45	0.35	3
0.70	0.30	0.80	1.40	0.40	0.30	2
0.60	0.25	0.75	1.20	0.35	0.25	1
Women						
0.90	0.50	0.85	2.70	0.70	0.60	10
0.85	0.45	0.80	2.50	0.65	0.55	9
0.80	0.42	0.75	2.30	0.60	0.52	8
0.70	0.38	0.73	2.10	0.55	0.50	7
0.65	0.35	0.70	2.00	0.52	0.45	6
0.60	0.32	0.65	1.80	0.50	0.40	5
0.55	0.28	0.63	1.60	0.45	0.35	4
0.50	0.25	0.60	1.40	0.40	0.30	3
0.45	0.21	0.55	1.20	0.35	0.25	2
0.35	0.18	0.50	1.00	0.30	0.20	1

Total points	Strength fitness category[a]
48-60	Excellent
37-47	Good
25-36	Average
13-24	Fair
0-12	Poor

[a]Based on data compiled by author for 250 college-age men and women.

sive isokinetic dynamometers lack this recording capability but are suitable for training and rehabilitation exercise.

Omnikinetic exercise dynamometers (see figure 6.5) provide maximum overload at every joint angle throughout the ROM at whatever speed the

Table 6.6 YMCA Bench Press Test Norms[a]

Percentile	Age group (years)					
	18-25	26-35	36-45	46-55	56-65	>65
Men						
95	42	40	34	28	24	20
75	30	26	24	20	14	10
50	22	20	17	12	8	6
25	13	12	10	6	4	2
5	2	2	2	1	0	0
Women						
95	42	40	32	30	30	22
75	28	25	21	20	16	12
50	20	17	13	11	9	6
25	12	9	8	5	3	2
5	2	1	1	0	0	0

[a]Score is number of repetitions completed in 1 min using 80-lb barbell for men and 35-lb barbell for women.

Data from YMCA of the USA (2000). *YMCA Fitness Testing and Assessment Manual* (4th ed.) Champaign, IL: Human Kinetics. Reprinted and adapted with permission of the YMCA of the USA, 101 N. Wacker Drive, Chicago, IL 60606.

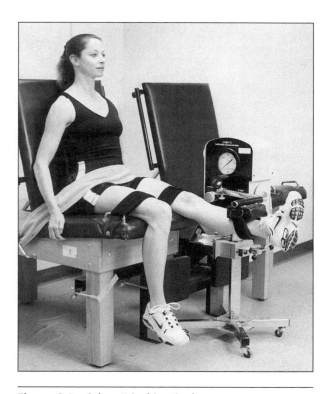

Figure 6.4 Cybex II isokinetic dynamometer.

individual is capable of generating. This testing system provides an accommodating resistance that adjusts to both the force and velocity output of the individual and is not limited to a preset velocity of limb movement. Thus, at any one setting, the individual maximally overloads both the force and velocity production capabilities of the contractile elements. The stronger the individual, the faster the speed of limb movement at any given setting. Also, increasing limb velocity results in increased resistance. Even as the muscle fatigues, the individual receives optimal overload with each repetition because the limb speed and resistance decrease. Theoretically, movement at slower speeds will allow recruitment of motor units that were not contributing to the total force production in earlier repetitions performed at faster speeds. Thus, self-accommodating, variable-resistance–variable-velocity exercise devices assess the isokinetic strength and endurance of both fast-twitch and slow-twitch motor units in the muscle group.

Table 6.8 summarizes isokinetic and omnikinetic test protocols for assessing strength, endurance, and power. For detailed descriptions of isokinetic

Table 6.7 Dynamic Muscular Endurance Test Battery

| Exercise | % Body mass to be lifted | | Repetitions (max = 15) |
	Men	Women	
Arm curl	0.33	0.25	_____
Bench press	0.66	0.50	_____
Lat pull-down	0.66	0.50	_____
Triceps extension	0.33	0.33	_____
Leg extension	0.50	0.50	_____
Leg curl	0.33	0.33	_____
Bent-knee sit-up			_____
	Total repetitions (max = 105) =		_____

Total repetitions	Fitness category[a]
91-105	Excellent
77-90	Very good
63-76	Good
49-62	Fair
35-48	Poor
<35	Very poor

[a]Based on data compiled by author for 250 college-age men and women.

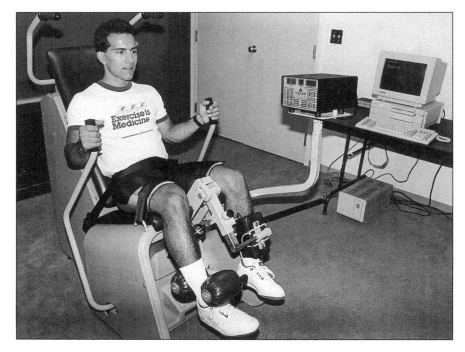

Figure 6.5 Omni-tron dynamometer.

Table 6.8   Isokinetic and Omnikinetic Test Protocols

Isokinetic tests	Speed setting	Protocol	Measure*
Strength	30° or 60°·sec⁻¹	2 submax practice trials, followed by 3 maximal trials	Peak torque (ft-lb or Nm)
Endurance	120° to 180°·sec⁻¹	1 maximal trial	Number of repetitions until torque reaches 50% of initial torque value
Power	120° to 300°·sec⁻¹	2 submax practice trials, followed by 3 maximal trials	Peak torque (ft-lb or Nm)

Omnikinetic tests	Resistance setting	Protocol	Measure*
Strength	10	3 submax trials at resistance setting 2, followed by 5 maximal trials	Peak torque (ft-lb)
Endurance	3	3 practice trials at resistance setting 2, followed by 20 maximal repetitions	Total work output (ft-lb)
Power	6	3 submax trials, followed by 1 maximal trial	Peak torque or total work (ft-lb)

*ft-lb = foot-pound; Nm = Newton-meter; 1 ft-lb = 0.138 Nm.

test protocols and test norms, see Perrin 1993. Appendix C.1, "Average Strength, Endurance, and Power Values for Isokinetic (Omni-tron) Tests" (p. 298), provides omnikinetic performance norms for young and middle-aged men and women, as well as male and female weight trainers.

Calisthenic-Type Strength and Muscular Endurance Tests

In certain field situations, you may not have access to dynamometers, free weights, or exercise machines to assess muscular fitness. As an alternative, you may use calisthenic-type strength and endurance tests to assess your client's strength and muscular endurance.

Dynamic Strength Tests

You can measure dynamic strength using calisthenic-type exercises by determining the maximum weight, in excess of body mass, that an individual can lift for one repetition of the movement. Because strength is related to the size and body mass of the individual, Johnson and Nelson (1986) recommend using relative strength scores. For each test, attach weight plates (2 1/2, 5, 10, and 25

lb or 1, 2.3, 4.5, and 11.4 kg) to the individual. The relative strength score is the amount of additional weight divided by the body mass. For example, if a 150-lb (68.2 kg) man successfully performs one pull-up with a 30-lb (13.6 kg) weight attached to the waist belt, his relative strength score is 0.20 (30 lb/150 lb). Test protocols and performance norms for the pull-up, dip strength, sit-up, and bench squat are described elsewhere (Johnson and Nelson 1986).

Dynamic Endurance Tests

You can assess dynamic muscular endurance by measuring the maximum number of repetitions for each calisthenic-type exercise. Test protocols and norms for some commonly used muscular endurance tests (e.g., pull-ups, sit-ups, and dips) are presented elsewhere (Johnson and Nelson 1986).

Because many women and children are unable to perform even one pull-up, the timed flexed arm hang is commonly used for these groups. However, the flexed arm hang measures isometric endurance. To assess dynamic endurance of the arm and shoulder girdle musculature, Baumgartner (1978) developed a modified pull-up test that uses an inclined board (30° angle to floor) with a pull-up bar at the top. A scooter board was modified to slide along garage door tracks attached to the inclined board (Baumgartner et al. 1984). While lying prone on the scooter board and grasping the pull-up bar, the individual pulls up until the chin is over the pull-up bar. Detailed testing procedures, equipment design, and performance norms for children, adolescents, and college-age men and women are available (Baumgartner 1978; Baumgartner et al. 1984).

The ACSM (2000) recommends using a push-up test to assess endurance of the upper-body musculature. If the client is a male, he assumes a standard push-up position, with back straight, head up, and hands placed shoulder-width apart. He lowers his body until his chin touches the mat; the abdomen should not touch the mat. The client must push up to a straight-arm position. For women, modify the standard push-up position by having the client assume a kneeling position with the lower legs in contact with the mat, ankles plantar flexed, and back straight. Score the push-up test for men and women as the maximum number of consecutive repetitions performed without rest. Table 6.9 provides norms for the push-up test.

Table 6.9   Age-Gender Norms for Push-Up Test

Percentile rankings* for men[a]	Age				
	20-29	30-39	40-49	50-59	60-69
90	41	32	25	24	24
80	34	27	21	17	16
70	30	24	19	14	11
60	27	21	16	11	10
50	24	19	13	10	9
40	21	16	12	9	7
30	18	14	10	7	6
20	16	11	8	5	4
10	11	8	5	4	2

Percentile rankings* for women[b]	Age					
	20-29	30-39	40-49	50-59	60-69	70+
90	31	27	25	19	18	24
80	27	22	21	17	15	17
70	21	20	17	13	13	11
60	19	17	16	12	11	9
50	18	16	14	11	9	7
40	14	13	11	9	6	2
30	13	10	10	6	4	0
20	10	7	8	3	0	0
10	6	1	4	0	0	0

*Descriptors for percentile rankings: 90 = well above average; 70 = above average; 50 = average; 30 = below average; 10 = well below average.

[a]Data for men from the Canada Fitness Survey, 1981. Reproduced, with permission, from *Canadian Standardized Test of Fitness Operations Manual-3rd Edition,* Health Canada, 1986. © Minister of Public Works and Government Services Canada, 2001.

[b]Data for modified push-up test for women provided by the Women's Exercise Research Center, The George Washington University Medical Center, Washington, D.C., 1998.

To assess the muscular endurance of the abdominal muscles, ACSM (2000) recommends using a partial curl-up (crunch) test. For this test, have the individual assume a supine position on a mat with the knees flexed to 90° and arms at the sides with fingers touching a piece of masking tape. Place a second piece of masking tape 8 cm (for individuals 45 years or older) or 12 cm (for individuals less than 45 years) beyond the first piece of tape. Set the metronome to 40 bpm (20 curl-ups per minute). Instruct clients to slowly lift their shoulder blades off the mat in time with the metronome. Clients should flex their trunks (curl up) until their fingertips touch the second tape mark or the trunk makes a 30° angle with the mat. Score the curl-up test as the number of consecutive curl-ups performed without pausing, up to a maximum of 75. Alternatively, you may have your client perform as many curl-ups as possible in 1 min (ACSM 2000). Table 6.10 provides norms for the partial curl-up test.

Table 6.10 Age-Gender Norms for Partial Curl-Up Test

Percentile rankings* for men	Age				
	20-29	30-39	40-49	50-59	60-69
90	75	75	75	74	53
80	56	69	75	60	33
70	41	46	67	45	26
60	31	36	51	35	19
50	27	31	39	27	16
40	24	26	31	23	9
30	20	19	26	19	6
20	13	13	21	13	0
10	4	0	13	0	0

Percentile rankings* for women	Age				
	20-29	30-39	40-49	50-59	60-69
90	70	55	50	48	50
80	45	43	42	30	30
70	37	34	33	23	24
60	32	28	28	16	19
50	27	21	25	9	13
40	21	15	20	2	9
30	17	12	14	0	3
20	12	0	5	0	0
10	5	0	0	0	0

*Descriptors for percentile rankings: 90 = well above average; 70 = above average; 50 = average; 30 = below average; 10 = well below average.

Data from the Canada Fitness Survey, 1981. Reproduced, with permission, from *Canadian Standardized Test of Fitness Operations Manual-3rd Edition*, Health Canada, 1986. © Minister of Public Works and Government Services Canada, 2001.

SOURCES OF MEASUREMENT ERROR IN MUSCULAR FITNESS TESTING

The validity and reliability of strength and muscular endurance measures are affected by client factors, equipment, technician skill, and environmental factors. You must control each of these factors to ensure the accuracy and precision of muscular fitness scores.

Client Factors

Before measuring your client's strength or muscular endurance, familiarize the individual with the equipment and testing procedures. Clients with limited or no prior weightlifting experience need time to practice each lift to control for the effects of learning on performance. You should give even experienced weight lifters time to practice so that you can correct any improper lifting techniques prior to testing.

Muscular fitness tests require clients to give a maximal effort. Therefore, clients should get adequate sleep before performing these tests, and you should restrict the use of drugs and medications that may adversely affect their performance. It is also important that you motivate your clients during testing by encouraging them to do their best and giving them positive feedback after each trial. Adequate rest between trials is necessary in order for clients to obtain scores that truly represent their maximal effort.

Equipment

The design of testing equipment may also affect your client's test scores. Most of the dynamic strength and muscular endurance protocols and norms presented in this chapter were developed using constant-resistance exercise machines. Therefore you should not use free weights and variable-resistance machines when administering these tests. It is also important to calibrate the equipment and make sure that it is in proper working condition prior to testing. Inspection and maintenance of equipment will increase accuracy and decrease risk of accidents. When selecting exercise machines, make sure that the equipment can be properly adjusted to accommodate varying limb lengths and body sizes. Use equipment specifically designed for smaller individuals when testing children and smaller adults.

Technician Skill

All strength testing should be done by qualified, trained technicians who are knowledgeable about proper lifting and spotting techniques and familiar with standardized testing procedures. Explain and demonstrate the proper lifting technique and then correct any performance errors you see as the client practices. During the test, clients may inadvertently "cheat" by moving extraneous body parts to help lift the weight. Carefully observe the client during the test, focusing on the grip used and the starting position. The type of grip (pronated vs. supinated) has a substantial effect on performance. For example, using a narrow grip instead of a wide grip during a lat pull-down exercise increases the amount of weight that can be lifted. Likewise, the client will be able to produce more force during an arm curl using a supinated grip compared to a pronated grip. The client's starting position may also affect strength scores. During the bench press, for example, eccentric movement (i.e., lowering the weight) prior to the concentric phase of the lift will increase maximal muscular force due to the stretch reflex and the tendency for the client to "bounce" the weight off the chest. To obtain accurate assessments of your client's strength, it is important to standardize starting positions and to follow all testing procedures carefully.

Environmental Factors

Factors such as room temperature and humidity may affect test scores. The room temperature should be 70° to 74° F (21° to 23° C) to maximize subject comfort during testing. Ideally, you want a quiet, clean environment with limited distractions (not an overcrowded weight room, for example). When assessing improvements due to training, remember to pretest and posttest your client at the same time of day to control for diurnal variations in strength.

ADDITIONAL CONSIDERATIONS FOR MUSCULAR FITNESS TESTING

This section addresses a number of additional factors and questions regarding the testing and evaluation of your client's muscular fitness.

■ *Is it safe to give 1-RM tests to children and older adults?*

It is safe to administer 1-RM tests to clients of all ages if appropriate procedures are used (Kraemer and Fleck 1993; Shaw, McCully, and Posner 1995). The risk of injury in older adults (55 to 80 years) is low, with only 2.4% of older adults experiencing an injury during 1-RM assessments (Shaw, McCully, and Posner 1995). However, some experts recommend using 6-RM tests to assess the strength of children (Kraemer and Fry 1995).

Alternatively, you can estimate the 1-RM of older clients, children, and adolescents from submaximal muscle endurance tests. Research demonstrates a strong relationship between muscle endurance (measured as the number of repetitions to fatigue) and the percentage of 1-RM lifted (Brzycki 1993). Muscular strength (1-RM) therefore can be predicted from muscular endurance tests with a fair degree of accuracy (Ball and Rose 1991; Braith, Graves, Leggett, and Pollock 1993; Invergo, Ball, and Looney 1991; Kuramoto and Payne 1995; Mayhew, Ball, Arnold, and Bowen 1992). The most frequently used prediction equations are based on the number of repetitions to fatigue in *one* set. For example, the Brzycki (1993) equation can be used to estimate 1-RM of men. This equation can be used for any combination of submaximal weights and repetitions to fatigue providing that the repetitions to fatigue do not exceed 10.

$$\text{1-RM} = \text{weight lifted (lb)}/[1.0278 \\ - (\text{reps to fatigue} \times 0.0278)]$$

For example, if your client completes seven repetitions to fatigue during a bench press exercise using a 100-lb barbell, the estimated 1-RM is calculated as follows:

$$\text{1-RM} = 100 \text{ lb}/[1.0278 - (7 \text{ reps} \times 0.0278)]$$

$$= 120 \text{ lb } (54.5 \text{ kg})$$

Alternatively, you can use the average number of repetitions corresponding to various percentages of 1-RM (see table 6.11). This technique and the Brzycki (1993) equation yield similar 1-RM estimates for lifts between 2-RM and 10-RM. To estimate the 1-RM from 2-RM to 10-RM values, divide the weight lifted by the respective % 1-RM, expressed as a decimal (% 1-RM/100). For example, a client lifting 100 lb (45.4 kg) for 8 repetitions would have an estimated 1-RM of 125 lb (56.7 kg):

$$\text{1-RM} - 100 \text{ lb}/0.80 = 125 \text{ lb } (56.7 \text{ kg})$$

For middle-aged and older women, Kuramoto and Payne (1995) developed prediction equations to estimate 1-RM from a submaximal muscular endurance test. For this endurance protocol, the client completes as many repetitions as possible

Table 6.11 Average Number of Repetitions and %1-RM Values

Repetitions	% 1-RM[a]
1	100
2	95
3	93
4	90
5	87
6	85
7	83
8	80
9	77
10	75

[a]These values may vary slightly for different muscle groups and ages. Data from Baechle, Earle, and Wathen (2000).

using a weight equivalent to 45% of her body mass. To estimate 1-RM, use the following equations:

Middle-aged women (40 to 50 years)

$$\text{1-RM} = (1.06 \times \text{weight lifted in kg}) \\ + (0.58 \times \text{reps}) - (0.20 \times \text{age}) - 3.41$$

$$R^2 = 0.89$$

standard error of estimate *(SEE)* = 1.85 kg

Older women (60 to 70 years)

$$\text{1-RM} = (0.92 \times \text{weight lifted in kg}) \\ + (0.79 \times \text{reps}) - 3.73$$

$$R^2 = 0.81, SEE = 2.04 \text{ kg}$$

Recently, Brzycki (2000) suggested using a prediction equation based on the number of repetitions to fatigue obtained in *two* submaximal sets to estimate 1-RM. Any two submaximal sets can be used as long as the number of reps to fatigue does not exceed 10. For example, you can determine your client's 5-RM value, or, the maximum weight that can be lifted for five reps (e.g., 120 lb for five reps) and the 10-RM value (e.g., 80 lb for 10 reps) and use them in the following equation:

$$\text{Predicted 1-RM} = [(SM_1 - SM_2)/(REP_2 - REP_1)] \\ \times (REP_1 - 1) + SM_1$$

$$= [(120 - 80)/(10 - 5)] \\ \times (5 - 1) + 120$$

$$= 152 \text{ lb}$$

In this equation, SM_1 and REP_1 represent the heavier submaximal weight (120 lb) and the respective number of repetitions (5 reps) completed, and SM_2 and REP_2 correspond to the lighter submaximal weight (80 lb) and the respective number of repetitions (10 reps) performed.

■ How is muscle balance assessed?

Muscle strength is important for joint stability; however, a strength imbalance between opposing muscle groups (e.g., quadriceps femoris and hamstrings) may compromise joint stability and increase the risk of musculoskeletal injury. For this reason, experts recommend maintaining a balance in strength between agonist and antagonistic muscle groups.

Muscle balance ratios differ among muscle groups and are affected by the force-velocity of muscle groups at specific joints. To control limb velocity during muscle balance testing, you will do best to use isokinetic dynamometers. In field settings, however, you may obtain a crude index of muscle balance by comparing 1-RM values of muscle groups. Based on isokinetic tests of peak torque production at slow speeds ($30°$ to $60°$· sec^{-1}), the following muscle balance ratios are recommended for agonist and antagonistic muscle groups:

Muscle groups	Muscle balance ratio
Hip extensors and flexors	1:1
Elbow extensors and flexors	1:1
Trunk extensors and flexors	1:1
Ankle inverters and everters	1:1
Shoulder flexors and extensors	2:3
Knee extensors and flexors	3:2
Shoulder internal and external rotators	3:2
Ankle plantar flexors and dorsiflexors	3:1

Muscle balance between other pairs of muscle groups is also important. The difference in strength between contralateral (right vs. left sides) muscle groups should be no more than 10% to 15%, and the strength-to-body mass (BM) ratio of the upper-body (bench press 1-RM/BM) should be at least 40% to 60% of the lower-body relative strength (leg press 1-RM/BM). If you detect imbalances, prescribe additional exercises for the weaker muscle groups.

■ Can strength or muscular endurance be assessed by a single test?

Strength and endurance are specific to the muscle group, the type of muscular contraction (static or dynamic), the speed of muscular contraction (slow or fast), and the joint angle being tested (static contraction). There is no single test to evaluate total body muscle strength or endurance. Minimally, the strength test battery should include a measure of abdominal, lower-extremity, and upper-extremity strength. In addition, if the individual trains dynamically, select a dynamic, not static, test to assess strength or endurance levels before and after training.

You should also use caution in selecting test items to measure muscle strength. The maximum number of sit-ups, pull-ups, or push-ups that an individual can perform measures muscular endurance, yet maximum-repetition tests have been included in some strength test batteries. This may lead to misinterpretation of the test results.

■ Should absolute or relative measures be used to classify a client's muscle strength?

There is a direct relationship between body size and muscle strength. Generally, larger individuals have more muscle mass, and therefore greater strength compared to smaller individuals with less muscle mass. Because strength is directly related to the body mass and lean body mass of the individual, you should express the test results in relative terms (i.e., 1-RM/BM). This is especially true for comparisons of groups that differ in body size and body composition (e.g., men vs. women or older vs. younger adults).

It is also important to use relative strength scores for assessing individual improvement due to training. As a result of resistance training, some individuals may gain body weight while others may lose weight, especially if they are using this form of training as part of a weight gain or weight loss program. If you compare the client's relative strength scores (pre- vs. posttest training), you will be able to evaluate the change in strength that is independent of changes in body weight.

■ How can the influence of strength on muscular endurance be controlled?

Performance on some endurance tests (e.g., pull-ups and push-ups) is highly dependent on the strength of the individual. It is recommended that you use relative endurance tests that are proportional to the body mass or maximum strength of the individual to assess muscle endurance. You cannot use a pull-up test to assess muscular endurance if the individual is not strong enough to lift the body weight for one repetition of that exercise. Therefore, select a modified or submaximal (percentage of body weight) endurance test.

■ *Are there comprehensive norms that can be used to classify muscular fitness levels of diverse population subgroups?*

Recently, strength norms for women (20 to 82 years) were developed for the bench press (1-RM), leg press (1-RM), static grip strength, and push-up tests (Brown and Miller 1998). These norms are based on data obtained from 304 independent-living women attending wellness classes at a university medical center. However, there is a lack of up-to-date endurance norms for men and strength/endurance norms for older men. New norms need to be established for this population in particular.

SOURCES FOR EQUIPMENT

Product	Manufacturer's Address
Body Masters (constant and variable resistance)	Body Masters Sports Industries, Inc. P.O. Box 259 Rayne, LA 70578 (800) 325-8964 www.body-masters.com
Cable tensiometer (static)	Pacific Scientific Co., Inc. 110 Fordham Rd. Wilmington, MA 01887 (888) 772-6284 www.pacsci.com
CAM II (variable resistance)	Keiser Corp. 2470 S. Cherry Ave. Fresno, CA 93706 (800) 888-7009 www.keiser.com
Cybex II, Orthotron (isokinetic)	Cybex International 10 Trotter Dr. Medway, MA 02053 (508) 533-4300 www.cybexintl.com
Free weights (constant resistance)	York Barbell Co. Box 1707 3300 Board Rd. York, PA 17405 (717) 767-6481 www.yorkbarbell.com
Handgrip dynamometer (static)	Creative Health Products 5148 Saddle Ridge Rd. Plymouth, MI 48170 (800) 742-4478 www.chponline.com
Leg/back dynamometer (static)	Best Priced Products P.O. Box 1174 White Plains, NY 10602 (800) 824-2939 www.best-priced-products.com

Nautilus (variable resistance)	Nautilus International 9800 W. Kincey Ave. Ste. 150 Huntersville, NC 28078 (800) 628-8458 www.nautilus.com
Omni-tron Total Power (omnikinetic)	Hydra-fitness 2121 Industrial Rd. Belton, TX 76513
Total Gym machines (variable resistance)	Total Gym/EFI 7755 Arjons Dr. San Diego, CA 92126 (800) 541-4900 www.totalgym.com
Universal Gym machines (constant and variable resistance)	Universal Gym Equipment P.O. Box 1270 Cedar Rapids, IA 52406 (800) 843-3906 www.universalgym.com

KEY POINTS

- Strength is the ability of a muscle group to exert maximal contractile force against a resistance in a single contraction.

- Muscular endurance is the ability of a muscle group to exert submaximal force for an extended duration.

- Both strength and muscular endurance are specific to the muscle group and to the type of muscle contraction—static, concentric, eccentric, or isokinetic.

- The greatest resistance that can be used during dynamic, concentric muscular contraction with a constant-resistance exercise mode is equal to the maximum weight that can be moved at the weakest point in the ROM.

- Dynamometers, cable tensiometers, and load cells are used to measure static strength and endurance.

- Constant-resistance modes of exercise (free weights and exercise machines) are used to assess dynamic (i.e., concentric and eccentric) strength and endurance.

- The accommodating-resistance mode of exercise is used to assess isokinetic and omnikinetic strength, endurance, and power.

- Calisthenic-type exercise tests provide a crude index of strength and endurance but can be used when other equipment is not available.

- Strength should be expressed relative to the body mass or lean body mass of the individual.

- Muscular endurance tests should take into account the body mass or maximal strength of the individual.

- Test batteries should include a minimum of three to four items that measure upper-body, lower-body, and abdominal strength or endurance.

- It is important to follow standardized testing procedures and to control for extraneous variables (e.g., motivation level, time of testing, isolation of body parts, and joint angles) when assessing strength and muscular endurance.

- It is safe to give 1-RM strength tests to children and older adults if appropriate testing procedures are followed.

- Although strength can be predicted from submaximal endurance tests, 1-RM assessments are preferable.

KEY TERMS

Learn the definition of each of the following key terms. Definitions of terms can be found in "Glossary of Terms," page 349.

accommodating-resistance exercise
concentric contraction
constant-resistance exercise
dynamic contraction
eccentric contraction
isokinetic contraction
isometric contraction

isotonic contraction
muscular endurance
muscular strength
omnikinetic exercise
one-repetition maximum (1-RM)
relative strength
static contraction
variable-resistance exercise

REVIEW QUESTIONS

In addition to being able to define each of the key terms, test your knowledge and understanding of the material by answering the following review questions.

1. During dynamic movement, why does muscle force production fluctuate throughout the ROM?

2. Name two methods for assessing static strength and muscular endurance.

3. How do constant-resistance, variable-resistance, and accommodating-resistance exercise machines differ?

4. Why are strength test scores typically expressed relative to the client's body mass?

5. Describe the recommended procedures for administering 1-RM strength tests.

6. Identify three sources of measurement error for muscular fitness testing. What can you do to control for these potential errors?

7. Is it safe to give 1-RM tests to children and older adults?

8. Why is it important to assess muscle balance?

9. In terms of the specificity principle, explain why a single test cannot be used to adequately assess your client's overall strength. Minimally, what muscle groups should be tested to evaluate overall strength?

10. Identify the test items recommended by ACSM for assessing your client's upper- and lower-body strength.

11. For certain clients, you may choose not to administer 1-RM strength tests. Describe how you could obtain an *estimate* of their strength instead.

REFERENCES

American College of Sports Medicine (ACSM). 2000. *ACSM's guidelines for exercise testing and prescription*. Philadelphia: Lippincott Williams & Wilkins.

Baechle, T.R., Earle, R.W., and Wathen, D. 2000. Resistance training. In *Essentials of strength training and conditioning,* eds. T.R. Baechle and R.W. Earle. Champaign, IL: Human Kinetics.

Ball, T.E., and Rose, K.S. 1991. A field test for predicting maximum bench press lift of college women. *Journal of Applied Sport Science Research* 5: 169–170.

Baumgartner, T.A. 1978. Modified pull-up test. *Research Quarterly* 49: 80–84.

Baumgartner, T.A., East, W.B., Frye, P.A., Hensley, L.D., Knox, D.F., and Norton, C.J. 1984. Equipment improvements and additional norms for the modified pull-up test. *Research Quarterly for Exercise and Sport* 55: 64–68.

Braith, R.W., Graves, J.E., Leggett, S.H., and Pollock, M.L. 1993. Effect of training on the relationship between maximal and submaximal strength. *Medicine & Science in Sports & Exercise* 25: 132–138.

Brown, D.A., and Miller, W.C. 1998. Normative data for strength and flexibility of women throughout life. *European Journal of Applied Physiology* 78: 77–82.

Brzycki, M. 1993. Strength testing—predicting a one-rep max from reps-to-fatigue. *Journal of Physical Education, Recreation and Dance* 64 (1): 88–90.

Brzycki, M. 2000. Assessing strength. *Fitness Management* 16(7): 34–37.

Canadian Society for Exercise Physiology. 1998. *The Canadian physical activity, fitness and lifestyle appraisal.* 2nd ed. Ottawa, ON: Author.

Clarke, D.H. 1975. *Exercise physiology.* Englewood Cliffs, NJ: Prentice Hall.

Clarke, H.H. 1966. *Muscular strength and endurance in man.* Englewood Cliffs, NJ: Prentice Hall.

Clarke, H.H., and Monroe, R.A. 1970. *Test manual: Oregon cable-tension strength test batteries for boys and girls from fourth grade through college.* Eugene, OR: University of Oregon.

Cooper Institute for Aerobics Research. 1994. *The physical fitness specialist certification manual.* Dallas, TX: author.

Corbin, C.B., Dowell, L.J., Lindsey, R., and Tolson, H. 1978. *Concepts in physical education.* Dubuque, IA: Brown.

Fess, E.E. 1992. Grip Strength. In *Clinical assessment recommendations,* American Society of Hand Therapists, 41–45, Chicago, IL: American Society of Hand Therapists.

Fitness Canada. 1986. *Canadian standardized test of fitness (CSTF) operations manual,* 3rd ed., Ottawa, ON: Fitness and Amateur Sport Canada.

Invergo, J.J., Ball, T.E., and Looney, M. 1991. Relationship of pushups and absolute muscular endurance to bench press strength. *Journal of Applied Sport Science Research* 5: 121–125.

Johnson, B.L., and Nelson, J.K., eds. 1986. *Practical measurements for evaluation in physical education.* Minneapolis: Burgess.

Knuttgen, H.G., and Kraemer, W.J. 1987. Terminology and measurement in exercise performance. *Journal of Applied Sport Science Research* 1: 1–10.

Kraemer, W.J., and Fleck, S.J. 1993. *Strength training for young athletes.* Champaign, IL: Human Kinetics.

Kraemer, W.J., and Fry, A.C. 1995. Strength testing: Development and evaluation of methodology. In *Physiological assessment of human fitness,* ed. P.J. Maud and C. Foster, 115–138. Champaign, IL: Human Kinetics.

Kreighbaum, E., and Barthels, K.M. 1981. *Biomechanics: A qualitative approach for studying human movement.* Minneapolis: Burgess.

Kuramoto, A.K., and Payne, V.G. 1995. Predicting muscular strength in women: A preliminary study. *Research Quarterly for Exercise and Sport* 66: 168–172.

Mayhew, J.L., Ball, T.E., Arnold, M.D., and Bowen, J.C. 1992. Relative muscular endurance performance as a predictor of bench press strength in college men and women. *Journal of Applied Sport Science Research* 6: 200–206.

Montoye, H.J., and Faulkner, J.A. 1964. Determination of the optimum setting of an adjustable grip dynamometer. *Research Quarterly* 35: 29–36.

Perrin, D.H. 1993. *Isokinetic exercise and assessment.* Champaign, IL: Human Kinetics.

Pollock, M.L., Wilmore, J.H., and Fox, S.M. III. 1978. *Health and fitness through physical activity.* New York: Wiley.

Shaw, C.E., McCully, K.K., and Posner, J.D. 1995. Injuries during the one repetition maximum assessment in the elderly. *Journal of Cardiopulmonary Rehabilitation* 15: 283–287.

Women's Exercise Research Center. 1998. Based on figures published by Brown, D.A., and Miller, W.C. 1998. Normative data for strength and flexibility of women throughout life. *European Journal of Applied Physiology* 78: 77–82.

YMCA of the USA. 2000. *YMCA fitness testing and assessment manual* (4th ed.), Champaign, IL: Human Kinetics.

chapter 7

Designing Resistance Training Programs

KEY QUESTIONS

- How do training principles specifically apply to the design of resistance training programs?

- How are resistance training programs modified to optimize the development of strength, muscular endurance, muscle tone, or muscle size?

- What factors do I need to consider when designing individualized exercise prescriptions?

- Is resistance training recommended for children, adolescents, and older adults?

- What methods can be used to design advanced resistance training programs?

- What are the outcomes and health benefits derived from resistance training?

- What is the cause of delayed-onset muscle soreness, and can it be prevented?

Muscular strength and endurance are important to the overall health and physical fitness of your clients, enabling them to engage in physically active leisure-time pursuits, to perform activities of daily living more easily, and to maintain functional independence later in life. Resistance training is a systematic program of exercise for development of the muscular system. Although the primary outcome of resistance training is improved strength and muscular endurance, a number of health benefits are also derived from this form of exercise. Resistance exercise builds bone mass, thereby counteracting the loss of bone mineral (osteoporosis) and risk of falls as one ages. This form of training also lowers blood pressure in hypertensive individuals, reduces body fat levels, and may prevent the development of low back syndrome.

While resistance training has long been widely used by bodybuilders, power lifters, and competitive athletes to develop strength and muscle size, participation in weightlifting by individuals of all ages and levels of athletic interest has increased dramatically over the past 20 years. The popularity and widespread appeal of weightlifting exercise for general muscle conditioning challenge exercise specialists and personal trainers to develop resistance training programs that can meet the diverse needs of their clients.

This chapter shows you how to apply basic training principles (see chapter 3) to the design of resistance training programs for novice, intermediate, and advanced weight lifters. The chapter also presents guidelines for developing general muscle toning and conditioning, strength and muscular endurance, and muscle size. The final section of the chapter is a discussion of common concerns and misconceptions about weightlifting.

TYPES OF RESISTANCE TRAINING

Muscular fitness can be improved using various types of resistance training—static (isometric), dynamic (concentric and eccentric), and isokinetic. Although there are general guidelines for designing static, dynamic, and isokinetic resistance training programs, each exercise prescription should be individualized to meet the specific needs and goals of your client.

Static (Isometric) Training

In 1953, Hettinger and Muller reported that people produce significant gains in static strength (5% per week) by holding one 6-sec contraction at two-thirds of maximum intensity, five days a week. This type of training became popular in the late 1950s and early 1960s because the exercises could be performed anywhere and at any time with little or no equipment. A major disadvantage is that strength gains are specific to the joint angle used during training (Gardner 1963). Thus, to increase strength throughout the range of motion, the exercise needs to be performed at a number of different joint angles (e.g., 30°, 60°, 90°, 120°, and 180° of knee flexion).

Static exercise is widely used in rehabilitation programs to counteract strength loss and muscle atrophy, especially in cases in which the limb is temporarily immobilized. This type of training, however, is contraindicated for coronary-prone and hypertensive individuals because the static contraction may produce large increases in intrathoracic pressure. This reduces the venous return to the heart, increases the work of the heart, and causes a substantial rise in blood pressure.

After further research, Hettinger and Muller modified their original exercise prescription. Table 7.1 presents the general guidelines for designing training programs for static strength and endurance development. For descriptions and illustrations of static exercises for various muscle groups, see appendix C.2, "Basic Static (Isometric) Exercises," page 300.

Dynamic Resistance Training

In recent years, the popularity of dynamic resistance training has risen in the United States. This type of training is suitable for developing muscular fitness of men and women of all ages, as well as children. Dynamic resistance training involves concentric and eccentric contractions of the muscle group performed against a constant or variable resistance. For this type of training, people typically use free weights (barbells and dumbbells) and constant- or variable-resistance machines.

Several important concepts used to prescribe dynamic resistance training programs are intensity, repetitions, set, training volume, and order of exercises (Fleck and Kraemer 1997). Intensity is expressed either as a percentage of the individual's one-repetition maximum (%1-RM) or as the **repetition maximum (RM)**, which is the maximum weight that the person can lift for a given number of repetitions of an exercise (e.g., 8-RM equals the maximum weight that the person can lift for eight repetitions). For the number of repetitions (i.e., 1 to 10 RM) corresponding to various percentages of 1-RM (i.e., 75 to 100% 1-RM), see table 6.11, page 128. The %1-RM values and number of repetitions for intensities less than 75% 1-RM are as follows:

$$60\% \text{ 1-RM} = 15\text{- to } 20\text{-RM}$$

$$65\% \text{ 1-RM} = 14\text{-RM}$$

$$70\% \text{ 1-RM} = 12\text{-RM}$$

Intensity is inversely related to repetitions. In other words, individuals are able to perform more **repetitions** using lighter resistance or weights and fewer repetitions using heavier resistance. A **set** consists of a given number of consecutive repetitions of the exercise. **Training volume** is the total amount of weight lifted during the workout and

Table 7.1 Guidelines for Designing Static (Isometric) Training Programs					
Type	**Intensity**	**Duration**	**Repetitions**	**Frequency (days/week)**	**Length of program**
Static strength	100% MVC*	5 sec/contraction	5-10	5	4 weeks or more
Static endurance	60% MVC or less	Until fatigued	1/session	5	4 weeks or more
*Maximal voluntary contraction.					

is calculated by summing the products of the weight lifted, repetitions, and sets for each exercise.

The optimal training stimulus for strength development is **high intensity-low repetitions**; whereas **low intensity-high repetitions** optimize muscular endurance gains. Although novice weight lifters experience muscular fitness gains from low training volumes (one to two sets using moderate resistance and repetitions, 2 days per week), you may need to prescribe larger training volumes (e.g., three to four sets, 3 to 4 days per week) for advanced resistance training programs.

Table 7.2 presents the ACSM (2000) guidelines for apparently healthy adults, older adults, and children who are beginning a resistance training program. For clients with resistance training experience, you need to modify these guidelines based on the client's goals, initial muscular fitness level, and time available for exercising.

You can tailor dynamic resistance training programs to optimize the development of muscle strength, tone, size (hypertrophy), or endurance by varying the intensity, repetitions, sets, and frequency of training. Table 7.3 presents guidelines for designing these types of resistance training programs for novice and advanced weight lifters. For descriptions of dynamic resistance training exercises, see appendix C.3, "Dynamic Resistance Training Exercises," page 303.

Intensity

To optimize strength gains, the intensity should be set at 75% to 90% 1-RM (Fleck and Kraemer 1997). At this intensity, most individuals are able to perform 4 to 10 repetitions (4- to 10-RM) of the exercise. For high-intensity strength training programs, the intensity usually ranges between 1- and 6-RM; for non-athletic populations, moderate-intensity programs (8- to 12-RM) are generally recommended (Feigenbaum and Pollock 1999). However, when your client's primary goal is to develop muscular endurance, prescribe an intensity of ≤60% 1-RM (15- to 20-RM). Although low-to-moderate intensity is best suited for muscle endurance and toning, your clients will also experience some strength gains. The degree and rate of strength gain, however, will be less than with a program designed specifically to optimize strength development (specificity principle). For advanced

---

Table 7.2 ACSM (2000) Guidelines for Resistance Training

Group	Intensity	Repetitions	Sets	Frequency	No. of exercises
Apparently healthy adults	70-80% 1-RM	8-12	≥1	2-3	8-10
Older adults[a]	60-75% 1-RM	10-15	≥1	2 minimum	8-10
Children[a,b]	70-80% 1-RM	8-12	1-2	2	8-10

[a]Multijoint exercises are recommended for older adults and children.
[b]Programs for children and adolescents should be closely supervised by trained personnel.

Table 7.3 Guidelines for Designing Dynamic Resistance Training Programs

Type	Intensity	Repetitions	Sets	Frequency	Length of program
Strength (novice)	70-80% 1-RM or 8- to 12-RM	8-12	≥1	3	6 weeks or more
Strength (advanced)	85-100% 1-RM or 1- to 6-RM	1-6	≥3	5-6	12 weeks or more
Toning	60-70% 1-RM or 12- to 15-RM	12-15	≥1	3	6 weeks or more
Endurance	≤60% 1-RM or 15- to 20-RM	15-20	≥1	3	6 weeks or more
Hypertrophy (advanced)	70-75% 1-RM or 10- to 12-RM	10-12	≥3	5-6	12 weeks or more

strength training and hypertrophy programs, individuals achieve large training volumes by increasing the number of sets, performing multiple exercises for each muscle group, and increasing the frequency of training. For programs designed specifically to increase muscle size, you also can maximize the client's training volume by using a combination of moderate intensities and repetitions (Fleck and Kraemer 1997).

Sets

The optimal number of sets for improving muscular strength is somewhat controversial and depends on your client's goals. Recent research studies suggest that single-set (one set per exercise) programs are just as effective as multiple-set (two to three sets per exercise) programs for increasing strength of untrained persons and recreational weight lifters during the first three to four months of resistance training (Feigenbaum and Pollock 1999; Hass, Garzarella, De Hoyas, and Pollock 2000). The ACSM (2000) recommends a minimum of one set for 8 to 10 different muscle groups to improve muscular strength of apparently healthy adults, older adults, and children. A major advantage of a single-set program is that the average amount of time required to complete the program is much less than for multiple-set programs (20 vs. 50 min, respectively), thereby potentially increasing your client's compliance. However, for serious athletes, power lifters, and bodybuilders engaging in advanced strength training and hypertrophy programs, you should prescribe multiple sets using periodization techniques to optimize strength gains (Fleck and Kraemer 1997; Kramer et al. 1997).

Frequency

Improvements in muscular fitness may result from exercising just one day per week, especially for clients with below-average muscular fitness. However, research suggests that training three days per week is superior to one to two days per week for optimizing strength gains of the chest, arms, and leg muscles (Feigenbaum and Pollock 1999). You should prescribe 48 hr of rest between workouts to allow the muscles to recuperate and to prevent injury from overtraining. Increasing the frequency of workouts is one way to achieve the high training volume necessary to stimulate gains in muscle strength and size for advanced resistance training programs.

Order of Exercises

A well-rounded resistance training program should include at least one exercise for each of the major muscle groups in the body. In this way, **muscle balance**—that is, the ratio of strength between opposing muscle groups (agonists vs. antagonists), contralateral muscle groups (right vs. left side), and upper- and lower-body muscle groups can be maintained. Order the exercises so that your client first executes multijoint exercises—such as the seated leg press, bench press, and lat pull-down—that involve larger muscles (e.g., gluteus maximus, pectoralis major, and latissimus dorsi) and more muscle groups. Then have your client progress to single-joint exercises for smaller muscle groups (see table 7.4). To avoid muscle fatigue in novice weight lifters, arrange the exercises so that successive exercises do not involve the same muscle group. This allows time for the muscle to recover.

Dynamic Resistance Training Methods

You can use a variety of methods to design dynamic resistance training programs. The majority of these methods are best suited for advanced programs. Each uses a different approach for prescribing sets, order of exercises, or frequency of workouts.

Variations for Sets

You can use either a single set or multiple sets of exercise. For multiple sets, you may choose to have your client consecutively perform a designated number of sets (usually three or more) at a constant intensity (e.g., 10-RM) for each exercise. Alternatively, you may have your client perform one set of three different exercises for the same muscle group. For example, instead of three consecutive sets of barbell curls for the elbow flexors, you may prescribe one set of incline dumbbell curls, one set of hammer curls, and one set of barbell curls. This adds variety to the program and changes the training stimulus because different muscles or parts of a muscle are used to perform each of these exercises.

A client performing multiple sets of a given exercise may choose to lift the same weight for each set or to vary the intensity of each set by lifting progressively heavier (light-to-heavy sets) or lighter (heavy-to-light sets) weights. **Pyramiding** is a light-to-heavy system in which the client per-

Table 7.4 Example of Exercise Order for a Basic Resistance Training Program

Body segment	Type of exercise*	Joint actions	Exercise
1. Hips and thighs	Multijoint	Hip extension and knee extension	Seated leg press
2. Chest	Multijoint	Shoulder horizontal flexion and elbow extension	Flat bench press
3. Upper and mid back	Multijoint	Shoulder extension/adduction and elbow flexion	Lat pull-down
4. Legs	Single joint	Knee extension	Leg extension
5. Shoulders and upper arms	Multijoint	Shoulder abduction and elbow flexion	Upright row
6. Lower back	Multijoint	Trunk extension and hip extension	Back extension
7. Upper arms	Single joint	Elbow extension	Triceps push-down
8. Leg	Single joint	Knee flexion	Leg curl
9. Upper arms	Single joint	Elbow flexion	Arm curl
10. Calves	Single joint	Ankle plantar flexion	Toe raise
11. Forearms	Single joint	Wrist flexion and extension	Wrist curl
12. Abdomen	Single joint	Trunk flexion	Curl-up

*Multijoint exercises involving larger muscle groups are followed by single-joint exercises for smaller muscle groups.

forms as many as six sets of each exercise. In the first set, the client lifts a relatively lighter weight for 10 to 12 repetitions (10- to 12-RM). In subsequent sets the individual lifts progressively heavier weights (i.e., 8-RM, 6-RM, and 4-RM). Because this involves such a large volume of work, you should prescribe the pyramid system for experienced weight lifters only. Bodybuilders commonly use this system to develop muscle size.

Variations for Order and Number of Exercises

Exercise scientists generally recommend ordering the exercises so that large muscle groups are exercised at the beginning of the workout with progression to smaller muscle groups later in the workout. To maximize the overload of muscle groups, however, some clients may choose to pre-exhaust muscle groups by reversing this order. To do this, the individual fatigues smaller muscles by using single-joint exercises prior to performing multijoint exercises.

When you prescribe two or more exercises for a specific muscle group, instruct the average individual to alternate muscle groups so that the muscle can rest and recover between exercises. For example, your client should not perform leg press and leg extension exercises consecutively because the quadriceps femoris is used in both of these exercises. Instead, intersperse one or more exercises using different muscle groups between these two exercises.

In contrast, many advanced weight lifters prefer to do **compound sets** or **tri-sets** in order to completely fatigue a targeted muscle group. To use this training system, the client performs two (compound sets) or three (tri-sets) exercises consecutively for the same muscle group, with little or no rest between the exercises. Many bodybuilders also use a training system called **supersetting**. For supersets, the client exercises agonistic and antagonistic muscle groups consecutively without resting. For example, to superset the quadriceps femoris and hamstrings, follow a leg extension set immediately with a leg curl set.

Variations for Frequency

Traditionally for advanced resistance training programs, exercise scientists have recommended resistance training three times per week on alternate days (e.g., M-W-F) to allow the muscles time to recover. For individuals who want to resistance train five to six days a week, prescribe a **split routine.** With a split routine, you are targeting different muscle groups on consecutive days, thereby allowing at least one day of recovery for each muscle group. For example, a bodybuilder may exercise the chest and shoulders on Monday and Thursday, the hips and legs on Tuesday and Friday, and the back and arms on Wednesday and Saturday.

Variations for Training Volume and Intensity: Periodization

Periodization is used in resistance training programs to avoid overtraining and to optimize strength and power gains for peak performance. Many athletes who train year-round use periodization models (i.e., traditional, stepwise, undulating, or overreaching) that systematically vary the volume and intensity of the resistance training exercises (Bompa 1999; Fleck 1999). Regardless of the model used, each **macrocycle** (usually 1 year) is divided into **mesocycles** that last anywhere from two weeks to several months (Frankel and Kravitz 2000). For the traditional or stepwise models, training volume progressively decreases as training intensity increases throughout the mesocycles (see table 7.5). The variation in training volume and intensity optimizes strength gains by systematically changing the training stimulus at regular intervals. Research comparing periodized to non-periodized (constant sets and reps throughout the program) single-set and multiple-set resistance training programs shows that even though the volume of training is reduced over time, periodized training produces significantly greater improvements in the strength of men (Baker, Wilson, and Carlyon 1994; Fleck 1999; Kraemer et al. 1997; Stone et al. 1999a; 1999b). More research is needed to assess the effectiveness of periodized training programs for women, older adults, and children.

Circuit Resistance Training

Circuit resistance training is a method of dynamic resistance training designed to increase strength, muscular endurance, and cardiorespiratory endurance (Gettman and Pollock 1981). Circuit resistance training compares favorably with the traditional resistance training programs for increasing muscle strength, especially if low-repetition, high-resistance exercises are used (Gettman, Ayres, Pollock, and Jackson 1978; Wilmore et al. 1978).

A circuit resistance training program usually has 10 to 15 stations per circuit (see figure 7.1). The circuit is repeated two to three times so that the total time of continuous exercise is 20 to 30 min. At each exercise station, select a resistance that fatigues the muscle group in approximately 30 sec (as many repetitions as possible at approximately 40% to 55% of 1-RM). Include a 15- to 20-sec rest period between exercise stations. Circuit resistance training is usually performed three days per week for at least six weeks. This method of training is ideal for clients with a limited amount of time for exercise. As mentioned in chapter 5, you can add aerobic exercise stations to the circuit between each weightlifting station (i.e., super circuit resistance training) to obtain additional cardiorespiratory benefits.

Isokinetic Training

Isokinetic exercise combines the advantages of dynamic (full range of motion) and static (maximum force exerted) exercise. Since the resistance is accommodating, isokinetic training overcomes the problems associated with using either a constant- or variable-resistance exercise mode. You can use isokinetic training to increase strength, power, and muscular endurance. Isokinetic training involves dynamic, shortening contractions of the muscle group against an accommodating resistance that matches the force produced by the muscle group throughout the entire range of motion. The speed of the movement is controlled mechanically by the isokinetic exercise device.

Table 7.5   Sample 16-Week Periodization Program

Mesocycle	Volume		Intensity % 1-RM	Frequency
	Sets	Reps		
I: weeks 1-4	5	10	75%	3
II: weeks 5-8	4	8	80%	3
III: weeks 9-12	3	6	85%	3
IV: weeks 13-16	3	4	90%	3

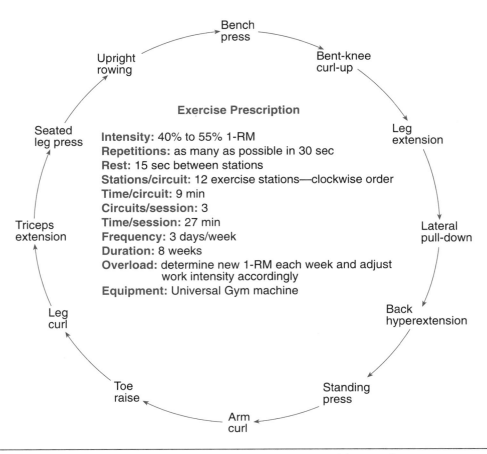

Exercise Prescription

Intensity: 40% to 55% 1-RM
Repetitions: as many as possible in 30 sec
Rest: 15 sec between stations
Stations/circuit: 12 exercise stations—clockwise order
Time/circuit: 9 min
Circuits/session: 3
Time/session: 27 min
Frequency: 3 days/week
Duration: 8 weeks
Overload: determine new 1-RM each week and adjust
work intensity accordingly
Equipment: Universal Gym machine

Figure 7.1 Sample circuit resistance training program. 1-RM = one-repetition maximum.

Isokinetic dynamometers are used for isokinetic training. If this equipment is not available, exercises can be done with a partner who offers accommodating resistance to the movement. The speed of the movement, however, is not precisely controlled.

Isokinetic training is done at speeds that vary between 24° and 300°·sec⁻¹, depending on the needs of the individual. The carryover effect appears to be greater when a person trains at faster speeds (180° to 300°·sec⁻¹) as compared to slower speeds (30° to 60°·sec⁻¹). In some studies, strength gains have been limited to velocities at or below the training velocity (Lesmes, Costill, Coyle, and

Fink 1978; Moffroid and Whipple 1970). Other researchers have reported significant strength gains at all testing velocities (30° to 300°·sec⁻¹) for high-velocity training groups (240° to 300°·sec⁻¹) (Coyle et al. 1981; Jenkins, Thackaberry, and Killian 1984). Additional research is needed to settle this issue. Table 7.6 presents general guidelines for designing isokinetic training programs for the development of strength and endurance.

A major advantage of isokinetic training over traditional forms of training is that little or no muscle soreness results because the muscles do not contract eccentrically. Isokinetic training is not the best choice, however, when the goal of training

Table 7.6 Guidelines for Designing Isokinetic Training Programs

Type	Intensity	Repetitions	Sets	Speed	Frequency	Length of program
Isokinetic strength	Maximum contraction	2-15	3	24-180°/sec	3-5 days/week	6 weeks or more
Isokinetic endurance	Maximum contraction	Until fatigued	1	≥180°/sec	3-5 days/week	6 weeks or more

is an increase in muscle size. Eccentric contractions are apparently essential for muscle hypertrophy (Cote et al. 1988; Hather, Tesch, Buchanan, and Dudley 1991). Cote et al. (1988) reported no change in muscle fiber cross-sectional area during isokinetic training even though the strength of the quadriceps femoris increased 54%.

DEVELOPING RESISTANCE TRAINING PROGRAMS

Before designing a resistance training program for your client, review training principles and determine how each of these principles can be incorporated into your client's program. The training program needs to be individualized. By varying the combination of intensity, duration, and frequency of exercise, you can develop programs that meet the unique goals and needs of each client. Be sure to follow guidelines and recommendations for resistance training programs (see tables 7.2 and 7.3, p. 137), as well as specific recommendations and precautions, when developing resistance training programs for children and older adults.

Application of Training Principles to Resistance Exercise

To develop effective resistance training programs, you must apply each of the training principles presented in chapter 3 (see p. 40). This section reviews some of the more pertinent training principles and outlines how these principles are applied to the design of resistance training programs.

Specificity Principle

The development of muscular fitness is specific to the muscle group that is exercised, the type of contraction, and training intensity. To increase the dynamic strength of the elbow flexors, for example, you must select exercises that involve the concentric and eccentric contraction of that particular muscle group. For strength, the person performs exercises at a high intensity with low repetitions; exercising at a low intensity with high repetitions stimulates the development of muscular endurance.

Strength and endurance gains are also specific to the speed and range of motion used during the training. With isometric training, strength gains at angles other than the training angle are typically 50% less than those at the exercised angle (Gardner 1963). Similarly, as previously noted,

strength gains in isokinetic training may be limited to velocities at or below the training velocity (Lesmes et al. 1978; Moffroid and Whipple 1970).

Overload Principle

To promote strength and endurance gains, the muscle group must be exercised at workloads that are greater than normal for the client. The exercise intensity should be at least 60% of maximum to stimulate the development of strength (McArdle, Katch, and Katch 1996). More rapid strength gains may be achieved, however, by exercising the muscle at or near maximum (80% to 100%) resistance. To stimulate endurance gains, intensities as low as 30% of maximum may be used; however, at low intensities the muscle group should be exercised to the point of fatigue.

Progression Principle

Generally, throughout the resistance training program, you must periodically increase the training volume, or total amount of work performed, to continue overloading the muscle so that the person can make further improvements in strength and muscular endurance. The progression needs to be gradual because doing too much too soon may cause musculoskeletal injuries and excessive muscle soreness. Typically you progressively overload muscle groups by increasing the resistance or amount of weight lifted. As clients adapt to the training stimulus, they will be able to perform more repetitions at the prescribed resistance. Thus, the number of repetitions a client is able to perform will indicate when it is necessary to increase the resistance throughout the training program.

Additional Principles

Individuals with lower initial strength will show greater relative gains and a faster rate of improvement in response to resistance training than those starting out with higher strength levels (principles of initial values and interindividual variability). However, the rate of improvement slows, and eventually plateaus, as clients progress through the program and move closer to their genetic ceiling (principle of diminishing returns). Also, when the individual stops resistance training, the physiological adaptations and improvements in muscle structure and function are reversed (principle of reversibility). Using periodization techniques (see "Variations for Training Volume and Intensity: Periodization" on p. 140), you can lessen the effects of detraining on athletes and maintain strength gains during the competitive period by manipulating the intensity and volume of the resistance training exercise (see Wathen 1994).

General Procedures and Sample Resistance Training Programs

After assessing your client's muscular fitness, you can individualize the resistance training exercise prescription to meet the needs and interests of each client by using the steps outlined below.

The first example, on page 144, describes a beginning resistance training program developed for an older man (70 years) with no previous weightlifting experience. The primary goal for this program is to develop adequate muscular fitness so that the client can retain functional independence. This program follows the guidelines suggested by ACSM (2000) for designing resistance training programs for older adults. During the first four weeks of training, low-intensity (30% to 40% 1-RM), high-repetition (15 to 20 repetitions) exercises familiarize the client with weightlifting exercise and reduce the chance of injury and excessive muscle soreness. The client gradually increases the resistance so that by the end of this phase, the exercise intensity is 50% 1-RM. After eight weeks, the intensity starts at 50% 1-RM and gradually increases to 75% 1-RM. The client does one to two sets of 10 to 15 repetitions for each exercise. To overload the muscles during this phase, he increases the resistance gradually, but only after he is able to complete 15 or more repetitions at the pre-scribed relative intensity. This program includes multijoint exercises using exercise machines only (no free weights). The client exercises two times a week, allowing at least two days of rest between each workout.

The second program (see p. 145) is for a 35-year-old woman whose primary goal is to improve muscle strength. Although this client has some previous weightlifting experience, she has not lifted weights for over two years. Results from her 1-RM tests indicated that her upper-body strength (particularly the shoulder flexor and forearm flexor muscle groups) is below average. Therefore, two exercises are prescribed for each of the weaker muscle groups. The strength of all other muscle groups is average or above average; therefore, only one exercise is prescribed for each of these muscle groups. Given her initial strength levels and previous weightlifting experience, the prescription is for three sets of each exercise; and the exercise intensity is set at 80% 1-RM to maximize the development of strength. The client completes about eight repetitions at the prescribed intensity for each set and gradually increases the weight when she is able to complete 10 to 12 repetitions at that intensity. She devotes 45 to 50 min, three days a week, to her workouts.

The third example (see p. 146) illustrates an advanced resistance training program developed for an experienced weight lifter (28-year-old male with superior strength) whose long-term goal is competitive bodybuilding. He engages in a high-volume training program, using moderate intensity (70% to 75% 1-RM) and moderate repetitions (10

STEPS FOR DEVELOPING A RESISTANCE TRAINING PROGRAM

These steps were used to design the sample dynamic resistance training programs on pages 144-147.

1. In consultation with your clients, identify the primary goal of the program (i.e., strength, muscular endurance, muscle size, or muscle toning) and ask clients how much time they are willing to commit to this program.

2. Based on your client's goal, time commitment, and access to equipment, determine the type of resistance training program (i.e., dynamic, static, or isokinetic).

3. Using results from your client's muscular fitness assessment, identify specific muscle groups that need to be targeted in the exercise prescription.

4. In addition to core exercises for the major muscle groups, select exercises for those muscle groups targeted in step 3.

5. For novice weight lifters, order the exercises so the same muscle group is not exercised consecutively.

6. Based on your client's goals, determine appropriate starting loads, repetitions, and sets for each exercise.

7. Set guidelines for progressively overloading each muscle group.

Sample Resistance Training Program for Older Adult

Client data

Age	70 years	*Intensity*	30-50% 1-RM for first 8 weeks; 50-75% 1-RM thereafter
Gender	Male		
Body weight	160 lb (72.7 kg)	*Frequency*	2 days/week; at least 48 hr between workouts
Program goal	Muscle fitness and functional independence		
		Duration	16 weeks or longer
		Overload	Increase reps first; only increase resistance when able to complete >15 reps
Time commitment	20-30 min/workout		
Equipment	Exercise machines		
		Rest	2-3 min between exercises

Training program

Exercise[a]	1-RM (lb)*	Weeks[b]	Intensity[c] (%1-RM)	Weight* (lb)	Reps	Sets	Muscle groups
Leg press (seated)	180	1-4	30-40	55-70	15-20	1	Hip extensors, knee extensors
		5-8	40-50	72-90	15-20	1	
		9-12	50-60	90-110	10-15	1	
		13-16	60-75	110-135	10-15	1	
Chest flys (seated)	90	1-4	30-40	30-36	15-20	1	Shoulder flexors and adductors
		5-8	40-50	36-45	15-20	1	
		9-12	50-60	45-54	10-15	1	
		13-16	60-75	54-68	10-15	1	
Leg curl (seated)	45	1-4	30-40	13-18	15-20	1	Knee flexors
		5-8	40-50	18-22	15-20	1	
		9-12	50-60	22-27	10-15	1	
		13-16	60-75	27-34	10-15	1	
Lat pull-down	100	1-4	30-40	30-40	15-20	1	Shoulder extensors and adductors, elbow flexors
		5-8	40-50	40-50	15-20	1	
		9-12	50-60	50-60	10-15	1	
		13-16	60-75	60-75	10-15	1	
Shoulder press (seated)	50	1-4	30-40	15-20	15-20	1	Shoulder flexors and abductors, elbow extensors
		5-8	40-50	20-25	15-20	1	
		9-12	50-60	25-30	10-15	1	
		13-16	60-75	30-38	10-15	1	
Heel (calf) raises (seated)	90	1-4	30-40	27-36	15-20	1	Ankle plantar flexors
		5-8	40-50	36-45	15-20	1	
		9-12	50-60	45-54	10-15	1	
		13-16	60-75	54-68	10-15	1	
Abdominal curls	–	1-4	–	Body weight	5-10	1-2	Trunk flexors
		5-8			10-15	1-2	
		9-12			15-20	1-2	
		13-16			20-25	1-2	

[a]Multijoint exercise machines are used for most exercises. Seated and lying (instead of standing) positions are recommended to stabilize the body during lifting. Exercises should be done in the order listed.

[b]During first 2 weeks, closely monitor and supervise workouts. Initial training lasts 8 weeks.

[c]Intensity is gradually increased every 2 weeks, only after client is able to do more than the prescribed number of repetitions at each target intensity.

*1 lb = 0.45 kg.

Sample Resistance Training Program for Novice

Client data

Age	35 years	*Intensity*	80% 1-RM
Gender	Female	*Frequency*	3 days/week, alternate days
Body weight	155 lb (70.4 kg)	*Duration*	12 weeks or longer
Program goal	Muscle strength	*Overload*	Increase weight when able to complete 10-12 reps at the prescribed intensity
Time commitment	40-50 min/workout		
Equipment	Variable-resistance machines and free weights	*Rest*	1 min between sets

Training program[a]

Exercise[b]	1-RM (lb)[c]	Intensity (%1-RM)	Weight (lb)[c]	Reps	Sets	Muscle groups
Leg press	200	80	160	8	3	Hip extensors, knee extensors
Bench press*	75	80	60	8	3	Shoulder flexors and adductors, elbow extensors
Leg curl (lying)	70	80	55	8	3	Knee flexors
Lat pull-down	125	80	100	8	3	Shoulder extensors and adductors, elbow flexors
Dumbbell fly* (flat bench)	20	80	15	8	3	Shoulder flexors and adductors
Heel (calf) raises (standing)	160	80	125	8	3	Ankle plantar flexors
Abdominal curls	–	–	–	15-20	3	Trunk flexors
Arm curl* (incline bench)	45	80	35	8	3	Elbow flexors
Lateral raises (dumbbell)	20	80	15	8	3	Shoulder abductors
Triceps press-down	60	80	45	8	3	Elbow extensors
Hammer curls* (dumbbells)	40	80	30	8	3	Elbow flexors

[a]Do exercises in order listed, using larger muscle groups first. Multijoint exercises are done before single-joint exercises.

[b]Other exercises that work the same muscle groups may be substituted to add variety to the program (see appendix C.3, "Dynamic Resistance Training Exercises," p. 303).

[c]1 lb = 0.45 kg.

*Two exercises prescribed for each of the weaker muscle groups (shoulder flexors and elbow flexors) identified from her strength assessment.

to 12 reps) to maximize the development of muscle size. To achieve a high training volume, he performs three exercises for each muscle group and three to four sets of each exercise. To effectively overload the muscles, he performs three exercises for each muscle group consecutively (tri-sets) with little or no rest between the sets. He lifts weights six days a week, splitting the routine so that he is not exercising the same muscle groups on con-

secutive days. With this routine, each muscle group is exercised two times a week. He increases the resistance when he is able to complete more than 12 repetitions in the set.

Several excellent references deal with the design of advanced resistance training programs (Baechle 1994; Fleck and Kraemer 1997; Zatsiorsky 1995) and give examples of sport-specific resistance training programs for athletes (Chu 1996).

Sample Advanced Resistance Training Program for Bodybuilder

Client	28-year-old male	Training methods	High volume; tri-sets; split routine
Body weight	190 lb		
Program goal	Muscle size for body-building	Intensity	70-75% 1-RM
		Frequency	6 days/week
Time commitment	90 min/workout	Duration	24 weeks or longer
Equipment	Free weights and exercise machines	Overload	Increase weight when able to complete >12 reps
		Rest	1 min between tri-sets

Exercise	1-RM (lb)	Intensity (% 1-RM)	Weight (lb)*	Repetitions	Sets	Muscles
Monday & Thursday[a]						
Chest [b]						
Flat bench press (barbell)	250	70-75	175-185	10-12	3-4	Pectoralis major (midsternal portion), triceps brachii
Incline dumbbell fly	80	70-75	55-60	10-12	3-4	Pectoralis major (clavicular portion), anterior deltoid
Decline bench press (barbell)	180	70-75	125-135	10-12	3-4	Pectoralis major (lower sternal portion)
Shoulders [b]						
Upright row (barbell)	140	70-75	100-105	10-12	3-4	Middle deltoid
Front dumbbell raises	80	70-75	55-60	10-12	3-4	Anterior deltoid
Posterior cable pull (horizontal plane)	100	70-75	70-75	10-12	3-4	Posterior deltoid
Tuesday & Friday[a]						
Hips and thighs [b]						
First tri-set						
Squats	300	70-75	210-225	10-12	3	Gluteus maximus, quadriceps femoris, upper hamstrings
Leg extension	150	70-75	105-110	10-12	3	Quadriceps femoris
Leg curl (standing, unilateral)	90	70-75	60-65	10-12	3	Hamstrings (mid-to-lower portions)
Second tri-set						
Leg press	400	70-75	280-300	10-12	3	Gluteus maximus, quadriceps femoris, upper hamstrings
Leg curl (lying)	130	70-75	90-100	10-12	3	Hamstrings (mid-to-lower portions)
Glut-ham raise	–	–	–	10-15	3	Gluteus maximus, hamstrings
Legs and calves [b]						
Standing calf (heel) raise	250	70-75	175-185	10-12	3-4	Gastrocnemius, soleus
Ankle flexion exercise (seated)	90	70-75	60-65	10-12	3-4	Tibialis anterior
Seated calf raise	180	70-75	125-135	10-12	3-4	Soleus, gastrocnemius

Exercise	1-RM (lb)	Intensity (% 1-RM)	Weight (lb)*	Repetitions	Sets	Muscles
Wednesday & Saturday[a]						
Back [b]						
Lat pull-down (wide grip)	225	70-75	155-170	10-12	3-4	Latissimus dorsi (lateral portions), biceps brachii, brachialis
Seated row (narrow grip)	240	70-75	170-180	10-12	3-4	Latissimus dorsi (mid portion), biceps brachii, brachialis
Dumbbell row	90	70-75	60-65	10-12	3-4	Latissimus dorsi (mid portion), biceps brachii, brachialis
Elbow flexors [b]						
Standing barbell curl	130	70-75	90-100	10-12	3-4	Biceps brachii, brachialis, brachioradialis
Preacher curl (dumbbells)	100	70-75	70-75	10-12	3-4	Biceps brachii (mid portion), brachialis
Hammer curl (dumbbells)	80	70-75	55-60	10-12	3-4	Brachioradialis, brachialis
Elbow extensors [b]						
Lying triceps extension (barbell)	120	70-75	85-90	10-12	3-4	Triceps brachii (long head)
Triceps push-down	150	70-75	105-110	10-12	3-4	Triceps brachii (short and lateral heads)
Triceps pull-down with lateral flair (cables)	130	70-75	90-100	10-12	3-4	Triceps brachii (lateral head)

[a]Other exercises that work the same muscles may be substituted on the second day to add variety to the program (see appendix C.3, "Dynamic Resistance Training Exercises," p. 303).

[b]For tri-sets, the three exercises listed are performed consecutively without rest, and then the tri-set is repeated for the prescribed number of sets for that body part.

*1 lb = 0.45 kg.

Designing Resistance Training Programs for Children

Children can safely participate in resistance training if special precautions and recommended guidelines (see table 7.2) are carefully followed (ACSM 2000). Because children are anatomically and physiologically immature, heavy weights may cause damage to the developing bones and joints. Exercise intensity should not exceed 80% 1-RM, which equates to 8 to 12 repetitions per set. Prescribe one to two sets of 8 to 10 multijoint (no single-joint) exercises and no more than two exercise sessions per week. To progressively overload the muscle groups, increase the number of repetitions before increasing the resistance. Instruct the child about proper weightlifting (e.g., no fast or jerky movements) and breathing techniques (no breath-holding). A trained exercise leader should closely supervise and monitor the weightlifting activity of the child during every workout.

Designing Resistance Training Programs for Older Adults

Resistance training provides many health benefits, especially for older adults. The primary goal of the resistance training program is to develop sufficient muscular fitness so that older adults may carry out activities of daily living without undue stress or fatigue and may retain their functional independence. In addition to the general guidelines for designing resistance training programs for older adults (see table 7.2), ACSM (2000) recommends these guidelines and precautions:

- During the first eight weeks of training, use minimal resistance (30% to 50% 1-RM) for all exercises.
- Instruct older adults about proper weightlifting and breathing techniques.
- Trained exercise leaders who have experience working with older adults should closely supervise and monitor the client's weightlifting techniques and resistance training program during the first few exercise sessions.
- Prescribe multijoint, rather than single-joint, exercises.
- Use exercise machines to stabilize body position and control the range of joint motion. Avoid using free weights with older adults.
- Each exercise session should be approximately 20 to 30 min and should never exceed 60 min.
- Older adults should rate their perceived exertion during exercise. Ratings of perceived exertion (RPEs) should be between 12 and 13 (somewhat hard).
- Allow at least 48 hr of rest between the exercise workouts.

- Never allow clients with arthritis to lift weights when they are actively experiencing joint pain or inflammation.
- When clients are returning to resistance training following a layoff of more than one month, they should start with a low resistance that is less than 50% of the weight they were lifting prior to the layoff.

EFFECTS OF RESISTANCE TRAINING PROGRAMS

Resistance training improves muscular fitness by increasing both strength and muscular endurance. This section addresses the morphological, neurological, and biochemical effects of resistance training.

Morphological Effects of Resistance Training on Skeletal Muscle

Resistance training leads to morphological adaptations in skeletal muscles. Structural changes in muscle fibers account for a large portion of the

---

Summary of Effects of Resistance Training

Morphological Factors

- Muscle hypertrophy due to increase in contractile proteins, number and size of myofibrils, connective tissues, and size of type II muscle fibers
- No change in relative amounts of type I and II muscle fibers
- Little or no change in the number of muscle fibers (<5%)
- Increase in size and strength of ligaments and tendons
- Increase in bone density and bone strength
- Increase in muscle capillary density

Neural Factors

- Increase in motor unit activation and recruitment
- Increase in discharge frequency of motor neurons
- Decrease in neural inhibition

Biochemical Factors

- Minor increase in ATP and CP stores
- Minor increase in CPK, myosin ATPase, and myokinase activity
- Decrease in mitochondrial volume density
- Increase in testosterone, growth hormone, IGF, and catecholamines during resistance training exercises

Additional Factors

- Little or no change in body mass
- Increase in fat-free mass
- Decrease in fat mass and relative body fat
- Improved bone health

strength gains resulting from resistance training. The following questions deal with these adaptations.

■ What is exercise-induced muscle hypertrophy?

One effect of strength training is an increase in the size of the muscle tissue. This adaptation, known as **exercise-induced hypertrophy,** results from an increase in the total amount of contractile protein, the number and size of myofibrils per fiber, and the amount of connective tissue surrounding the muscle fibers (Goldberg, Etlinger, Goldspink, and Jablecki 1975).

■ Is it possible to increase the number of muscle fibers by resistance training?

Heavy resistance training has been reported to produce an increase in the number of muscle fibers (i.e., hyperplasia) in animals due to longitudinal splitting and satellite cell proliferation (Antonio and Gonyea 1993; Edgerton 1970; Gonyea, Ericson, and Bonde-Petersen 1977). Such processes, however, have not been clearly demonstrated in human skeletal muscle tissue (Taylor and Wilkinson 1986; Tesch 1988). Although some data suggest that human skeletal muscle has the potential to increase muscle fiber number (Alway, Grumbt, Gonyea, and Stray-Gundersen 1989; Sjostrom, Lexell, Eriksson, and Taylor 1992), hyperplasia probably contributes less than 5% to overall muscle growth in response to heavy resistance training (Kraemer, Fleck, and Evans 1996). The major factor contributing to exercise-induced hypertrophy for humans apparently is an increase in the size of existing muscle fibers.

■ Does resistance training alter muscle fiber type from slow-twitch to fast-twitch?

Although strength training produces greater hypertrophy in fast-twitch (type II) muscle fibers than in slow-twitch (type I) fibers (Tesch 1988; Thorstensson, Hulten, vonDobeln, and Karlsson 1976), there is no evidence to support the conversion of slow-twitch to fast-twitch fibers (Costill, Coyle, Fink, Lesmes, and Witzmann 1979; Dons, Bollerup, Bonde-Petersen, and Hancke 1979; Mikesky, Giddings, Matthews, and Gonyea 1991). Resistance training does not alter the percentage of type I and II muscle fibers. However, heavy resistance training affects the proportion of fibers comprising subgroups of type II muscle fibers, increasing the percentage of type IIA (fast-twitch—glycolytic) muscle fibers while decreasing the percentage of type IIB (fast-twitch—oxidative) fibers

in both men and women (Kraemer et al. 1995; Staron et al. 1994).

■ Is the relationship between muscle size and strength the same for men and women?

Muscle strength is directly related to the cross-sectional area of the muscle tissue. Ikai and Fukunaga (1968) noted that the static strength per unit of cross-sectional area of the elbow flexors was similar for young men and women. These values ranged between 4.5 and 8.9 kg/cm^2; average values were 6.2 and 6.7 kg/cm^2 for women and men, respectively. Cureton, Collins, Hill, and McElhannon (1988) also reported that the dynamic strength per unit of cross-sectional area (CSA) was similar for men and women. Posttraining ratios of elbow flexor/extensor strength to upper arm CSA were 1.65 kg/cm^2 and 1.85 kg/cm^2, respectively, for men and women. Likewise, the posttraining ratios for leg strength to thigh CSA were 1.10 kg/cm^2 for men and 0.90 kg/cm^2 for women.

■ How much do women's muscles hypertrophy in response to resistance training?

In the past, researchers believed that resistance training produced less muscle hypertrophy in women than in men even though their relative strength gains were similar (Brown and Wilmore 1974; Mayhew and Gross 1974; Wilmore 1974). These studies assessed muscle hypertrophy indirectly using anthropometric and body composition measures. Cureton et al. (1988), however, using computerized tomography to directly assess muscle hypertrophy in a heavy resistance training program (70% to 90% 1-RM, three days per week for 16 weeks), found significant increases in CSA of the upper arms of women (5 cm^2 or 23%) as well as men (7 cm^2 or 15%). Although the absolute change was slightly larger in men, the relative degree of hypertrophy was similar for men and women.

■ Is it possible for older adults to increase the size of their muscles by resistance training?

Electromyographic evidence led Mortani and deVries (1979) to conclude that increased strength in older men who engaged in resistance training was highly dependent on neural changes, such as increased frequency of motor neuron discharge and recruitment of motor units. Because of studies such as this, it was long believed that strength gains from resistance training in older individuals were due primarily to neural adaptation rather than muscle hypertrophy.

However, Frontera, Meredith, O'Reilly, Knuttgen, and Evans (1988) reported that resistance training produces muscle hypertrophy in men ages 60 to 72 years. The men trained in a high-intensity program for the knee extensors and flexors (three sets at 80% 1-RM) for 12 weeks. Computerized tomography revealed significant increases in total thigh area (4.8%), total muscle area (11.4%), and quadriceps area (9.3%). The relative increase in total muscle area was similar to values reported for young men (Luthi et al. 1986). Research also shows significant increases in muscle size in older women, as well as in very old (87 to 96 years) men and women, due to high-intensity (80% 1-RM) resistance training (Charette et al. 1991; Fiatarone et al. 1990).

Exercise-induced hypertrophy appears to be an important mechanism underlying strength gains in older women and men. This implies that older adults can effectively counter age-related loss in muscle mass by participating in a vigorous resistance training program.

Biochemical Effects of Resistance Training

The morphological changes in skeletal muscles due to resistance training are caused by hormones. This section addresses questions regarding hormonal responses to resistance exercise, as well as changes in the metabolic profile of skeletal muscles.

■ *What causes the increase in muscle size with resistance training?*

Exercise-induced hypertrophy occurs through hormonal mechanisms. Anabolic (protein-building) hormones such as testosterone, growth hormone, and insulin-like growth hormone increase in response to heavy resistance exercise and interact to promote protein synthesis. The magnitude of testosterone and growth hormone release, however, appears to be related to the size of the muscle groups used, the exercise intensity (% 1-RM), and the length of rest between sets, with larger increases observed for high-intensity (5- to 10-RM) exercise and short (1 min) rest periods involving large muscle groups (Kraemer et al. 1991). In men, high-intensity resistance training produces significant increases in testosterone and growth hormone (Fahey, Rolph, Moungmee, Nagel, and Mortara 1976; vanHelder, Radomski, and Goode 1984; Weiss, Cureton, and Thompson 1983). Levels of catecholamines (norepinephrine, epinephrine, and dopamine), which augment the release of testosterone and insulin-like growth fac-

tor, also increase in men in response to heavy resistance exercise (Kraemer, Noble, Clark, and Culver 1987). In women, the growth hormone response to resistance exercise varies over stages of the menstrual cycle (Kraemer et al. 1991).

■ *Does resistance training alter the metabolic profile of skeletal muscles?*

Although high-intensity resistance training results in substantial increases in muscle proteins, it appears to have little or no effect on muscle substrate stores and enzymes involved with the generation of adenosine triphosphate (ATP). Although stores of ATP and creatine phosphate (CP) may increase significantly in response to strength training (MacDougall et al. 1979), the changes are not large enough to have practical significance. Strength training produces only minor alterations in myosin adenosinetriphosphatase (ATPase) activity (Tesch 1992) and other ATP turnover enzymes, such as creatine phosphokinase (CPK), in response to strength training (Costill, Coyle, Fink, Lesmes, and Witzmann 1979; Komi, Viitasalo, Rauramaa, and Vihko 1978; Thorstensson, Hulten, vonDobeln, and Karlsson 1976). Strength training using heavy resistance and explosive exercises results in decreased activities for hexokinase, myofibrillar ATPase, and citrate synthase (Tesch 1988).

■ *Does resistance training decrease aerobic capacity and endurance performance?*

The mitochondrial volume density following heavy resistance training has been reported to decrease as a consequence of a disproportionate increase of contractile protein in comparison with mitochondria. In theory, this could be detrimental to aerobic capacity and endurance performance. A review of studies of this phenomenon, however, concluded that participation in heavy resistance training does not negatively affect aerobic power (Dudley and Fleck 1987; Sale, MacDougall, Jacobs, and Garner 1987). Also, capillary density has been shown to increase, which in turn enhances the potential to remove lactate produced by the muscles during moderate-intensity, high-volume resistance exercise (Kraemer, Fleck, and Evans 1996).

Neurological Effects of Resistance Training

The nervous system also responds to resistance training. Neurological adaptations account for much of the improvement in muscle strength in the early stages of resistance training, leading to the following question: How long does it take to show substantial improvements in muscle strength and size?

The answer is somewhat complex. Increased muscle size alone cannot account for the rate of strength gain due to resistance training (Dons, Bollerup, Bonde-Petersen, and Hancke 1979; Moritani and deVries 1979). In the early stages (2 to 8 weeks) of resistance training, neural factors are also involved. These factors include learning to disinhibit motor neurons and to increase activation levels of motor units (Kraemer, Deschenes, and Fleck 1988; Sale 1988). At about 8 to 10 weeks of resistance training, muscle hypertrophy contributes more than neural adaptations to strength gains but eventually levels off (Sale 1988). Staron et al. (1994) noted that at least 16 resistance training workouts are needed in order to produce substantial increases in muscle contractile proteins (hypertrophy).

Additional Effects of Resistance Training

Resistance training also positively affects bone health and overall body composition. The following questions address these adaptations.

▪ Does resistance training improve bone health and joint integrity?

Resistance training has beneficial effects on bone health that may decrease the risk of osteoporosis and bone fractures, particularly in women. This form of training may help to achieve the highest possible peak bone mass in premenopausal women and may aid in maintaining and increasing bone in postmenopausal women and older adults (Layne and Nelson 1999). Bone mineral density of the lumbar spine and femur in premenopausal women significantly increased after 12 to 18 months of strength training (Lohman et al. 1995). Also, lumbar bone mineral density of early-postmenopausal women was improved following nine months of strength training (Pruitt, Jackson, Bartels, and Lehnhard 1992). However, in a study of older women (65 to 79 years), 12 months of high-intensity (80% 1-RM) and low-intensity (40% 1-RM) resistance training did not significantly improve the bone mineral density of the lumbar spine and hip (Pruitt, Taaffe, and Marcus 1995). Still, evidence suggests that resistance training and higher-intensity weight-bearing activities (not walking) may slow the decline in bone loss even if there is no significant increase in bone mineral density. Physical activity, however, should not

be substituted for hormonal replacement therapy at the time of menopause (ACSM 1995).

Resistance training also improves the size and strength of ligaments and tendons (Edgerton 1973; Fleck and Falkel 1986; Tipton, Matthes, Maynard, and Carey 1975). These changes may increase joint stability, thereby reducing the risk of sprains and dislocations.

▪ Is resistance training effective for weight control?

Resistance training positively alters body composition and preserves lean body tissues. Although total body weight undergoes little change, the lean body mass increases as the absolute and relative amounts of body fat decrease (Brown and Wilmore 1974; Mayhew and Gross 1974; Ross 1997; Wilmore 1974). Given that muscle tissue is more metabolically active than fat tissue, the increase in muscle size and lean body mass due to resistance training helps to maintain the resting metabolic rate of individuals on weight loss diets. For weight loss programs, exercise science and nutrition professionals recommend using resistance training, in combination with aerobic exercise, to maximize the loss of body fat while maintaining lean body tissues (see chapter 9).

MUSCULAR SORENESS

Muscular soreness may develop as a result of resistance training because isolated muscle groups are being overloaded beyond normal use. **Acute-onset muscle soreness** occurs during or immediately following the exercise and is usually caused by ischemia and the accumulation of metabolic waste products in the muscle tissue. The pain and discomfort may persist up to 1 hr after the cessation of the exercise.

In **delayed-onset muscle soreness (DOMS)**, the pain occurs 24 to 48 hr after exercise. Although the causes of DOMS are not known (Armstrong 1984; Smith 1991), it appears to be related to the type of muscle contraction. Eccentric exercise produces a greater degree of delayed muscular soreness than either concentric or isometric exercise (Byrnes, Clarkson, and Katch 1985; Schwane, Johnson, Vandenakker, and Armstrong 1983; Talag 1973). Little or no muscular soreness occurs with isokinetic exercise (Byrnes, Clarkson, and Katch 1985). This most likely relates to the fact that isokinetic exercise devices offer no resistance to the recovery phase of the movement and therefore the muscle does not contract eccentrically.

Theories of Delayed-Onset Muscle Soreness

Although the precise causes of DOMS remain unclear, several theories have been proposed. The more widely recognized theories suggest that exercise, particularly eccentric exercise, causes damage to skeletal muscle cells and connective tissues, producing an acute inflammation.

Connective Tissue Damage

Abraham (1977) extensively studied the factors related to DOMS produced by resistance training. He suggested that DOMS most likely results from disruption in the connective tissue of the muscle and its tendinous attachments. Abraham noted that urinary excretion of hydroxyproline, a specific by-product of connective tissue breakdown, was higher in subjects who experienced muscular soreness than in those who did not. Because a significant rise in urinary hydroxyproline levels indicates an increase in both collagen degradation and synthesis, he concluded that more strenuous exercise damages the connective tissue, which increases the degradation of collagen and creates an imbalance in collagen metabolism. To compensate for this imbalance, the rate of collagen synthesis increases.

Skeletal Muscle Damage

Researchers have assessed skeletal muscle damage induced through exercise by examining micrographs of the myofibrils obtained from biopsy samples. Friden, Sjostrom, and Ekblom (1983) observed structural damage to myofibrillar Z bands resulting from intense eccentric exercise. The damage to fast-twitch fibers was more extensive than that to slow-twitch fibers.

Researchers also have examined markers of muscle damage such as serum CPK, lactate dehydrogenase, and myoglobin. Schwane, Johnson, Vandenakker, and Armstrong (1983) noted a significant increase in plasma CPK levels produced by downhill running. They suggested that the mechanical stress from eccentric exercise causes cellular damage that results in an enzyme efflux. Clarkson, Byrnes, McCormick, Turcotte, and White (1986) reported similar increases in serum CPK levels following concentric (37.6%), eccentric (35.8%), and isometric (34%) arm curl exercises. They concluded that muscle damage occurred with all three types of contraction; however, the subjects perceived greater muscle soreness with eccentric and isometric exercises. Likewise, Byrnes et al. (1985) observed that both concentric and eccentric resistance training elevated serum CPK levels but that individuals who trained concentrically did not develop DOMS.

Armstrong's Model of Delayed-Onset Muscle Soreness

On the basis of an extensive literature review, Armstrong (1984) proposed the following model of the development of DOMS:

1. The structural proteins in muscle cells and connective tissue are disrupted by high mechanical forces produced during exercise, especially eccentric exercise.

2. Structural damage to the sarcolemma alters the permeability of the cell membrane, allowing a net influx of calcium from the interstitial space. Abnormally high levels of calcium inhibit cellular respiration, thereby lessening the cell's ability to produce ATP for active removal of calcium from the cell.

3. High calcium levels within the cell activate a calcium-dependent proteolytic enzyme that degrades Z discs, troponin, and tropomyosin.

4. This progressive destruction of the sarcolemma (postexercise) allows intracellular components to diffuse into the interstitial space and plasma. These substances attract monocytes and activate mast cells and histocytes in the injured area.

5. Histamine, kinins, and potassium accumulate in the interstitial space because of the active phagocytosis and cellular necrosis. These substances, as well as increased tissue edema and temperature, may stimulate pain receptors resulting in the sensation of DOMS.

Acute Inflammation Theory

Smith (1991) suggested that acute inflammation, in response to muscle cell and connective damage caused by eccentric exercise, is the primary mechanism underlying DOMS. Many of the signs and symptoms of acute inflammation, such as pain, swelling, and loss of function, are also present with DOMS. Based on research about acute inflammation and DOMS, Smith proposed the following sequence of events:

1. Connective tissue and muscle tissue disruption occurs during eccentric exercise, especially when the individual is not accustomed to eccentric exercise.

2. Within a few hours, neutrophils in the blood are elevated and migrate to the site of injury for several hours postinjury.

3. Monocytes also migrate to the injured tissues at 6 to 12 hr postinjury.

4. Macrophages synthesize prostaglandins (series E).

5. The prostaglandins sensitize type III and IV pain afferents, resulting in the sensation of pain in response to intramuscular pressure caused by movement or palpation.

6. The combination of increased pressure and hypersensitization produces the sensation of DOMS.

Prevention of Muscular Soreness

To prevent muscular soreness due to resistance training, you should prescribe warm-up and cooldown exercises for your clients. For many years, slow static stretching exercises were recommended to warm up major muscle groups at the start of the resistance training workout. It was believed that this form of stretching prevented muscle injury and soreness (deVries 1961). However, recent evidence suggests that stretching prior to physical activity does not prevent injury (Pope, Herbert, Kirwan, and Graham 2000). Instead of performing static stretching, your client should warm up by completing 5 to 10 repetitions of the exercise at a low intensity (e.g., 40% 1-RM). Have clients use slow static stretching as part of the cool-down segment of the resistance training workout.

Using a gradual progression of exercise intensity at the beginning of a resistance training program also may help to prevent muscular soreness. McArdle et al. (1996) suggest using 12- to 15-RM during the beginning phases of strength training. After two weeks, have clients increase the exercise intensity to 6- to 8-RM. Avoiding eccentric contractions during dynamic resistance training also may lessen the chance of muscular soreness. An assistant or exercise partner should return the weight to the starting position.

COMMON MISCONCEPTIONS AND QUESTIONS ABOUT RESISTANCE TRAINING

Because of the overwhelming amount of misinformation about resistance training in popular magazines, your clients will have many questions and concerns.

■ *Will my muscles be stiff and sore after I lift weights?*

It is highly likely that you will experience some muscle soreness one to two days after your workout, especially if you are a beginning weight lifter or have not been lifting weights on a regular basis. To lessen the chance of developing sore muscles, warm up before each workout by exercising at a low intensity. If you have never lifted weights, you should begin by using light weights (≤60% of your 1-RM) during the first few weeks of training. As your muscles get stronger, progressively but gradually increase the amount of weight for each exercise. Avoid doing too much, too soon.

■ *What can I do to relieve my muscle soreness?*

If your muscles are sore, you should not lift weights. Sometimes slow static stretching of the sore muscles will help to relieve some of the pain. Nonprescription painkillers such as aspirin and ibuprofen often help. If the soreness persists for more than 48 hr, you should contact your physician.

■ *Is it okay to lift weights every day?*

During weightlifting, your muscles are exercised at greater-than-normal workloads, producing microscopic tears in the muscle cells and connective tissues. Your body responds by producing new muscle proteins. This causes muscle growth and increased strength. For these changes to occur, you need to rest the exercised muscles between workouts. Also, most people can show substantial improvements in strength when they lift weights every other day, just two to three times a week. If you lift weights every day, you run the risk of overtraining your muscles. This may cause muscle strains, tendinitis, bursitis, and other injuries to your muscles and joints. Experienced weight lifters who work out every day split their exercise routine so that they are not exercising the same muscle groups on consecutive days. This type of routine reduces the risk of developing excessive muscle soreness and overuse injuries if you lift weights every day.

■ Can I use calisthenic exercises, like push-ups and pull-ups, to improve my strength?

Calisthenic exercises can be used to increase your strength. Exercise professionals often prescribe push-ups and pull-ups, in addition to free-weight and machine exercises, to build the strength of chest, arm, and back muscles.

When you do calisthenic exercises, your body weight provides the resistance. Therefore, if you are unable to lift your body weight, you will need to modify the calisthenic exercise. For example, doing push-ups with your body weight supported by the knees and hands is easier than doing standard push-ups with your body fully extended and the weight supported by the hands and feet. As your strength improves, you may increase the difficulty of the push-up by placing the hands farther than shoulder-width apart.

If you are unable to lift your body weight, you can modify pull-ups by using a spotter. As you pull up, you can assist your movement by extending your knees as the spotter supports your lower legs or ankles. To increase the difficulty of a pull-up, place your hands farther apart than shoulder-width and use an overhand (pronated) grip instead of an underhand (supinated) grip.

■ Are exercise devices more effective than just calisthenic exercises for strengthening my abdominal muscles?

No scientific evidence currently justifies claims that doing calisthenic exercises with the aid of an abdominal exercise device is more effective than simply doing calisthenic exercises, like abdominal curls, without these devices. As your strength improves, you can modify abdominal exercises to overload the muscles by changing your body position (e.g., abdominal curls done on a decline bench are more difficult than on a flat bench), holding weight plates across your chest, or changing your arm position. Abdominal exercises get progressively more difficult as your arms are moved from along your sides to behind your head and overhead.

■ Will I get "muscle-bound" and lose joint flexibility if I lift weights?

It is a common misconception that resistance training decreases your joint flexibility. Studies of elite bodybuilders and power lifters indicate that these athletes have excellent levels of flexibility.

The key to remaining flexible while you are doing resistance training is to perform each exercise throughout the entire range of motion. Also, you should statically stretch muscle groups after each workout to ensure the maintenance of flexibility.

■ Will my strength improve if I train aerobically at the same time that I am resistance training?

If you do aerobic training concurrently with resistance training, your muscle growth and strength improvement may be lessened because of the increased energy demands and protein requirements for endurance training. Although this is an important consideration for competitive bodybuilders and power athletes, the decision to participate in both forms of training depends on your overall exercise program goal. If your goal is improved health or weight loss, experts recommend including both aerobic training and resistance training in your exercise program.

■ Are protein and amino acid supplements necessary to maximize my muscle growth and strength during resistance training?

Provided that your diet is well balanced and nutritionally sound, you do not need to use protein or amino acid supplements. Although the protein needs of resistance-trained individuals (1.2 to 1.6 g/kg per day) are slightly higher than the recommended dietary allowance for inactive individuals (0.9 g/kg per day), a well-balanced diet containing 12% to 15% protein is adequate to meet the increased protein need while an individual is weightlifting. Protein intake in excess of this level does not increase protein synthesis. Instead, excess protein is metabolized by the body. So your muscle size and strength will not be enhanced by a high protein intake. Also, there is no scientific evidence to justify the claim that amino acid supplements stimulate muscle growth or increase muscle strength and performance.

■ Will creatine supplements enhance my strength and muscle size during resistance training?

Studies show that creatine supplementation increases muscular strength, body mass, fat-free mass, muscle fiber size, and training volume in healthy, young adults; however, it may not enhance the performance and body composition of older men and women (67 to 80 years) who resistance train (Terjung et al. 2000; Volek 1999). Research shows that creatine supplements increase muscle creatine, thereby enhancing the training intensity and volume. The increased training stimulus results in an improved physiological adaptation to resistance training (i.e., a greater gain in muscle mass and strength). Increases in muscle creatine, however, may be limited to those who have low to average muscle creatine levels.

■ *Is it safe to take creatine supplements?*

Although there are anecdotal reports of an association between creatine supplementation and nausea, muscle cramping, and minor gastrointestinal distress, short-term creatine supplementation does not appear to have an adverse effect on kidney, liver, or cardiovascular function (Volek 1999). The lack of adverse effects, however, does not mean it is safe to take creatine; more research on the potential deleterious side effects of creatine supplementation over long periods of time is needed.

■ *I have followed my exercise prescription closely; but over the last several weeks, I haven't seen any change in my strength. What should I do?*

At the beginning of your program, your strength gains were dramatic and rapid because your initial strength level was less than it is now. As you get closer to your genetic limit, the rate and degree of improvement in strength decrease, and eventually you reach a plateau. It may be helpful if you periodically change the training stimulus by using a different combination of intensity, repetitions, and sets. For example, if you are presently doing high-intensity, low-repetition exercises, you may want to try decreasing your intensity (from 80% to 70% 1-RM) and increasing your repetitions from 6-8 to 10-12 reps for several weeks. Selecting different exercises for the muscle groups may also help.

KEY POINTS

- The specificity principle states that muscular fitness development is specific to the muscle group, type of contraction, training intensity, speed, and range of movement.

- The overload principle states that the muscle group must be exercised at greater-than-normal workloads to promote muscular strength and endurance development.

- For non-periodized resistance training programs, the training volume must be progressively increased to overload the muscle groups for continued gains in strength and muscular endurance.

- In most programs, resistance training exercises should be ordered so that successive exercises do not involve the same muscle group. For advanced programs, however, exercises for the same muscle group should be done consecutively.

- Dynamic resistance training can be used to develop muscular strength, tone, size, or endurance by modifying the intensity, repetitions, sets, and frequency of the exercise.

- Periodization programs can result in greater changes in strength than non-periodized resistance training programs.

- Strength and endurance gains resulting from resistance training are due to morphological, neurological, and biochemical changes in the muscle tissue.

- Eccentric exercise produces a greater degree of DOMS than either concentric, isometric, or isokinetic exercise.

- Little or no muscular soreness is produced by isokinetic training.

- The precise cause of DOMS is unknown; however, connective tissue and muscle damage, as well as acute inflammation, has been proposed as a possible cause.

KEY TERMS

Learn the definition of each of the following key terms. Definitions of terms can be found in "Glossary of Terms," page 349.

acute-onset muscle soreness	high intensity-low repetitions
compound sets	low intensity-high repetitions
delayed-onset muscle soreness (DOMS)	macrocycle
exercise-induced hypertrophy	mesocycles

muscle balance   set
periodization   split routine
pyramiding   supersetting
repetition maximum (RM)   training volume
repetitions   tri-sets

REVIEW QUESTIONS

In addition to being able to define each of the key terms, test your knowledge and understanding of the material by answering the following review questions.

1. What are the health benefits of resistance training?

2. Name three general types of resistance training. Which one is best suited for physical therapy rehabilitation programs?

3. What is the major advantage of isokinetic training compared to traditional forms of resistance training?

4. Describe the ACSM guidelines for designing resistance training programs for healthy adults. What modifications are necessary when you are planning resistance training programs for children and older adults?

5. Describe how the basic exercise prescriptions for strength training and muscular endurance training programs differ.

6. Describe how you can increase training volume for advanced strength training and hypertrophy programs.

7. Describe two methods of varying sets for advanced strength training programs.

8. Explain two methods that an advanced weight lifter can use to completely fatigue a targeted muscle group.

9. What is the purpose of periodization? How is this purpose accomplished?

10. Explain how the specificity, overload, and progression principles are applied in designing resistance training programs.

11. Explain what causes the exercise-induced hypertrophy resulting from resistance training. In the time course of a resistance training program, when is this morphological adaptation most likely to occur?

12. What neural adaptations account for initial strength gains during resistance training? When are these changes most likely to observed during the time course of resistance training?

13. Describe the potential effects of resistance training on bone health.

14. Describe one theory of DOMS. What can you instruct your clients to do to help prevent and relieve muscle soreness caused by resistance training?

15. What will you tell your clients if they ask about supplementing their resistance training with creatine?

REFERENCES

Abraham, W.M. 1977. Factors in delayed muscle soreness. *Medicine and Science in Sports* 9: 11–20.

Alway, S.E., Grumbt, W.H., Gonyea, W.J., and Stray-Gundersen, J. 1989. Contrasts in muscle and myofibers of elite male and female bodybuilders. *Journal of Applied Physiology* 67: 24–31.

American College of Sports Medicine (ACSM). 1995. ACSM position stand on osteoporosis and exercise. *Medicine & Science in Sports & Exercise* 27(4): i–vii.

American College of Sports Medicine. 2000. *ACSM's guidelines for exercise testing and prescription.* Philadelphia: Lippincott Williams & Wilkins.

Antonio, J., and Gonyea, W.J. 1993. Skeletal muscle fiber hyperplasia. *Medicine & Science in Sports & Exercise* 25: 1333–1345.

Armstrong, R.B. 1984. Mechanisms of exercise-induced delayed onset muscular soreness: A brief review. *Medicine & Science in Sports & Exercise* 16: 529–538.

Baechle, T.R. 1994. *Essentials of strength training and conditioning.* Champaign, IL: Human Kinetics.

Baker, D., Wilson, G., and Carlyon, R. 1994. Periodization: The effect on strength of manipulating volume and intensity. *Journal of Strength and Conditioning Research* 8: 235–242.

Bompa, T.O. 1999. *Periodization training for sports.* Champaign, IL: Human Kinetics.

Brown, C.H., and Wilmore, J.H. 1974. The effects of maximal resistance training on the strength and body composition of women athletes. *Medicine and Science in Sports* 6: 174–177.

Byrnes, W.C., Clarkson, P.M., and Katch, F.I. 1985. Muscle soreness following resistive exercise with and without eccentric contraction. *Research Quarterly for Exercise and Sport* 56: 283–285.

Charette, S.L., McEvoy, L., Pyka, G., Snow-Harter, C., Guido, D., Wiswell, R.A., and Marcus, R. 1991. Muscle hypertrophy response to resistance training in older women. *Journal of Applied Physiology* 70: 1912–1916.

Chu, D.A. 1996. *Explosive power and strength.* Champaign, IL: Human Kinetics.

Clarkson, P.M., Byrnes, W.C., McCormick, K.M., Turcotte, L.P., and White, J.S. 1986. Muscle soreness and serum creatine kinase activity following isometric, eccentric and concentric exercise. *International Journal of Sports Medicine* 7: 152–155.

Costill, D.L., Coyle, E.F., Fink, W.F., Lesmes, G.R., and Witzmann, F.A. 1979. Adaptations in skeletal muscle following strength training. *Journal of Applied Physiology* 46: 96–99.

Cote, C., Simoneau, J.A., Lagasse, P., Bouley, M., Thibault, M.C., Marcotte, M., and Bouchard, C. 1988. Isokinetic strength training protocols: Do they induce skeletal muscle fiber hypertrophy? *Archives of Physical Medicine and Rehabilitation* 69: 281–285.

Coyle, E.F., Feiring, D.C., Rotkis, T.C., Cote, R.W. III, Roby, F.B., Lee, W., and Wilmore, J.H. 1981. Specificity of power improvements through slow and fast isokinetic training. *Journal of Applied Physiology* 51: 1437–1442.

Cureton, K.J., Collins, M.A., Hill, D.W., and McElhannon, F.M. Jr. 1988. Muscle hypertrophy in men and women. *Medicine & Science in Sports & Exercise* 20: 338–344.

deVries, H.A. 1961. Prevention of muscular distress after exercise. *Research Quarterly* 32: 177–185.

Dons, B., Bollerup, K., Bonde-Petersen, F., and Hancke, S. 1979. The effect of weight-lifting exercise related to muscle fiber composition and muscle cross-sectional area in humans. *European Journal of Applied Physiology* 40: 95–106.

Dudley, G.A., and Fleck, S.J. 1987. Strength and endurance training: Are they mutually exclusive? *Sports Medicine* 4: 79–85.

Edgerton, V.R. 1970. Morphology and histochemistry of the soleus muscle from normal and exercised rats. *American Journal of Anatomy* 127: 81–88.

Edgerton, V.R. 1973. Exercise and the growth and development of muscle tissue. In *Physical activity, human growth and development,* ed. G.L. Rarick, 1–31. New York: Academic Press.

Fahey, T.D., Rolph, R., Moungmee, P., Nagel, J., and Mortara, S. 1976. Serum testosterone, body composition, and strength of young adults. *Medicine and Science in Sports* 8: 31–34.

Feigenbaum, M.S., and Pollock, M.L. 1999. Prescription of resistance training for health and disease. *Medicine & Science in Sports & Exercise* 31: 38–45.

Fiatarone, M.A., Marks, E.C., Ryan, N.D., Meredith, C.N., Lipstiz, L.A., and Evans, W.J. 1991. High-intensity strength training in nonagenarians. Effects on skeletal muscle. *Journal of the American Medical Association* 263: 3029–3034.

Fleck, S.J. 1999. Periodized strength training: A critical review. *Journal of Strength and Conditioning Research* 13(1): 82–89.

Fleck, S.J., and Falkel, J.E. 1986. Value of resistance training for the reduction of sports injuries. *Sports Medicine* 3: 61–68.

Fleck, S.J., and Kraemer, W.J. 1997. *Designing resistance training programs.* Champaign, IL: Human Kinetics.

Frankel, C., and Kravitz, L. 2000. Periodization. *IDEA Personal Trainer* 11(1): 15–17.

Friden, J., Sjostrom, M., and Ekblom, B. 1983. Myofibrillar damage following intense eccentric exercise in man. *International Journal of Sports Medicine* 4: 170–176.

Frontera, W.R., Meredith, C.N., O'Reilly, K.P., Knuttgen, H.G., and Evans, W.J. 1988. Strength conditioning in older men: Skeletal muscle hypertrophy and improved function. *Journal of Applied Physiology* 64: 1038–1044.

Gardner, G.W. 1963. Specificity of strength changes of the exercised and non-exercised limb following isometric training. *Research Quarterly* 34: 98–101.

Gettman, L.R., Ayres, J.J., Pollock, M.L., and Jackson, A. 1978. The effect of circuit weight training on strength, cardiorespiratory function, and body composition of adult men. *Medicine and Science in Sports* 10: 171–176.

Gettman, L.R., and Pollock, M.L. 1981. Circuit weight training: A critical review of its physiological benefits. *The Physician and Sportsmedicine* 9: 44–60.

Goldberg, A., Etlinger, J., Goldspink, D., and Jablecki, C. 1975. Mechanism of work-induced hypertrophy of skeletal muscle. *Medicine and Science in Sports* 7: 185–198.

Gonyea, W.J., Ericson, G.C., and Bonde-Petersen, F. 1977. Skeletal muscle fiber splitting induced by weight-lifting exercise in cats. *Acta Physiologica Scandinavica* 99: 105–109.

Hass, C.J., Garzarella, L., De Hoyas, D., and Pollock, M. 2000. Single versus multiple sets in long-term recreational weightlifters. *Medicine & Science in Sports & Exercise* 32: 235–242.

Hather, B.M., Tesch, P.A., Buchanan, P., and Dudley, G.A. 1991. Influence of eccentric actions on skeletal muscle adaptations to resistance training. *Acta Physiologica Scandinavica* 143: 177–185.

Hettinger, T., and Muller, E.A. 1953. Muskelleistung und muskeltraining. *European Journal of Applied Physiology* 15: 111–126.

Ikai, M., and Fukunaga, T. 1968. Calculation of muscle strength per unit cross-sectional area of human muscle by means of ultrasonic measurement. *European Journal of Applied Physiology* 26: 26–32.

Jenkins, W.L., Thackaberry, M., and Killian, C. 1984. Speed-specific isokinetic training. *Journal of Orthopaedic and Sports Physical Therapy* 6: 181–183.

Komi, P.V., Viitasalo, J.T., Rauramaa, R., and Vihko, V. 1978. Effect of isometric strength training on mechanical, electrical, and metabolic aspects of muscle function. *European Journal of Applied Physiology* 40: 45–55.

Kraemer, W.J. 1997. A series of studies—the physiological basis for strength training in American football: Fact over philosophy. *Journal of Strength and Conditioning Research* 11: 131–142.

Kraemer, W.J., Deschenes, M.R., and Fleck, S.J. 1988. Physiological adaptations to resistance exercise: Implications for athletic conditioning. *Sports Medicine* 6: 246–256.

Kraemer, W.J., Fleck, S.J., and Evans, W.J. 1996. Strength and power training: Physiological mechanisms of adaptation. In *Exercise and Sport Sciences Reviews*, ed. J.O. Holloszy, 24: 363–397. Baltimore: Williams & Wilkins.

Kraemer, W.J., Gordon, S.J., Fleck, S.J., Marchitelli, L.J., Mello, R., Dziados, J.E., Friedl, K., Harman, E., Maresh, C., and Fry, A.C. 1991. Endogenous anabolic hormonal and growth factor responses to heavy resistance exercise in males and females. *International Journal of Sports Medicine* 12: 228–235.

Kraemer, W.J., Noble, B.J., Clark, M.J., and Culver, B.W. 1987. Physiologic responses to heavy-resistance exercise with very short rest periods. *International Journal of Sports Medicine* 8: 247–252.

Kraemer, W.J., Patton, J., Gordon, S.E., Harman, E.A., Deschenes, M.R., Reynolds, K., Newton, R.U., Triplett, N.T., and Dziados, J.E. 1995. Compatibility of high intensity strength and endurance training on hormonal and skeletal muscle adaptations. *Journal of Applied Physiology* 78: 976–989.

Kramer, J.B., Stone, M.H., O'Bryant, H.S., Conley, M.S., Johnson, R.L., Nieman, D.C., Honeycutt, D.R., and Hoke, T.P. 1997. Effects of single vs. multiple sets of weight training: Impact of volume, intensity, and variation. *Journal of Strength and Conditioning Research* 11: 143–147.

Layne, J.E., and Nelson, M.E. 1999. The effects of progressive resistance training on bone density: A review. *Medicine & Science in Sports & Exercise* 31:25–30.

Lesmes, G.R., Costill, D.L., Coyle, E.F., and Fink, W.J. 1978. Muscle strength and power changes during maximal isokinetic training. *Medicine and Science in Sports* 10: 266–269.

Lohman, T.G., Going, S., Pamenter, R., Hall, M., Boyden, T., Houtkooper, L., Ritenbaugh, C., Bare, L., Hill, A., and Aickin, M. 1995. Effects of resistance training on regional and total bone mineral density in premenopausal women: A randomized prospective study. *Journal of Bone Mineral Research* 10: 1015–1024.

Luthi, J.M., Howald, H., Claasen, H., Rosler, K., Vock, P., and Hoppeler, H. 1986. Structural changes in skeletal muscle tissue with heavy resistance exercise. *International Journal of Sports Medicine* 7: 123–127.

MacDougall, J.D., Sale, D.G., Moroz, J.R., Elder, G.C., Sutton, J.R., and Howalk, H. 1979. Mitochondrial volume density in human skeletal muscle following heavy resistance training. *Medicine and Science in Sports* 11: 164–166.

Mayhew, J.L., and Gross, P.M. 1974. Body composition changes in young women with high resistance weight training. *Research Quarterly* 45: 433–440.

McArdle, W.D., Katch, F.I., and Katch, V.L. 1996. *Exercise physiology.* Baltimore: Williams & Wilkins.

Mikesky, A.E., Giddings, C.J., Matthews, W., and Gonyea, W.J. 1991. Changes in fiber size and composition in response to heavy-resistance exercise. *Medicine & Science in Sports & Exercise* 23: 1042–1049.

Moffroid, M.T., and Whipple, R.H. 1970. Specificity of speed of exercise. *Physical Therapy* 50: 1699–1704.

Moritani, T., and deVries, H.A. 1979. Neural factors versus hypertrophy in the time course of muscle strength gain. *American Journal of Physical Medicine* 58: 115–130.

Pope R.P., Herbert, R.D., Kirwan, J.D., and Graham, B.J. 2000. A randomized trial of preexercise stretching for prevention of lower limb injury. *Medicine & Science in Sports & Exercise* 32: 271–277.

Pruitt, L.A., Jackson, R.D., Bartels, R.L., and Lehnhard, H.J. 1992. Weight-training effects on bone mineral density in early postmenopausal women. *Journal of Bone Mineral Research* 7: 179–185.

Pruitt, L.A., Taaffe, D.R., and Marcus, R. 1995. Effects of a one-year high-intensity versus low-intensity resistance training program on bone mineral density in older women. *Journal of Bone Mineral Research* 10: 1788–1795.

Ross, R. 1997. Effects of diet- and exercise-induced weight loss on visceral adipose tissue in men and women. *Sports Medicine* 24: 55–64.

Sale, D. 1988. Neural adaptation to resistance training. *Medicine & Science in Sports & Exercise* 20: S135–S145.

Sale, D., MacDougall, J.D., Jacobs, I., and Garner, S. 1987. Interaction between concurrent strength and endurance training. *Journal of Applied Physiology* 68: 260–270.

Schwane, J.A., Johnson, S.R., Vandenakker, C.B., and Armstrong, R.B. 1983. Delayed-onset muscular soreness and plasma CPK and LDH activities after downhill running. *Medicine & Science in Sports & Exercise* 15: 51–56.

Sjostrom, M., Lexell, J., Eriksson, A., and Taylor, C.C. 1992. Evidence of fiber hyperplasia in human skeletal muscles from healthy young men? *European Journal of Applied Physiology* 62: 301–304.

Smith, L.L. 1991. Acute inflammation: The underlying mechanism in delayed onset muscle soreness? *Medicine & Science in Sports & Exercise* 23: 542–551.

Staron, R.S., Karapondo, D.L., Kraemer, W.J., Fry, A.C., Gordon, S.E., Falkel, J.E., Hagerman, F.C., and Hikida, R.S. 1994. Skeletal muscle adaptations during the early phase of heavy-resistance training in men and women. *Journal of Applied Physiology* 76: 1247–1255.

Stone, M.H., Pierce, K.C., Haff, G.G., Koch, A.J., and Stone, M. 1999a. Periodization: Effects of manipulating volume and intensity. Part 1. *Strength and Conditioning Journal* 21(2): 56–62.

Stone, M.H., Pierce, K.C., Haff, G.G., Koch, A.J., and Stone, M. 1999b. Periodization: Effects of manipulating volume and intensity. Part 2. *Strength and Conditioning Journal* 21(3): 54–60.

Talag, T.S. 1973. Residual muscular soreness as influenced by concentric, eccentric, and static contractions. *Research Quarterly* 44: 458–469.

Taylor, N.A.S., and Wilkinson, J.G. 1986. Exercise-induced skeletal muscle growth: Hypertrophy or hyperplasia? *Sports Medicine* 3: 190–200.

Terjung, R.L., Clarkson, P., Eichner, R., Greenhaff, P.L., Hespel, P.J., Israel, R.G., Kraemer, W.J., Meyer, R.A., Spriet, L.L., Tarnopolsky, M.A., Wagenmakers, A., and Williams, M.H. 2000. The American College of Sports Medicine roundtable on physiological and health effects of oral creatine supplementation. *Medicine & Science in Sports & Exercise* 32: 706–717.

Tesch, P.A. 1988. Skeletal muscle adaptations consequent to long-term heavy resistance exercise. *Medicine & Science in Sports & Exercise* 20: S132–S134.

Tesch, P.A. 1992. Short- and long-term histochemical and biochemical adaptations in muscle. In *Strength and power in sports. The encyclopaedia of sports medicine,* ed. P. Komi, 239–248. Oxford: Blackwell.

Thorstensson, A., Hulten, B., vonDobeln, W., and Karlsson, J. 1976. Effect of strength training on enzyme activities and fibre characteristics in human skeletal muscle. *Acta Physiologica Scandinavica* 96: 392–398.

Tipton, C.M., Matthes, R.D., Maynard, J.A., and Carey, R.A. 1975. The influence of physical activity on ligaments and tendons. *Medicine and Science in Sports* 7: 165–175.

vanHelder, W.P., Radomski, M.W., and Goode, R.C. 1984. Growth hormone responses during intermittent weight lifting exercise in men. *European Journal of Applied Physiology* 53: 31–34.

Volek, J. 1999. Update: What we know about creatine. *ACSM's Health & Fitness Journal* 3(3): 27–33.

Wathen, D. 1994. Periodization: Concepts and applications. In *Essentials of strength training and conditioning,* ed. T.R. Baechle, 459–472. Champaign, IL: Human Kinetics.

Weiss, L.W., Cureton, K.J., and Thompson, F.N. 1983. Comparison of serum testosterone and androstenedione responses to weight lifting in men and women. *European Journal of Applied Physiology* 50: 413–419.

Wilmore, J.H. 1974. Alterations in strength, body composition and anthropometric measurements consequent to a 10-week weight training program. *Medicine and Science in Sports* 6: 133–138.

Wilmore, J.H., Parr, R.B., Girandola, R.N., Ward, P., Vodak, P.A., Barstow, T.J., Pipes, T.V., Romero, G.T., and Leslie, P. 1978. Physiological alterations consequent to circuit weight training. *Medicine and Science in Sports* 10: 79–84.

Zatsiorsky, V.M. 1995. *Science and practice of strength training.* Champaign, IL: Human Kinetics.

chapter **8**

Assessing Body Composition

| KEY QUESTIONS |

- Why is it important to measure body composition, and how are body composition measures used by health and fitness professionals?

- What are the standards for classifying body fat levels?

- What is the difference between two-component and multicomponent body composition models?

- What are the guidelines and limitations of the hydrostatic weighing method?

- Is dual-energy X-ray absorptiometry considered to be a "gold standard" method for measuring body composition?

- What are the guidelines, limitations, and sources of measurement error for the skinfold method?

- What is bioelectrical impedance analysis? What factors affect the accuracy of this method?

- Can circumferences and skeletal diameters be used to accurately assess body composition?

- Is near-infrared interactance a viable alternative to skinfolds and bioimpedance analysis for measuring body composition in field settings?

Body composition is a key component of an individual's health and physical fitness profile. Obesity is a serious health problem that reduces life expectancy by increasing one's risk of developing coronary artery disease, hypertension, type 2 diabetes, obstructive pulmonary disease, osteoarthritis, and certain types of cancer. Too little body fat also poses a health risk because the body needs a certain amount of fat for normal physiological functions. Essential lipids, such as phospholipids, are needed for cell membrane formation; nonessential lipids, like triglycerides found in adipose tissue, provide thermal insulation and store metabolic fuel (free fatty acids). In addition, lipids are involved in the transport and storage of fat-soluble vitamins (A, D, E, and K) and in the functioning of the nervous system, the menstrual cycle, and the reproductive system, as well as in growth and maturation during pubescence. Thus, too little body fatness, as found in individuals with eating disorders (anorexia nervosa), exercise addiction,

and certain diseases such as cystic fibrosis, can lead to serious physiological dysfunction.

This chapter describes standardized testing procedures for laboratory (hydrostatic weighing, air displacement plethysmography, and dual X-ray absorptiometry) and field (skinfold, bioimpedance, and anthropometry) methods for assessing body composition. For each method, you will learn to identify potential sources of measurement error, as well as ways to minimize these errors.

CLASSIFICATION AND USES OF BODY COMPOSITION MEASURES

To classify level of body fatness, the **relative body fat** (%BF) is used. Table 8.1 presents recommended %BF standards for men, women, and children, as well as physically active adults. The minimal, average, and obesity fat values vary with age, gender, and activity status. For example, the average or median %BF values for adult men and women (18 to 34 years) are 13% for men and 28% for women; the minimal fat values are 8% and 20%, respectively; and the standard for obesity is >22% BF for men and >35% BF for women.

In addition to classifying your client's %BF and disease risk, body composition measures are useful for

- estimating a healthy body weight and formulating nutritional recommendations and exercise prescriptions (see chapter 9);
- estimating competitive body weight for athletes participating in sports that use body

weight classifications for competition (e.g., wrestling and bodybuilding);

- monitoring the growth of children and adolescents and identifying those at risk because of under- or overfatness; and
- assessing changes in body composition associated with aging, malnutrition, and certain diseases, and assessing the effectiveness of nutrition and exercise interventions in counteracting these changes.

BODY COMPOSITION MODELS

In order to make the most valid assessment of body composition for your client, it is necessary

---

Table 8.1   Percent Body Fat Standards for Adults, Children, and Physically Active Adults

	Recommended %BF levels for adults and children				
	NR*	Low	Mid	Upper	Obesity
Males					
18-34 years	<8	8	13	22	>22
35-55 years	<10	10	18	25	>25
55+ years	<10	10	16	23	>23
6-17 years	<5	5-10	11-25	26-31	>31
Females					
18-34 years	<20	20	28	35	>35
35-55 years	<25	25	32	38	>38
55+ years	<25	25	30	35	>35
6-17 years	<12	12-15	16-30	31-36	>36

	Recommended %BF levels for physically active adults		
	Low	Mid	Upper
Males			
18-34 years	5	10	15
35-55 years	7	11	18
55+ years	9	12	18
Females			
18-34 years	16	23	28
35-55 years	20	27	33
55+ years	20	27	33

*NR = not recommended; %BF = percent body fat.
Data from Lohman, Houtkooper, and Going (1997).

to understand the underlying theoretical models. You may recall that the body is composed of water, protein, minerals. and fat. The two-component model of body composition (Brozek, Grande, Anderson, and Keys 1963; Siri 1961) divides the body into a fat component and a **fat-free body** (FFB) component. The FFB consists of all residual chemicals and tissues including water, muscle (protein), and bone (mineral). The **two-component model** of body composition makes the following five assumptions:

1. The density of fat is 0.901 g·cc^{-1}.
2. The density of the FFB is 1.100 g·cc^{-1}.
3. The densities of fat and the FFB components (water, protein, mineral) are the same for all individuals.
4. The densities of the various tissues composing the FFB are constant within an individual, and their proportional contribution to the lean component remains constant.
5. The individual being measured differs from the reference body only in the amount of fat; the FFB of the reference body is assumed to be 73.8% water, 19.4% protein, and 6.8% mineral.

This two-component model has served as the foundation for the **hydrodensitometry** (underwater weighing) method. With use of the assumed proportions of water, mineral, and protein and their respective densities, equations were derived to convert the individual's total body density (Db) from hydrostatic weighing into relative body fat proportions (%BF). Two commonly used equations are the Siri (1961) equation, %BF = (4.95/Db − 4.50) × 100, and the Brozek, Grande, Anderson, and Keys (1963) equation, %BF = (4.57/Db − 4.142) × 100. These two equations yield similar %BF estimates for body densities ranging from 1.0300 to 1.0900 g/cc. For example, if a client's measured Db is 1.0500 g/cc, the %BF estimates, obtained by plugging this value into the Siri and Brozek equations, are 21.4% and 21.0%, respectively.

Generally, two-component model equations provide accurate estimates of %BF as long as the basic assumptions of the model are met. However, there is no guarantee that the FFB composition of an individual within a certain population subgroup will exactly match the values assumed for the reference body. Researchers have reported that FFB density varies with age, gender, ethnicity, level of body fatness, and physical activity level, depending mainly on the relative proportion of water and

mineral composing the FFB (Baumgartner, Heymsfield, Lichtman, Wang, and Pierson 1991; Williams et al. 1993). For example, the average FFB density of black women and black men (~1.106 g/cc) is greater than 1.10 g/cc because of their higher mineral content (~7.3% FFB) and/or relative body protein (Cote and Adams 1993; Ortiz et al. 1992; Wagner and Heyward 2001). Because of this difference in FFB density, the body fat of blacks will be systematically underestimated when two-component model equations are used to estimate %BF. In fact, negative %BF values were reported for professional football players whose measured Db exceeded 1.10 g·cc^{-1} (Adams, Mottola, Bagnall, and McFadden 1982). Likewise, the FFB density of children is estimated to be only 1.084 g/cc because of their relative lower mineral (5.2% FFB) and higher body water values (76.6% FFB) compared to the reference body (Lohman, Boileau, and Slaughter 1984). Also, the average density of the FFB of elderly men and women is 1.096 g/cc because of the relatively low body mineral value (6.2% FFB) in this population (Heymsfield et al. 1989). Thus, the relative body fat of children and persons who are elderly will be systematically overestimated using two-component model equations.

For certain population subgroups, therefore, scientists have applied **multicomponent models** of body composition based on measured total body water and bone mineral values. With the multicomponent approach, you can avoid systematic errors in estimating body fat by replacing the reference man with population-specific reference bodies that take into account the age (e.g., for children, for persons who are elderly), gender, and ethnicity of the individual. Table 8.2 provides population-specific formulas for converting Db to %BF. You will note that population-specific conversion formulas do not yet exist for all age groups within each ethnic group. You may have to use the age-specific conversion formula developed for white males and females in these cases. Also, you can use the population-specific conversion formulas for anorexic and obese females only when it is obvious that your client is either anorexic or obese.

LABORATORY METHODS FOR ASSESSING BODY COMPOSITION

In many laboratory and clinical settings, **densitometry** and dual-energy X-ray absorptiometry are used to obtain reference measures of body

Table 8.2   Population-Specific Formulas for Conversion of Body Density to Percent Body Fat

Population	Age	Gender	%BF	FFB$_d$ (g/cc)*
Ethnicity				
American Indian	18-60	Female	(4.81)/Db − 4.34	1.108
Black	19-45	Male	(4.86)/Db − 4.39	1.106
	24-79	Female	(4.85)/Db − 4.39	1.106
Hispanic	20-40	Female	(4.87)/Db − 4.41	1.105
Japanese native	18-48	Male	(4.97)/Db − 4.52	1.099
		Female	(4.76)/Db − 4.28	1.111
	61-78	Male	(4.87)/Db − 4.41	1.105
		Female	(4.95)/Db − 4.50	1.100
White	7-12	Male	(5.30)/Db − 4.89	1.084
		Female	(5.35)/Db − 4.95	1.082
	13-16	Male	(5.07)/Db − 4.64	1.094
		Female	(5.10)/Db − 4.66	1.093
	17-19	Male	(4.99)/Db − 4.55	1.098
		Female	(5.05)/Db − 4.62	1.095
	20-80	Male	(4.95)/Db − 4.50	1.100
		Female	(5.01)/Db − 4.57	1.097
Levels of body fatness				
Anorexic	15-30	Female	(5.26)/Db − 4.83	1.087
Obese	17-62	Female	(5.00)/Db − 4.56	1.098

*FFB$_d$ = fat-free body density; Db = body density; %BF = percent body fat.
Data from Heyward and Stolarczyk 1996, *Applied body composition assessment.* Champaign, IL: Human Kinetics.

composition. For densitometric methods, total **body density** (Db) is estimated from the ratio of body mass to body volume (Db = BM/BV). Body volume can be measured using either hydrostatic weighing or air displacement plethysmography.

Hydrostatic Weighing

Hydrostatic weighing (HW) is a valid, reliable, and widely used laboratory method for assessing total Db. Hydrostatic weighing provides an estimate of total body volume (BV) from the water displaced by the body's volume. According to **Archimedes' principle**, weight loss under water is directly proportional to the volume of water displaced by the body volume. For calculating Db, body mass is divided by body volume. The total Db is a function of the amounts of muscle, bone, water, and fat in the body.

Using Hydrostatic Weighing

Determine BV by totally submerging the body in an underwater weighing tank or pool and measuring the **underwater weight** (UWW) of the body. To measure UWW, you can use either a chair attached to an HW scale (see figure 8.1) or a platform attached to load cells (see figure 8.2). Given that the weight loss under water is directly proportional to the volume of water displaced by the body's volume, the BV is equal to the body mass (BM) minus the UWW (see figure 8.3). The net UWW is the difference between the UWW and the weight of the chair or platform and its supporting equipment (i.e., tare weight). The BV must be corrected for the volume of air remaining in the lungs after a maximal expiration (i.e., **residual volume** or RV), as well as the volume of air in the gastrointestinal tract (GV). The GV is assumed to be 100 ml.

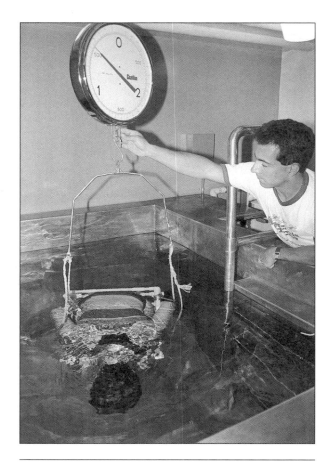

Figure 8.1 Hydrostatic weighing using scale and chair.

The RV is commonly measured using helium dilution, nitrogen washout, or oxygen dilution techniques. The RV is measured in liters and must be converted to kilograms (kg) in order to correct UWW. This is easy to do because 1 L of water weighs approximately 1 kg; therefore, the water weight per liter of RV is 1 kg. The BV is corrected by subtracting the equivalent weight of the RV and the GV (100 ml or 0.1 kg). Since water density varies with water temperature, the BV is corrected for water density (see appendix D.1, "Density of Water at Different Temperatures," p. 310). Under normal circumstances, the water temperature of the underwater weighing tank or swimming pool will be between 34 and 36 °C. The resulting equation for BV is

$$BV = [(BM - net\ UWW)/density\ of\ water] - (RV + GV)$$

Calculate body density (Db in g/cc) by dividing BM by BV: Db = BM/BV. After you calculate Db, you can convert it into **percent body fat (%BF)** by using the appropriate population-specific conversion formula (see table 8.2).

You should adhere to the following guidelines when using the HW technique:

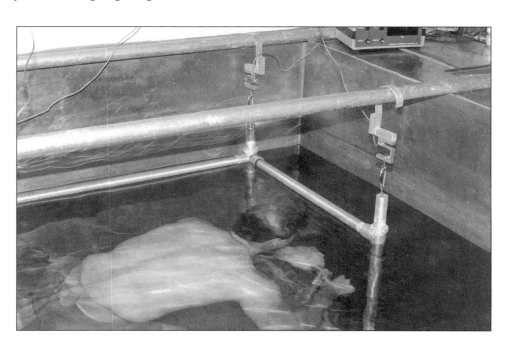

Figure 8.2 Hydrostatic weighing using load cells and platform.

Hydrostatic Weighing Data

Name _____   Date _____

Gender _____   Body mass_____ lb _____ kg   Age_____

I.   Residual volume (average 2 trials within 100 ml)

Trial 1 _____   Trial 2 _____   Trial 3 _____

Average RV = _____ L

II. Water temperature _____ °C

Water density _____ g/cc
(see appendix D.1)

III. Gross underwater weight (in kg)

Trial 1 _____   Trial 6 _____

Trial 2 _____   Trial 7 _____

Trial 3 _____   Trial 8 _____

Trial 4 _____   Trial 9 _____

Trial 5 _____   Trial 10 _____

Average (3 trials within 0.1 kg) = _____ kg

IV. Tare weight (chair, platform, and
supporting equipment) _____ kg

V.   Net underwater weight
gross UWW _____ – tare weight _____
= _____ kg

VI. Body volume

[(BM in kg – net UWW in kg)/water density]
– (RV + GV)   BV = _____ L
Note. GV assumed value = 100 ml or 0.1 L

VII. Body density = BM (kg)/BV (L) (carry out to 5
or 6 decimal places)   Db = _____ g/cc

VIII. % body fat (select conversion formula from
table 8.2)   BF = _____ %

IX. Fat mass = BM × % BF (decimal)
_____ × _____   FM = _____ kg

X.   Fat-free mass = BM – FM
_____ – _____   FFM = _____ kg

Figure 8.3 Hydrostatic weighing data collection form.

GUIDELINES FOR HYDROSTATIC WEIGHING

1. The client should wear a lightweight swimming suit.

2. The client must urinate and eliminate as much gas and feces as possible before testing.

3. Determine the accuracy of the HW scale prior to use by hanging calibrated weights from the scale and checking the corresponding scale values. To calibrate a load cell system, place the weights on the platform and check the recorded values.

4. Weigh the chair or platform, as well as all of the supporting equipment, under water; this is the *tare weight.*

5. Check the water temperature just prior to the test; it should range between 34 and 36 °C.

6. Have the client kneel on the underwater weighing platform or assume a sitting posi-

tion in the chair after removing all air bubbles from swimming suit and hair. You may need to add a scuba diving belt around your client's waist to facilitate this position.

7. The client should exhale as much air as possible when totally submerged in the tank. The highest weight at the end of maximal exhalation is the gross UWW. The client should try to remain as still as possible during this procedure.

8. Administer at least 3 to 10 trials. Average the highest 3 trials within 0.1 kg, and record this figure as the gross UWW.

9. Determine the net UWW by subtracting the weight of the chair or platform, its supporting equipment, the swimsuit, and the scuba diving belt (if used) from the gross UWW.

Special Considerations

Some clients may have difficulty performing the HW test using these standardized procedures. Accurate test results are highly dependent on the client's skill, cooperation, and motivation. The following section addresses the use of modified HW procedures, as well as other questions and concerns about the use of this method.

■ *What should I do when my client is unable to blow out all of the air from the lungs or remain still while under water?*

You will likely come across clients who are uncomfortable expelling all of the air from their lungs during HW. In such cases, you can weigh these individuals at functional residual capacity (FRC) or total lung capacity (TLC) instead of RV. Thomas and Etheridge (1980) underwater-weighed 43 males, comparing the body densities measured at FRC (taken at the end of normal expiration while the person was submerged) and at RV (at the end of maximal expiration). The two methods yielded similar results. Similarly, Timson and Coffman (1984) reported that Db measured by HW at TLC (vital capacity + RV) was similar (less than 0.3% BF difference) to that measured at RV if TLC was measured in the water. However, when the TLC was measured out of the water, the method significantly overestimated Db. When using these modifications of the HW method, you must still measure RV in order to calculate the FRC or TLC of your client. Also, be certain to substitute the appropriate lung volume (FRC or TLC) for RV in the calculation of BV.

Because of their lower Db, clients with greater amounts of body fat are more buoyant than leaner individuals; therefore, they have more difficulty remaining motionless while under the water. To correct this problem, place a weighted scuba belt around the client's waist. Be certain to include the weight of the scuba belt when measuring and subtracting the tare weight of the HW system.

■ *What should I do when my clients are afraid to put their face in the water or are not flexible enough to get their backs and heads completely submerged?*

Occasionally, you will encounter clients who are extremely fearful of being submerged, who dislike facial contact with water, or who are unable to bend forward to assume the proper body position for HW. In such cases, a satisfactory alternative would be to weigh your clients at TLC while their heads remain above water level. Donnelly et al.

(1988) compared this measure (i.e., TLCNS or total lung capacity with head not submerged) to the criterion Db obtained from HW at RV for 75 men and 67 women. Vital capacity was measured with the subject submerged in the water to shoulder level. Regression analysis yielded the following equations for predicting Db at RV, using the Db determined at TLCNS as the predictor:

Males

$$Db \text{ at } RV = 0.5829(Db \text{ at TLCNS}) + 0.4059$$

$$r = 0.88, SEE = 0.0067 \text{ g·cc}^{-1}$$

Females

$$Db \text{ at } RV = 0.4745(Db \text{ at TLCNS}) + 0.5173$$

$$r = 0.85, SEE = 0.0061 \text{ g·cc}^{-1}$$

The correlations *(r)* between the actual Db at RV and the predicted Db at RV were high, and the standard errors of estimate *(SEE)* were within acceptable limits. These equations were cross-validated for an independent sample of 20 men and 20 women. The differences between the Db from HW at RV and the predicted Db from weighing at TLCNS were quite small (less than 0.0014 g·cc^{-1} or 0.7% BF). This method may be especially useful for HW of older adults, obese individuals with limited flexibility, and people with physical disabilities.

■ *Will the accuracy of the HW test be affected if I estimate RV instead of measuring it?*

Several prediction equations have been developed to estimate RV based on the individual's age, height, gender, and smoking status (see appendix D.2, "Prediction Equations for Residual Volume (RV)," p. 311). However, these RV prediction equations have large prediction errors (*SEE* = 400 to 500 ml). When RV is measured, the precision of the HW method is excellent (≤1% BF). However, this precision error increases substantially (±2.8% to 3.7% BF) when RV is estimated (Morrow, Jackson, Bradley, and Hartung 1986). Therefore, always measure RV when you are using the HW method.

■ *When is the best time during the menstrual cycle to hydrostatically weigh my female clients?*

Some women, particularly those whose body weight fluctuates widely during their menstrual cycles, may have significantly different estimates of Db and %BF when weighed hydrostatically at different times in their cycles. Bunt, Lohman, and Boileau (1989) reported that changes in total body water values due to water retention during the menstrual cycle partly explain the differences in body weight and Db during a menstrual cycle. On the average, the relative body fat of the women was 24.8% BF at their lowest body weights, compared to an average of 27.6% BF at their peak body weights during their menstrual cycles. Because their low and peak body weights occurred at different times during the menstrual cycle (varied from 0 to 14 days prior to the onset of the next menses), the effect of total body water fluctuations cannot be routinely controlled by using the same day of the menstrual cycle for all women. However, when you are monitoring changes in body composition over time or establishing healthy body weight for a female client, it is recommended that you hydrostatically weigh her at the same time within her menstrual cycle and outside of the period of her perceived peak body weight.

Air Displacement Plethysmography

Air displacement plethysmography is a densitometric method used in laboratory and clinical settings to measure BV and to estimate Db. Compared to HW, this method is relatively expensive, requiring the use of a whole-body plethysmograph (e.g., Bod Pod). The Bod Pod is a large, egg-shaped fiberglass chamber that uses air displacement and pressure-volume relationships to derive BV (see figure 8.4). The BV is equal to the volume of air in the empty chamber minus the volume of air remaining in the chamber after the client enters the chamber. This method is quick (usually takes 5 to 10 min) and requires minimal compliance by the client. For this test, the client sits in the chamber and breathes normally. Although residual lung volume does not have to be measured, thoracic gas volume is assessed during this procedure using a gentle "puffing" maneuver. This value is used to correct BV. For detailed descriptions of test procedures and operating principles, see Dempster and Aitkens 1995.

Although the Bod Pod has been commercially available for several years, there is a limited amount of research validating this device. Early studies showed good test-retest reliability and acceptable validity ($r^2 = 0.93$, *SEE* = 1.8% BF) compared to HW (McCrory, Gomez, Bernauer, and Mole 1995). However, more recent research has produced mixed results. The Bod Pod significantly overestimated the average Db of children (Lockner, Heyward, Baumgartner, and Jenkins

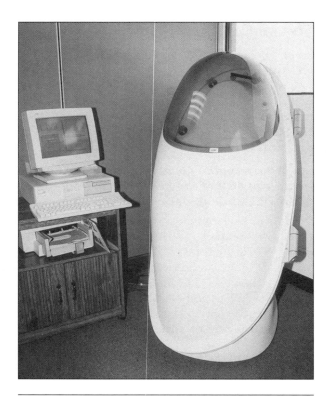

Figure 8.4 Air displacement plethysmograph.

2000) and collegiate football players (Collins et al. 1999) who were hydrostatically weighed; in contrast, the average Db of black men and an ethnically mixed sample of physically active men and women was systematically underestimated (Janot et al. 2001; Wagner, Heyward, and Gibson 2000). Still, some researchers have reported good agreement between the Bod Pod and HW methods for estimating Db of healthy adults (Biaggi et al. 1999; Nunez et al. 1999). Certainly more research is needed to firmly establish the validity of the Bod Pod.

Dual-Energy X-Ray Absorptiometry

Dual-energy X-ray absorptiometry (DXA) is gaining recognition as a reference method for body composition research (see figure 8.5). This method yields estimates of bone mineral, fat, and lean soft-tissue mass. Dual-energy X-ray absorptiometry is highly reliable, and there is a high degree of agreement between %BF estimates obtained by HW and by DXA (Going et al. 1993; Van Loan and Mayclin 1992). Dual-energy X-ray absorptiometry is an attractive alternative to HW as a reference method because it is safe and rapid

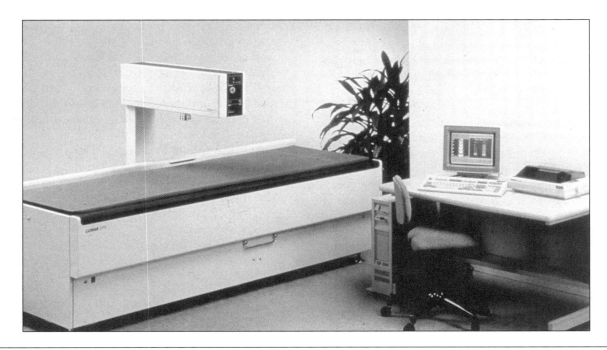

Figure 8.5 Dual-energy X-ray absorptiometer.
Photo courtesy of Lunar Corporation, Madison, WI.

(a total body scan takes 10 to 20 min), requires minimal subject cooperation, and, most importantly, accounts for individual variability in bone mineral content. Although some body composition prediction equations have been developed and validated using DXA as a reference method, further research is needed before DXA can be firmly established as the best reference method (Kohrt 1995; Roubenoff, Kehayias, Dawson-Hughes, and Heymsfield 1993).

FIELD METHODS FOR ASSESSING BODY COMPOSITION

In field settings, you can use more practical methods to estimate your client's body composition. Your choices include bioelectrical impedance, skinfold, and other types of anthropometric prediction equations. To use these methods and equations appropriately, you need to understand the basic assumptions and principles, as well as the potential sources of measurement error for each method. You must closely follow standardized testing procedures, and you must practice in order to perfect your measurement techniques for each method. For more detailed information about

these field methods and how they are applied to various population subgroups, see Heyward and Stolarczyk (1996).

Skinfold Method

A **skinfold** (SKF) indirectly measures the thickness of subcutaneous adipose tissue. When you use the SKF method to estimate total Db in order to calculate relative body fat (%BF), certain basic relationships are assumed:

■ **The SKF is a good measure of subcutaneous fat.** Research has demonstrated that the subcutaneous fat, assessed by SKF measurements at 12 sites, is similar to the value obtained from magnetic resonance imaging (Hayes, Sowood, Belyavin, Cohen, and Smith 1988).

■ **The distribution of fat subcutaneously and internally is similar for all individuals within each gender.** The validity of this assumption is questionable. There are large interindividual differences in the patterning of subcutaneous adipose tissue within and between genders (Martin, Ross, Drinkwater, and Clarys 1985). Older subjects of the same gender and Db have proportionately less subcutaneous fat than their younger counterparts. Also, lean individuals have a higher proportion of internal fat, and the proportion of fat located internally decreases as overall body fatness increases (Lohman 1981).

- **Because there is a relationship between subcutaneous fat and total body fat, the sum of several SKFs can be used to estimate total body fat.** Research has established that SKF thicknesses at multiple sites measure a common body fat factor (Jackson and Pollock 1976; Quatrochi et al. 1992). It is assumed that approximately one-third of the total fat is located subcutaneously in men and women (Lohman 1981). However, there is considerable biological variation in subcutaneous, intramuscular, intermuscular, and internal organ fat deposits (Clarys, Drinkwater, and Marfell-Jones 1987), as well as essential lipids in bone marrow and the central nervous system. Age, gender, and degree of fatness all affect variation in fat distribution (Lohman 1981).

- **There is a relationship between the sum of SKFs (ΣSKF) and Db.** This relationship is linear for homogenous samples (population-specific SKF equations) but nonlinear over a wide range of Db (generalized SKF equations) for both men and women. A linear regression line depicting the relationship between the ΣSKF and Db will fit the data well only within a narrow range of body fatness values. Thus, you will get an inaccurate estimate if you use a population-specific equation to estimate the Db of a client who is not representative of the sample used to develop that equation (Jackson 1984).

- **Age is an independent predictor of Db for both men and women.** Using age and the quadratic expression of the sum of skinfolds (ΣSKF^2) accounts for more variance in Db of a heterogeneous population than using the ΣSKF^2 alone (Jackson 1984).

Using the Skinfold Method

Skinfold prediction equations are developed using either linear (population specific) or quadratic (generalized) regression models. There are well over 100 population-specific equations for predicting Db from various combinations of SKFs, circumferences, and bony diameters (Jackson and Pollock 1985). These equations were developed for relatively homogeneous populations and are assumed to be valid only for individuals having similar characteristics, such as age, gender, ethnicity, or level of physical activity. For example, an equation derived specifically for 18- to 21-year-old sedentary men would not be valid for predicting the Db of 35- to 45-year-old sedentary men. Population-specific equations are based on a linear relationship between SKF fat and Db (linear model); however, research shows that there is a curvilinear relationship (quadratic model) between SKFs and Db across a large range of body fatness (see figure 8.6). Population-specific equations will tend to underestimate %BF in fatter subjects and overestimate it in leaner subjects.

Using the quadratic model, Jackson and colleagues (Jackson and Pollock 1978; Jackson, Pollock, and Ward 1980) developed generalized equations applicable to individuals varying greatly in age (18 to 60 years) and body fatness (up to 45% BF). These equations also take into account the effect of age on the distribution of subcutaneous and internal fat. An advantage of the generalized equations is that you can use one equation, instead of several, to accurately estimate your clients' %BF.

Most equations use two or three SKFs to predict Db. Experts recommend using equations that have SKF measures from a variety of sites, including both upper- and lower-body sites (Martin et al. 1985). The Db is then converted to %BF using the appropriate population-specific conversion formula (see table 8.2). Table 8.3 presents commonly used population-specific and generalized SKF prediction equations. Calculating the Db and %BF is tedious and time consuming, especially when you are assessing the body composition of many clients. You will save time by using computer software (Ng 1997) developed for the SKF equations included in this book. This software selects the appropriate SKF equation and population-specific conversion formula in table 8.2 to estimate %BF based on physical demographics (e.g., age, gender, ethnicity, and physical activity level) of your client. Using these equations, you can accurately estimate the %BF of your clients within the recommended value, ±3.5% BF (Lohman 1992).

Alternatively, nomograms exist for some SKF prediction equations. The nomogram in figure 8.7 was specifically developed for the Jackson sum of three SKF equations. To use this nomogram, plot the sum of three skinfolds (Σ3SKF) and age in the appropriate columns and use a ruler to connect these two points. The corresponding %BF is read at the point where the connecting line intersects the %BF column on the nomogram.

Although nomograms are potential time-savers, you should be aware that this nomogram is based on a two-component body composition model, using the Siri equation to convert Db to %BF. In general, use this nomogram only to calculate %BF of white males.

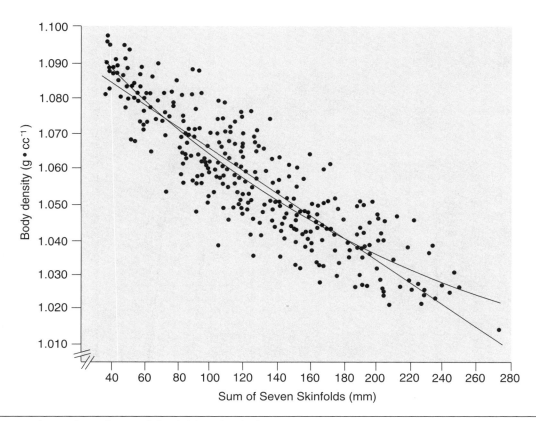

Figure 8.6 Relationship of sum of skinfolds to body density.

Reprinted, by permission, from A.S. Jackson and M.L. Pollock, 1978, "Generalized equations for predicting body density of men," *British Journal of Nutrition* 40: 502.

Table 8.3 Skinfold Prediction Equations

SKF sites	Population subgroups	Equation	Reference
Σ7SKF (chest + abdomen + thigh + triceps + subscapular + suprailiac + midaxilla)	Black or Hispanic women, 18-55 years	Db (g/cc)[a] = 1.0970 − 0.00046971(Σ7SKF) + 0.00000056(Σ7SKF)^2 − 0.00012828(age)	Jackson et al. (1980)
	Black men or male athletes, 18-61 years	Db (g/cc)[a] = 1.1120 − 0.00043499(Σ7SKF) + 0.00000055(Σ7SKF)^2 − 0.00028826(age)	Jackson and Pollock (1978)
Σ4SKF (triceps + anterior suprailiac + abdomen + thigh)	Female athletes, 18-29 years	Db (g/cc)[a] = 1.096095 − 0.0006952(Σ4SKF) + 0.0000011(Σ4SKF)^2 − 0.0000714(age)	Jackson et al. (1980)
Σ3SKF (triceps + suprailiac + thigh)	White or anorexic women, 18-55 years	Db (g/cc)[a] = 1.0994921 − 0.0009929(Σ3SKF) + 0.0000023(Σ3SKF)^2 − 0.0001392(age)	Jackson et al. (1980)
(chest + abdomen + thigh)	White men, 18-61 years	Db (g/cc)[a] = 1.109380 − 0.0008267(Σ3SKF) + 0.0000016(Σ3SKF)^2 − 0.0002574(age)	Jackson and Pollock (1978)
Σ2SKF (triceps + calf)	Black or white boys, 6-17 years	%BF = 0.735(Σ2SKF) + 1.0	Slaughter et al. (1988)
	Black or white girls, 6-17 years	%BF = 0.610(Σ2SKF) + 5.1	Slaughter et al. (1988)

ΣSKF = sum of skinfolds (mm).

[a]Use population-specific conversion formulas to calculate %BF (percent body fat) from Db (body density).

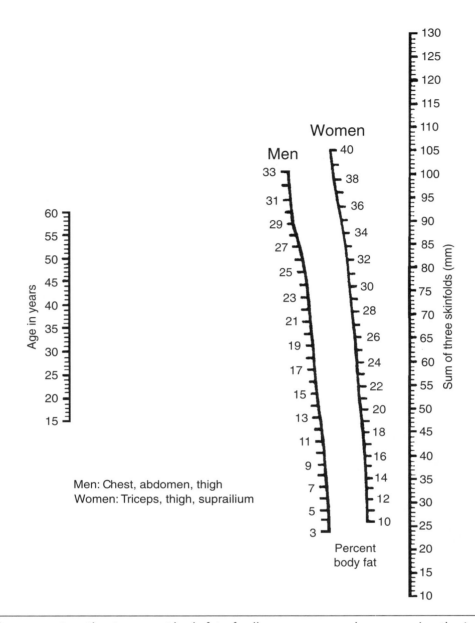

Figure 8.7   Nomogram to estimate percent body fat of college-age men and women using the Jackson sum-of-three skinfold equations.

From "A Nomogram for the Estimate of Percent Body Fat From Generalized Equations" by W.B. Baun and M.R. Baun, 1981. Reprinted with permission from *Research Quarterly for Exercise and Sport,* 52, p. 382. Copyright 1981 by American Alliance for Health, Physical Education, and Dance, 1900 Association Drive, Reston, VA 20191.

Skinfold Technique

It takes a great deal of time and practice to develop your skill as a SKF technician. Following standardized procedures (p. 173) will increase the accuracy and reliability of your measurements (Harrison et al. 1988).

You will also be able to increase your skill as a SKF technician by following the recommendations (p. 173) made by experts in the field (Jackson and Pollock 1985; Lohman, Pollock, Slaughter, Brandon, and Boileau 1984; Pollock and Jackson 1984).

Sources of Measurement Error

The accuracy and precision of SKF measurements and the SKF method are affected by the technician's skill, the type of SKF caliper, and client factors. The following questions and responses address these sources of measurement error.

STANDARDIZED PROCEDURES FOR SKINFOLD MEASUREMENTS

1. Take all SKF measurements on the right side of the body.

2. Carefully identify, measure, and mark the SKF site, especially if you are a novice SKF technician (see appendix D.3, "Standardized Sites for Skinfold Measurements," p. 312).

3. Grasp the SKF firmly between the thumb and index finger of your left hand. Lift the fold 1 cm (0.4 in.) above the site to be measured.

4. Lift the fold by placing the thumb and index finger 8 cm (~3 in.) apart on a line that is perpendicular to the long axis of the SKF. The long axis is parallel to the natural cleavage lines of the skin. For individuals with extremely large SKFs, you will need to separate your thumb and finger more than 8 cm in order to lift the fold.

5. Keep the fold elevated while you take the measurement.

6. Place the jaws of the caliper perpendicular to the fold, approximately 1 cm below the thumb and index finger and halfway between the crest and the base of the fold. Release the jaw pressure slowly.

7. Take the SKF measurement 4 sec after the pressure is released. The ACSM (2000) recommends that you wait only 1 to 2 sec before reading the caliper.

8. Open the jaws of the caliper to remove it from the site. Close the jaws slowly to prevent damage or loss of calibration.

RECOMMENDATIONS FOR SKINFOLD TECHNICIANS

- Be meticulous when locating the anatomical landmarks used to identify the SKF site, when measuring the distance, and when marking the site with a surgical marking pen.

- Read the dial of the caliper to the nearest 0.1 mm (Harpenden or Holtain), 0.5 mm (Lange), or 1 mm (plastic calipers).

- Take a minimum of two measurements at each site. If values vary from each other by more than ±10%, take additional measurements.

- Take SKF measurements in a rotational order (circuits) rather than taking consecutive readings at each site.

- Take the SKF measurements when the client's skin is dry and lotion free.

- Do not measure SKFs immediately after exercise because the shift in body fluid to the skin tends to increase the size of the SKF.

- Practice taking SKFs on 50 to 100 clients.

- Avoid using plastic calipers if you are an inexperienced SKF technician. Instead use metal calipers.

- Train with skilled SKF technicians and compare your results.

- Use a SKF training videotape that demonstrates proper SKF techniques (Lohman 1987).

- Seek additional training at workshops held at state, regional, and national conferences.

■ *Is there high agreement among SKF values when the measurements are taken by two different technicians?*

A major source of measurement error is differences between SKF technicians. Objectivity, or between-technician reliability, is improved when SKF technicians follow standardized testing procedures, practice taking SKFs together, and mark the SKF site (Pollock and Jackson 1984). A major cause of low intertester reliability is improper location and measurement of the SKF sites (Lohman, Pollock, Slaughter, Brandon, and Boileau 1984).

■ *Are the anatomical descriptions for specific SKF sites the same for all SKF equations?*

In the past, for some SKF sites, the anatomical location and direction of the fold have varied. For example, Behnke and Wilmore (1974) recommend measuring the abdominal SKF using a horizontal fold adjacent to the umbilicus; Jackson and Pollock (1978), however, recommend measuring a vertical fold taken 2 cm (0.8 in.) lateral to the umbilicus. Inconsistencies such as this have led to confusion and lack of agreement among SKF technicians. As a result, groups of experts in the field of anthropometry have developed standardized testing procedures and detailed descriptions for identification and measurement of SKF sites (Harrison et al. 1988; Ross and Marfell-Jones 1991). Appendix D.3, "Standardized Sites for Skinfold Measurements" (p. 312), summarizes some of the most commonly used sites, as described in the *Anthropometric Standardization Reference Manual.*

Although the objective is to have all SKF technicians follow standardized procedures and recommendations for site location and SKF measurements, you may not be able to do so under all circumstances. For example, if you are using the generalized equations of Jackson and Pollock (1978) and Jackson et al. (1980), the chest, midaxillary, subscapular, abdominal, and suprailiac SKFs will be located at sites that differ from those described in the *Anthropometric Standardization Reference Manual.* The descriptions for the sites used in these equations are presented in appendix D.4, "Skinfold Sites for Jackson's Generalized Skinfold Equations," page 317.

■ *How many measurements do I need to take at each SKF site?*

A lack of intra-technician reliability or consistency of measurements by the SKF technician is another source of error for the SKF method. You need to practice your SKF technique on 50 to 100 clients to develop a high degree of skill and proficiency (Jackson and Pollock 1985). Take a minimum of two measurements at each site using a

rotational order. If values vary from each other by more than ±10%, take additional measurements and average the two trials that meet this criterion. Use this average value in the SKF prediction equation. The ±10% value for duplicate measurements at each site is recommended as the standardized procedure in the *Anthropometric Standardized Reference Manual.*

However, if you are preparing to take an ACSM certification examination, you will need to modify this standardized procedure slightly by using the ACSM-recommended criterion for duplicate SKF measurements. The ACSM (2000) also suggests taking at least two measurements at each site in rotational order; however, these two measurements at a given site need to be within 1 to 2 mm of each other. If you take more than two measurements to meet this criterion, average the two trials that are within ±1 to 2 mm of each other and use this value in the prediction equation to estimate Db and %BF. On the other hand, some researchers suggest taking three SKF measurements at each site and using the median (middle score) instead of the mean (average) (Ward and Anderson 1998).

■ *What types of SKF calipers are available and how do these calipers differ?*

When selecting a SKF caliper for use in the field, you should consider factors such as cost, durability, and degree of precision needed, as well as your skill and experience as a SKF technician. You

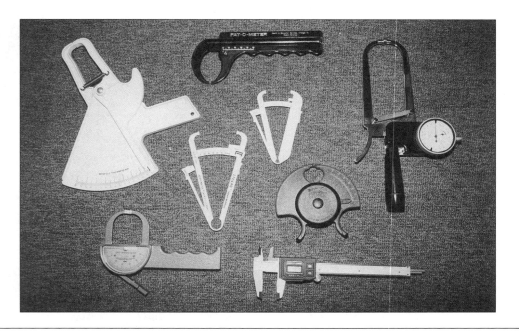

Figure 8.8 Skinfold calipers.

can use either high-quality metal calipers or plastic calipers to measure SKF thickness (see figure 8.8). The cost of SKF calipers varies in relation to the materials used in construction (metal or plastic) and the caliper's accuracy and precision throughout the range of measurement. High-quality instruments, such as Harpenden, Lange, Holtain, and Lafayette calipers, exert constant pressure (~10 g/mm^2) throughout the range of measurement (0 mm to 60 mm). Calipers should not vary in tension more than 2.0 g/mm^2 over the range, and the jaw pressure should not exceed 15 g/mm^2 (Edwards, Hammond, Healy, Tanner, and Whitehouse 1955). Excessive tension and force cause client discomfort (a pinching sensation) and significantly reduce the SKF measurement (Gruber, Pollock, Graves, Colvin, and Braith 1990). High-quality calipers also have excellent scale precision (0.2 mm and 1.0 mm for Harpenden and Lange calipers, respectively). The accuracy of your caliper should be checked periodically using a high-precision Vernier caliper or SKF calibration blocks.

Although the Harpenden and Lange SKF calipers have similar pressure characteristics, a number of researchers have reported that SKFs measured with Harpenden calipers produce smaller values than those measured with the Lange calipers (Gruber et al. 1990; Lohman, Pollock, et al. 1984). Even though the pressure is similar for the Lange (9.3 g/mm^2) and Harpenden (9.36 g/mm^2) calipers, researchers noted that opening the jaws of the Harpenden caliper requires three times more force. Therefore, it is more likely that the Harpenden caliper will compress adipose tissue to a greater extent, resulting in smaller SKF measurements than the Lange caliper would yield.

■ Are plastic SKF calipers as accurate as metal SKF calipers?

Compared to high-quality calipers such as the Harpenden, Lange, Holtain, and Skyndex metal calipers, plastic SKF calipers (i.e., Body Caliper, McGaw caliper, Fat-O-Meter, Ross adipometer, and Slim-Guide) have less scale precision (~2 mm), nonconstant tension throughout the range of measurement (Hawkins 1983), a smaller measurement scale (~40 mm), and less consistency when used by inexperienced SKF technicians (Lohman, Pollock, et al. 1984). Despite these differences, several researchers (Cataldo and Heyward 2000; Hawkins 1983; Lohman, Pollock, et al. 1984) reported only small differences (≤0.5 mm) between SKFs measured with high-quality metal calipers (Harpenden, Holtain, or Lange) and plastic calipers (Body Caliper, McGaw caliper, Ross adipometer, or Fat-O-Meter).

Other researchers comparing a variety of both metal and plastic calipers reported that SKFs measured with Harpenden, McGaw, Slim-Guide, and Skyndex calipers were significantly smaller than those measured with Lange calipers (Burgert and Anderson 1979; Gruber et al. 1990; Hawkins 1983; Lohman, Pollock, et al. 1984; Zando and Robertson 1987). Lohman, Pollock, et al. (1984) noted that differences among instruments (Harpenden, Lange, Holtain, and Ross adipometer calipers) varied depending on the SKF technician. Differences among technicians were less for the Harpenden and Holtain calipers compared to the Lange caliper and Ross adipometer. Given that the caliper's type may be a potential source of measurement error, be sure you use the same caliper when monitoring changes in your client's SKF thicknesses.

■ Will my client's hydration level affect the SKF measurements?

Skinfold measurements may also be affected by compressibility of the adipose tissue and hydration levels of your clients (Ward, Rempel, and Anderson 1999). Martin, Drinkwater, and Clarys (1992) reported that variation in SKF compressibility may be an important limitation of the SKF method. In addition, an accumulation of extracellular water (edema) in the subcutaneous tissue—caused by factors such as peripheral vasodilation or certain diseases—may increase SKF thicknesses (Keys and Brozek 1953). This suggests that you should not measure SKFs immediately after exercise, especially in hot environments. Also, most of the weight gain experienced by some women during their menstrual cycles is caused by water retention (Bunt et al. 1989). This theoretically could increase SKF thicknesses, particularly on the trunk and abdomen; but there are no empirical data to support or refute this hypothesis.

■ Should SKFs be measured on the right or left side of the body?

There are only small differences (1 to 2 mm) between SKF thicknesses on the right and left sides of the body for the typical individual. The standard practice in the United States, as well as in European and developing countries, however, is to take SKF measurements on the right side of the body, as recommended in the *Anthropometric Standardization Reference Manual* (Lohman, Roche, and Martorell 1988) and by the International Society for the Advancement of Kinanthropometry (Norton et al. 2000).

■ *Should I use SKFs to measure the body fat of obese clients?*

It is difficult, even for highly skilled SKF technicians, to measure the SKF thickness of extremely obese individuals accurately. Sometimes the client's SKF thickness exceeds the maximum aperture of the caliper, and the jaws of the caliper may slip off the fold during the measurement, resulting in a potentially embarrassing and awkward situation for you and your client. Therefore, avoid using the SKF method to measure body fat of extremely obese clients.

Bioelectrical Impedance Method

Bioelectrical impedance analysis (BIA) is a rapid, noninvasive, and relatively inexpensive method for evaluating body composition in field settings. With this method, a low-level electrical current is passed through the client's body, and the **impedance** (Z), or opposition to the flow of current, is measured with a BIA analyzer. You can estimate the individual's total body water (TBW) from the impedance measurement because the electrolytes in the body's water are excellent conductors of electrical current. When the volume of TBW is large, the current flows more easily through the body with less resistance (R). The resistance to current flow is greater in individuals with large amounts of body fat, since adipose tissue, with its relatively low water content, is a poor conductor of electrical current. Because the water content of the FFB component is relatively large (~73% water), **fat-free mass** (FFM) can be predicted from TBW estimates. Individuals with large FFM and TBW have less resistance to current flowing through their bodies than those with a smaller FFM.

Bioelectrical impedance indirectly estimates FFM and TBW. Therefore, the following assumptions are made about the geometric shape of the body and the relationship of impedance to the length and volume of the conductor.

■ **The human body is shaped like a perfect cylinder with a uniform length and cross-sectional area.** Of course, this assumption is not entirely true. Because the body segments are not uniform in length or cross-sectional area, resistance to the flow of current through these body segments will differ.

■ **Assuming the body is a perfect cylinder, at a fixed signal frequency (e.g., 50 kHz), the impedance (Z) to current flow through the body is** directly related to the length (L) of the conductor (height) and inversely related to its cross-sectional area [$Z = p(L/A)$, where **p** is the specific resistivity of the body's tissues and is assumed to be constant]. To express this relationship in terms of Z and the body's volume, instead of its cross-sectional area, the equation is multiplied by L/L: $Z = p(L/A)(L/L)$. $A \times L$ is equal to volume (V), so rearranging this equation yields $V = pL^2/Z$. Thus, the volume of the FFM or TBW of the body is directly related to L^2, or height squared (ht^2), and indirectly related to Z.

■ **Biological tissues act as conductors or insulators, and the flow of current through the body will follow the path of least resistance.** Because the FFM contains large amounts of water (~73%) and electrolytes, it is a better conductor of electrical current than fat. Fat is anhydrous and a poor conductor of electrical current. The total body impedance, measured at the constant frequency of 50 kHz, primarily reflects the volumes of the water and muscle compartments composing the FFM and the extracellular water volume (Kushner 1992).

■ **Impedance is a function of resistance and reactance, where $Z = \sqrt{(R^2 + X_c^2)}$. Resistance** (R) is a measure of pure opposition to current flow through the body; **reactance** (X_c) is the opposition to current flow caused by capacitance produced by the cell membrane (Kushner 1992). R is much larger than X_c (at a 50-kHz frequency) when whole-body impedance is measured; therefore, R is a better predictor of FFM and TBW than Z (Lohman 1989). For these reasons, the **resistance index** (ht^2/R), instead of ht^2/Z, is often used in many BIA models to predict FFM or TBW.

Using the Bioelectrical Impedance Analysis Method

Bioelectrical impedance analysis prediction equations are based on either population-specific or generalized models. These equations provide acceptable estimates of FFM and TBW because of theoretical and empirical relationships among FFM, TBW, and bioimpedance measures. Many population-specific BIA equations have been developed for homogenous subgroups to account for differences due to age, ethnicity, gender, physical activity level, and level of body fatness. These equations are valid only for individuals whose physical characteristics are similar to those in the specific population subgroup. For example, an equation developed for younger men will systematically overestimate the FFM of older men (Deurenberg, van der Kooy, Evers, and Hulshof 1990).

As an alternative to population-specific equations, you can use generalized BIA equations developed for heterogeneous populations varying in age, gender, and body fatness. This approach accounts for the biological variability among population subgroups by including factors such as age and gender as predictor variables in BIA equations estimating FFM or TBW (Deurenberg et al. 1990; Gray, Bray, Gemayel, and Kaplan 1989; Kushner and Schoeller 1986; Van Loan and Mayclin 1987).

Table 8.4 presents commonly used population-specific and generalized BIA equations. With these equations, you can accurately estimate the FFM of your clients within the recommended values, ±2.8 kg for women and ±3.5 kg for men (Lohman 1992). To use these equations, obtain R and X_c directly from your BIA analyzer. Computer software exists that allows you to select an appropriate BIA equation to estimate your client's FFM based on physical characteristics (i.e., age, gender, ethnicity, physical activity level, and level of body fatness) (Ng 1997). Using this software will save time and prevent errors in calculating FFM from these equations. Estimate the %BF of your client by determining the **fat mass** (FM = BM – FFM) and dividing FM by the client's body mass [%BF = (FM/BM) × 100].

Experts recommend not using the FFM and %BF estimates obtained directly from your BIA analyzer (e.g., BMR, Holtain, RJL, or Valhalla) unless you know for sure which equations are programmed in the analyzer's computer software, obtain information from the manufacturer regarding the validity and accuracy of these equations, and determine that these equations are applicable to your clients.

Although the relative predictive accuracy of the BIA method is similar to that of the SKF method, BIA may be preferable in some settings for the following reasons:

- It does not require a high degree of technician skill.

- It is generally more comfortable and does not intrude as much upon the client's privacy.

- It can be used to estimate body composition of obese individuals (Gray, Bray, Gemayel, and Kaplan 1989; Segal, Van Loan, Fitzgerald, Hodgdon, and Van Itallie 1988).

Table 8.4 Bioelectrical Impedance Analysis Prediction Equations

Population subgroup	%BF level[a]	Equation	Reference
American Indian, Hispanic, or white men, 17-62 years	<20% BF	FFM (kg) = 0.00066360(ht²) – 0.02117(R) + 0.62854(BM) – 0.12380(age) + 9.33285	Segal et al. (1988)
	≥20% BF	FFM (kg) = 0.00088580(ht²) – 0.02999(R) + 0.42688(BM) – 0.07002(age) + 14.52435	Segal et al. (1988)
American Indian, black, Hispanic, or white women, 17-62 years	<30% BF	FFM (kg) = 0.000646(ht²) – 0.014(R) + 0.421(BM) + 10.4	Segal et al. (1988)
	≥30% BF	FFM (kg) = 0.00091186(ht²) – 0.01466(R) + 0.29990(BM) – 0.07012(age) + 9.37938	Segal et al. (1988)
White boys and girls, 8-15 years	NA	FFM (kg) = 0.62(ht²/R) + 0.21(BM) + 0.10(X_c) + 4.2	Lohman (1992)
White boys and girls, 10-19 years	NA	FFM (kg) = 0.61(ht²/R) + 0.25(BM) + 1.31	Houtkooper et al. (1992)
Female athletes, age range not reported	NA	FFM (kg) = 0.73(ht²/R) + 0.16(BM) + 2.0	Houtkooper et al. (1989)
Male athletes, 19-40 years	NA	FFM (kg) = 0.186(ht²/R) + 0.701(BM) + 1.949	Oppliger et al. (1991)

NA = not applicable.

[a]For clients who are obviously lean, use the <20% BF (men) and <30% BF (women) equations. For clients who are obviously obese, use the ≥20% BF (men) and ≥30% BF (women) equations. For clients who are not obviously lean or obese, calculate their FFM using *both* the lean and obese equations and then average the two FFM estimates.

%BF = percent body fat; FFM = fat-free mass; BM = body mass; R = resistance; X_c = reactance.

Bioelectrical Impedance Analysis Technique

The tetrapolar method uses four electrodes applied to the hand, wrist, foot, and ankle (see figure 8.9). An excitation current (500 µÅ to 800 µÅ) at 50 kHz is applied at the source (distal) electrodes on the hand and foot, and the voltage drop due to impedance is detected by the sensor (proximal) electrodes on the wrist and ankle. The total resistance to current flow through the arm, trunk, and leg is measured using this type of electrode configuration.

The accuracy of the BIA method depends on controlling factors that may increase the measurement error. Therefore, it is important to determine whether your client meets all BIA guidelines outlined below. In addition, you need to closely follow the standardized testing procedures for the BIA method presented on p. 179.

Sources of Measurement Error

The accuracy and precision of the BIA measurements are affected by instrumentation, technician skill, client factors, and environmental factors. The following questions and responses deal with these sources of measurement error.

■ *Can different types of bioimpedance analyzers be used interchangeably?*

Two commonly used impedance analyzers are the RJL System (Detroit, MI) and the Vahalla Scientific analyzer (San Diego, CA). Research demonstrates that the whole-body resistance (hand to foot) measured by different brands of single-

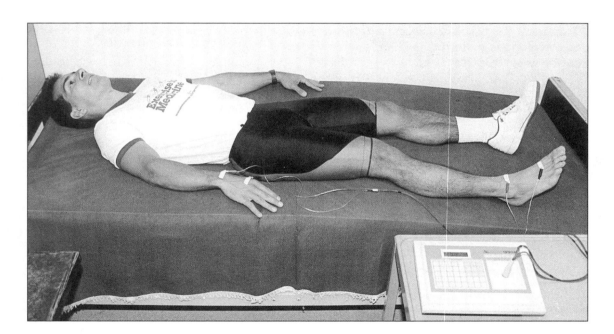

Figure 8.9 Bioelectrical impedance analysis electrode placement and client positioning.

BIOELECTRICAL IMPEDANCE ANALYSIS CLIENT GUIDELINES

■ Client should not eat or drink anything within 4 hr of the test.

■ Client should not engage in moderate or vigorous exercise within 12 hr of the test.

■ Client should void completely within 30 min of the test.

■ Client should abstain from alcohol consumption within 48 hr of the test.

■ Client should ingest no diuretics, including caffeine, prior to the assessment, unless prescribed by a physician.

■ You should postpone testing of female clients who perceive they are retaining water during the stage of the menstrual cycle they are in.

STANDARDIZED TESTING PROCEDURES FOR BIOELECTRICAL IMPEDANCE ANALYSIS METHOD

1. Bioimpedance measures are taken on the right side of the body, with the client lying supine on a nonconductive surface, in a room with normal ambient temperature (~22 °C or 72 °F).

2. Clean the skin at the electrode sites with an alcohol pad.

3. Place the sensor (proximal) electrodes (see figure 8.9) (a) on the dorsal surface of the wrist so that the upper border of the electrode bisects the head of the ulna and (b) on the dorsal surface of the ankle so that the upper border of the electrode bisects the medial and lateral malleoli. You can use a measuring tape and surgical marking pen to mark these points for electrode placement.

4. Place the source (distal) electrodes at the base of the second or third metacarpophalangeal joints of the hand and foot (see figure 8.9). Make certain the proximal and distal electrodes are separated by at least 5 cm (2 in.).

5. Attach the lead wires to the appropriate electrodes. Attach the red leads to the wrist and ankle, and the black leads to the hand and foot.

6. Make certain that the client's legs and arms are abducted approximately 45° to each other. There should be no contact between the thighs or between the arms and the trunk.

frequency analyzers differs by as much as 36 Ω (Graves, Pollock, Colvin, Van Loan, and Lohman 1989). For example, the average %BF estimated for men from one BIA equation differed by 6.3% BF with use of the Valhalla and Bioelectrical Sciences (BES, La Jolla, CA) analyzers to measure R. In general, the Valhalla analyzer produced significantly higher resistances (~16 to 19 Ω) than the RJL analyzer for men and women, causing a systematic underestimation of FFM (Graves et al. 1989). To control for this potential source of measurement error, always use the same instrument when monitoring changes in your client's body composition.

Recently, less expensive bioimpedance analyzers have been marketed for home use. The Tanita™ analyzer measures lower-body resistance between the right and left legs as the individual stands on the analyzer's electrode plates. The Omron Body Logic™ analyzer, which is handheld, measures upper-body resistance between the right and left arms (see figure 8.10). The upper-body or lower-body resistance measured by these analyzers will be larger than whole-body resistance (right arm-trunk-right leg) given the relatively smaller volumes of these body segments compared to the trunk.

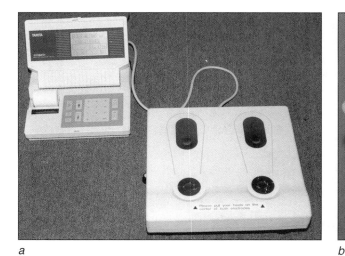
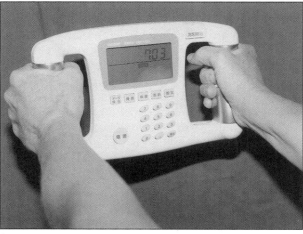

a b

Figure 8.10 Tanita *(a)* and Omron *(b)* bioelectrical impedance analyzers.

There is limited research verifying the validity and applicability of equations programmed into these newer analyzers for assessing body composition of diverse subgroups of the population. Some studies reported that the Tanita analyzers (Model TBF-105, TBF-515, and TBF-531) significantly overestimate the %BF of young adults (Ashley and Tonery 2000; Rodd, Ho, and Enzler 1999; Whatley, Florence, Ransdell, Yates, and Clasey 1999). The Omron analyzers (Model HBF-300 and HBF-301), on the other hand, provide an accurate estimate of %BF for young and middle-aged adults (19 to 59 years) from black, Hispanic, and white ethnic groups; the prediction errors for the Omron analyzers were similar to those reported for whole-body BIA equations (Ashley and Tonery 2000; Gibson, Heyward, and Mermier 2000; Loy et al. 1998; Whatley, Florence, Ransdell, Yates, and Clasey 1999).

■ *Does eating or being dehydrated have any effect on bioimpedance measures?*

A major source of error for the BIA method is variability due to the client's state of hydration. Eating, drinking, and dehydration alter the individual's hydration state, thereby affecting total body resistance and the estimate of FFM. Taking resistance measures 2 to 4 hr after a meal decreases R and is likely to overpredict the FFM of your client by almost 1.5 kg (Deurenberg, Westrate, Paymans, and van der Kooy 1988). Dehydration, on the other hand, increases resistance ($\sim$40 Ω), resulting in a 5.0-kg underestimate of FFM (Lukaski 1986).

■ *Will bioimpedance test results be affected if I measure my client immediately after exercise?*

The degree to which test results are affected depends on the intensity and duration of the exercise workout. Researchers have reported that jogging and cycling at moderate intensities ($\sim$70% $\dot{V}O_2$max) for 90 to 120 min substantially decrease resistance (50 to 70 Ω), resulting in a large overestimate of FFM ($\sim$12 kg) (Khaled et al. 1988; Lukaski 1986). The decrease in resistance after strenuous exercise most likely reflects the relatively greater loss of body water in the sweat and expired air, compared to the loss of electrolytes. This leads to a higher electrolyte concentration in the body's fluids, thereby lowering resistance values (Deurenberg et al. 1988). Increases in core body temperature and skin temperature also may contribute to the sharp decline in resistance after exercising because increased skin temperature (33.4 °C compared to 24 °C) decreases resistance (Caton, Mole, Adams, and Heustis 1988).

■ *Are bioimpedance measures affected by the menstrual cycle?*

Although the menstrual cycle alters the TBW value, the ratio of extracellular to intracellular water, and body mass (Mitchell et al. 1993), there are only small changes in bioimpedance measures (Z and R) between the follicular and premenstrual stages ($\sim$5 to 8 Ω) and between menses and the follicular stage ($\sim$7 Ω) (Deurenberg et al. 1988; Gleichauf and Rose 1989). In women experiencing relatively large body weight gains (2 to 4 kg) during the menstrual cycle, a substantial part of this weight gain is due to an increase in TBW (Bunt et al. 1989). Until there are more conclusive data dealing with this issue, you should take BIA measurements at a time during the menstrual cycle when the client perceives that she is not experiencing a large weight gain. This practice should minimize error and yield a more accurate estimate of FFM for your clients.

■ *Is there a high degree of agreement in bioimpedance values when measurements are taken by two different technicians?*

Technician skill is not a major source of measurement error for the BIA method. There is virtually no difference in resistance measurements taken by different technicians, provided that each follows standardized procedures for electrode placement and client positioning (Jackson, Pollock, Graves, and Mahar 1988). The proximal sensor electrodes, in particular, need to be correctly positioned at the wrist and ankle. For example, a 1-cm displacement of the sensor electrodes may result in a 2% error in resistance (Elsen, Siu, Pineda, and Solomons 1987). As a standard practice, you should take bioimpedance measures on the right side of the body.

Other Anthropometric Methods

Anthropometry refers to the measurement of the size and proportion of the human body. You can use circumferences, SKF thicknesses, skeletal breadths, and segment lengths to assess the size and proportions of body segments. In addition to body size and proportions, anthropometric measures have been used to assess total body and regional body composition. Anthropometric indexes such as body mass index (BMI) and **waist-to-hip circumference ratio (WHR)** are used to identify individuals at risk for disease. Compared to SKF measures, these anthropometric methods are relatively simple, are inexpensive, and do not require a high degree of technical skill and training.

Several basic principles are associated with the use of anthropometric measures such as BMI, circumferences, and skeletal diameters to estimate body composition:

■ **Circumferences are affected by fat mass, muscle mass, and skeletal size; therefore, these measures are related to fat mass and lean body mass.** Jackson and Pollock (1978) reported that circumference and bony diameter measures are markers of lean body mass (muscle mass and skeletal size); however, some circumferences are also highly associated with the fat component. Waist circumference, for example, is strongly related to total abdominal fat (Despres, Prud'homme, Pouliot, Tremblay, and Bouchard, 1991). These findings confirm the fact that circumference measures reflect both the fat and fat-free components of body composition.

■ **Skeletal size is directly related to lean body mass.** Behnke (1961) proposed that lean body mass could be accurately estimated from skeletal diameters, and subsequently developed equations for predicting lean body mass. Cross-validation of these equations yielded a moderately high (r = 0.80) relationship and closely estimated the average lean body mass obtained from hydrodensitometry (Wilmore and Behnke 1969, 1970). Behnke's hypothesis was also supported by the observation that skeletal diameters, along with circumference measures, are strong markers of lean body mass (Jackson and Pollock 1978).

■ **To estimate total body fat from weight-to-height indexes, the index should be highly related to body fat but independent of height.** On the basis of data from two large-scale epidemiological surveys (National Health and Nutrition Examination Surveys I and II), Micozzi, Albanes, Jones, and Chumlea (1986) reported that BMI (body mass divided by height squared) is not significantly related to height of men and women, but is directly related to SKF thickness and the estimated fat area of the arm in adults. However, the relationship to body fat varies with age and gender (Deurenberg, Westrate, and Seidell 1991; Ross et al. 1988; Wagner, Heyward, and Stolarczyk 1997). Body mass index is not totally independent of height, especially in younger children (<15 years of age).

Using Anthropometric Methods

You can use various combinations of SKFs, circumferences, and skeletal diameters to estimate your client's body composition. This section includes only those equations using circumferences and diameters as predictors, for the following reasons:

■ The predictive accuracy of anthropometric (circumference and diameter) equations is not greatly improved by the addition of SKF measures.

■ Anthropometric equations using only circumferences as predictors estimate the body fatness of obese individuals more accurately than SKF prediction equations (Seip and Weltman 1991).

■ Compared to SKFs, circumferences and skeletal diameters can be measured with less error (Bray and Gray 1988a).

■ Some practitioners may not have access to SKF calipers.

Population-specific anthropometric equations are valid for, and can be applied only to, individuals whose physical characteristics (age, gender, and level of body fatness) are similar to those in a specific population subgroup. For example, anthropometric equations developed to estimate the body composition of obese individuals (Weltman, Levine, Seip, and Tran 1988; Weltman, Seip, and Tran 1987) should not be applied to non-obese individuals. On the other hand, generalized equations, applicable to individuals varying in age and body fatness, have been developed for heterogeneous populations of women (15 to 79 years of age; 13% to 63% BF) and men (20 to 78 years of age; 2% to 49% BF) (Tran and Weltman 1988, 1989). Table 8.5 provides anthropometric prediction equations that are applicable to various population subgroups. You can also use computer software to obtain body composition estimates from these equations for your clients (Ng 1997).

Anthropometric measures have other uses besides estimating your client's body composition. For example, in epidemiological studies, BMI is used as a crude index of obesity, and ACSM (2000) recommends using BMI to evaluate obesity (BMI ≥ 30 kg/m^2) as a risk factor for coronary heart disease. The BMI is the ratio of body mass to height squared: BMI (kg/m^2) = BM (kg)/ht^2 (m). Alternatively, you can use a nomogram (see figure 8.11) to calculate and classify BMI (Bray 1978). To use this nomogram, plot your client's height and BM in the appropriate columns and connect these two

Table 8.5 Circumference and Skeletal Diameter Prediction Equations

Population subgroup	Equation	Reference
White women, 15-79 years	Db (g/cc)[a] = 1.168297 − 0.002824(abdom C[b]) + 0.0000122098(abdom C[b])^2 − 0.000733128(hip C) + 0.000510477(ht) − 0.00021616(age)	Tran and Weltman (1989)
White men, 18-40 years	FFM (kg) = 39.652 + 1.0932(BM) + 0.8370(bi-iliac D) + 0.3297(AB$_1$ C) − 1.0008(AB$_2$ C) − 0.6478(knee C)	Wilmore and Behnke (1969)
White, obese women, 20-60 years	%BF = 0.11077(abdom C[b]) − 0.17666(ht) + 0.14354(BM) + 51.033	Weltman et al. (1988)
White, obese men, 24-68 years	%BF = 0.31457(abdom C[b]) − 0.10969(BM) + 10.834	Weltman et al. (1987)

[a]Use population-specific conversion formula to calculate %BF from Db.

[b]abdom C (cm) is the average abdominal circumference measured at two sites: (1) anteriorly midway between the xiphoid process of sternum and the umbilicus and laterally between the lower end of the rib cage and iliac crests; (2) at the umbilicus level.

Db = body density; FFM = fat-free mass; %BF = percent body fat; BM = body mass.

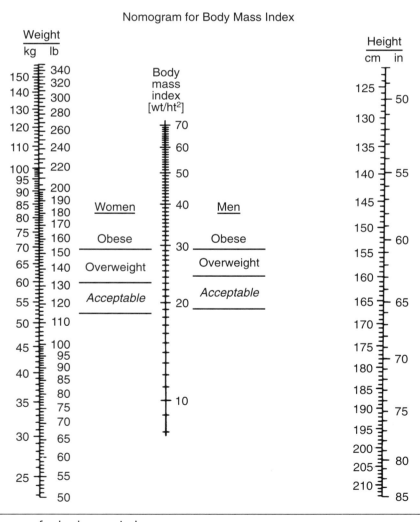

Figure 8.11 Nomogram for body mass index.

Reprinted, by permission, from G.A. Bray, 1978, "Definitions, measurements, and classifications of the syndromes of obesity," *International Journal of Obesity* 2(2): 99-112.

points with a ruler. Read the corresponding BMI at the point where the connecting line intersects the BMI column on the nomogram.

Table 8.6 describes standards for classifying BMI. The use of BMI in health risk appraisals assumes that people who are disproportionately heavy are so because of excess fat mass. It is important to remember that BMI is only a crude index of obesity and that it should not be used to estimate body fatness of your clients because the prediction error is unacceptable ($\geq 5.0\%$ BF).

The waist circumference and WHR can help you distinguish between patterns of fat distribution in the upper and lower body. These measures are strongly associated with visceral fat and appear to be acceptable indexes of intra-abdominal fat (Despres et al. 1991; Seidell et al. 1987). The National Cholesterol Education Program (NCEP 2001) recommends using waist circumference (>100 cm for men and >88 cm for women) to evaluate obesity as a risk factor for coronary heart disease and metabolic diseases. Also, young adults with WHR values in excess of 0.94 for men and 0.82 for women are at high risk for adverse health consequences (Bray and Gray 1988b). However, the WHR is not valid for evaluating fat distribution in prepubertal children (Peters, Fox, Armstrong, Sharpe, and Bell 1992). The WHR norms (see table 8.7) were established using the standardized measurement procedures described in the *Anthropometric Standardization Reference Manual.* Calculate the WHR by dividing waist circumference (cm) by hip circumference (cm). Alternatively, you can use a nomogram (figure 8.12) to obtain WHR. Plot the client's waist and hip circumferences in the corresponding columns of the nomogram and connect the points with a ruler. Read the WHR at the point where this line intersects the WHR column.

When you are evaluating the body weight of your client using height-weight tables, you can improve their usefulness by classifying frame size according to skeletal diameters. Skeletal breadths are important estimators of the bone and muscle

Table 8.6 Classification of Overweight and Obesity Based on Body Mass Index (BMI)

Classification	BMI value
Underweight	<18.5
Normal weight	18.5-24.9
Overweight	25.0-29.9
Obesity	
Class I	30.0-34.9
Class II	35.0-39.9
Class III	≥ 40.0

Data from WHO Report. 1998. Obesity: Preventing and managing the global epidemic. *Report of a WHO Consultation on Obesity.* Geneva: World Health Organization.

Table 8.7 Waist-to-Hip Circumference Ratio Norms for Men and Women

	Age	Risk			
		Low	Moderate	High	Very high
Men	20-29	<0.83	0.83-0.88	0.89-0.94	>0.94
	30-39	<0.84	0.84-0.91	0.92-0.96	>0.96
	40-49	<0.88	0.88-0.95	0.96-1.00	>1.00
	50-59	<0.90	0.90-0.96	0.97-1.02	>1.02
	60-69	<0.91	0.91-0.98	0.99-1.03	>1.03
Women	20-29	<0.71	0.71-0.77	0.78-0.82	>0.82
	30-39	<0.72	0.72-0.78	0.79-0.84	>0.84
	40-49	<0.73	0.73-0.79	0.80-0.87	>0.87
	50-59	<0.74	0.74-0.81	0.82-0.88	>0.88
	60-69	<0.76	0.76-0.83	0.84-0.90	>0.90

Adapted from Bray and Gray (1988b) "Obesity – Part I – Pathogensis", *Western Journal of Medicine* 149: 432.

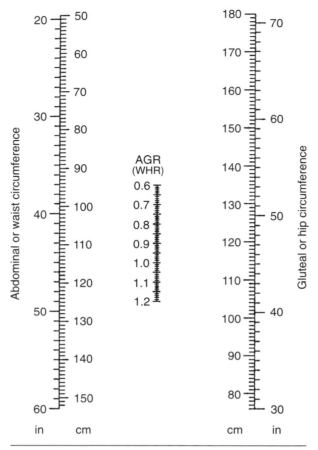

Figure 8.12 Nomogram for waist-to-hip ratio (WHR).
Reprinted by permission of *The Western Journal of Medicine*, G.A. Bray and D.S. Gray, "Obesity: Part I—Pathogenesis," 1988, 149: 432. ©BMJ Publishing Group.

components of FFM; therefore, an estimate of frame size allows you to differentiate between those who weigh more because of a large musculoskeletal mass and those who are overweight because of a large fat mass. You can classify frame size by using reference data for elbow breadth (see table 8.8). The anatomical landmarks for measuring elbow breadth are described in appendix D.6, "Standardized Sites for Bony Breadth Measurements," page 319.

Anthropometric Techniques

You must practice in order to become proficient in measuring skeletal diameters and circumferences. Following the standardized procedures (see p. 185) will increase the accuracy and reliability of your measurements (Callaway et al. 1988; Wilmore et al. 1988).

Sources of Measurement Error

The accuracy and reliability of anthropometric measures are potentially affected by equipment, technician skill, and client factors (Bray 1978; Callaway et al. 1988). The following questions and responses concern these sources of measurement error.

■ *What equipment will I need to measure bony widths?*

Use skeletal anthropometers and sliding or spreading calipers to measure bony widths and

Table 8.8	Elbow Breadth Norms (in cm) for Men and Women in the United States			
		Frame size		
	Age (years)	Small	Medium	Large
Men	18-24	≤6.6	>6.6 and <7.7	≥7.7
	25-34	≤6.7	>6.7 and <7.9	≥7.9
	35-44	≤6.7	>6.7 and <8.0	≥8.0
	45-54	≤6.7	>6.7 and <8.1	≥8.1
	55-64	≤6.7	>6.7 and <8.1	≥8.1
	65-74	≤6.7	>6.7 and <8.1	≥8.1
Women	18-24	≤5.6	>5.6 and <6.5	≥6.5
	25-34	≤5.7	>5.7 and <6.8	≥6.8
	35-44	≤5.7	>5.7 and <7.1	≥7.1
	45-54	≤5.7	>5.7 and <7.2	≥7.2
	55-64	≤5.8	>5.8 and <7.2	≥7.2
	65-74	≤5.8	>5.8 and <7.2	≥7.2

From A.R. Frisancho, 1984, "New Standards for Weight and Body Composition by Frame Size and Height for Assessment of Nutritional Status of Adults and the Elderly." *American Journal of Clinical Nutrition* 40: 810. Copyright 1984 by the *American Journal of Clinical Nutrition*. Reprinted by permission.

STANDARDIZED PROCEDURES FOR ANTHROPOMETRIC MEASUREMENTS

1. Take all circumference and bony diameter measurements of the limbs on the right side of the body.

2. Carefully identify and measure the anthropometric site. Be meticulous about locating anatomical landmarks used to identify the measurement site (see appendix D.5, "Standardized Sites for Circumference Measurements," p. 318; and appendix D.6, "Standardized Sites for Bony Breadth Measurements," p. 319), and instruct your clients to relax their muscles during the measurement.

3. Take a minimum of three measurements at each site in rotational order.

4. To measure the breadth of smaller segments, like the elbow or wrist, use small sliding calipers (range of 30 cm or 11.8 in.) with greater scale precision instead of larger skeletal anthropometers (range of 60 to 80 cm or 23.6 to 31.5 in.).

5. Hold the skeletal anthropometer or caliper in both hands so the tips of the index fingers are adjacent to the tips of the caliper.

6. Place the caliper on the bony landmarks and apply firm pressure to compress the underlying muscle, fat, and skin. Apply pressure to a point where the measurement no longer continues to decrease.

7. Use an anthropometric tape to measure circumferences. Hold the zero end of the tape in your left hand, positioned below the other part of the tape that is held in your right hand.

8. Apply tension to the tape so that it fits snugly around the body part but does not indent the skin or compress the subcutaneous tissue.

9. For some circumferences (e.g., waist, hip, and thigh), you should align the tape in a horizontal plane, parallel to the floor.

body breadths (see figure 8.13). The precision characteristics (0.05 to 0.50 cm) and range of measurement (0 to 210 cm) depend on the type of skeletal anthropometer or caliper you are using (Wilmore et al. 1988). The instruments must be carefully maintained and must be calibrated periodically so that their accuracy can be checked and restored.

■ *Can I use any type of tape measure to measure body circumferences?*

Use an anthropometric tape measure to measure circumferences (see figure 8.13). The tape measure should be made from a flexible material that does not stretch with use. You can use a plastic-coated tape measure if an anthropometric tape measure is not available. Some anthropometric tapes have a spring-loaded handle (i.e., Gulick handle) that allows a constant tension to be applied to the end of the tape during the measurement.

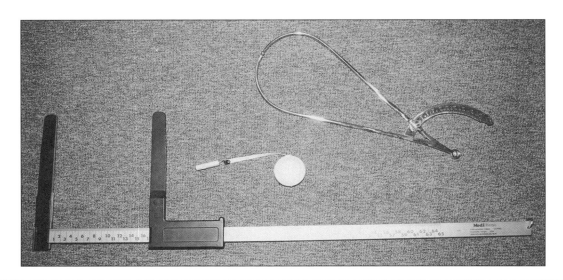

Figure 8.13 Skeletal anthropometers and anthropometric tape measure.

■ *How much skill and practice are required to ensure accurate circumference and skeletal diameter measurements?*

Compared to the SKF method, technician skill is not a major source of measurement error. However, you need to practice in order to perfect the identification of the measurement sites and your measurement technique. Experts recommend practicing on at least 50 people and taking a minimum of three measurements for each site in rotational order (Callaway et al. 1988). Closely follow standardized testing procedures for locating measurement sites, positioning the anthropometer or tape measure, and applying tension during the measurement. Appendix D.5 ("Standardized Sites for Circumference Measurements," p. 318) and appendix D.6 ("Standardized Sites for Bony Breadth Measurements," p. 319) describe some of the most commonly used circumference and skeletal diameter sites.

■ *Is there good agreement in circumference and skeletal diameter values when the measurements are taken by two different technicians?*

Variability in circumference measurements taken by different technicians is relatively small (0.2 to 1.0 cm), with some sites differing more than others (Callaway et al. 1988). Skilled technicians can obtain similar values even when measuring circumferences of obese individuals (Bray and Gray 1988a).

■ *Are the circumferences of obese clients more easily measured than SKFs?*

As with the SKF method, it is more difficult to obtain consistent measurements of circumference for obese compared to lean individuals (Bray and Gray 1988a). However, circumferences are preferable to SKFs for measuring obese clients, for several reasons:

■ You can measure circumferences of obese individuals regardless of their size, whereas the maximum aperture of the SKF caliper may not be large enough to allow measurement.

■ Measurement of circumferences requires less technician skill.

■ Differences between technicians are smaller for circumferences compared to SKF measurements (Bray and Gray 1988a).

■ *Is it possible to accurately measure bony widths of heavily muscled and obese clients?*

Accurate measurement of bony diameters in heavily muscled or obese individuals may be difficult because the underlying muscle and fat tissues must be firmly compressed. It may be difficult to identify and palpate bony anatomical landmarks, leading to error in locating the measurement site.

Near-Infrared Interactance Method

Although **near-infrared interactance** (NIR) has been commercially available for several years, research suggests that the equations programmed in the Futrex analyzers (Futrex-5000, Futrex-5000A, and Futrex-1000) have poor validity and unacceptable prediction errors (*SEE* = 3.7% to 6.3% BF). Many studies show that these equations systematically underestimate %BF of adults and overestimate the %BF of children (Eaton, Israel, O'Brien, Hortobagyi, and McCammon 1993; Elia, Parkinson, and Diaz 1990; Heyward, Cook, et al. 1992; Heyward, Jenkins, et al. 1992; Israel et al. 1989; McLean and Skinner 1992; Nielsen et al. 1992; Wilmore, McBride, and Wilmore 1994). Therefore, avoid using these equations to assess the body composition of your clients. Further research is needed to develop and cross-validate gender-specific NIR equations and to determine whether this method is valid for assessing body composition.

SOURCES FOR EQUIPMENT

Product	Manufacturer's Address
Air displacement plethysmograph BOD POD Body Composition System	LMI, Inc. 1980 Oliveri Rd. Suite C Concord, CA 94520 (800) 426-3763 www.bodpod.com

Anthropometers

Spreading calipers
Sliding calipers
Standard skeletal anthropometer

Pfister Import-Export, Inc.
450 Barell Ave.
Carlstadt, NJ 07072
(202) 939-4606

Rosscraft Industries
14732 16A Ave.
Surrey, BC Canada V4A 5M7
(604) 531-5049
tep2000.com/Rosscraft.htm

Anthropometric tape measure

Country Technology, Inc.
P.O. Box 87
Gays Mills, WI 54631
(608) 735-4718
www.fitnessmart.com

Bioimpedance analyzers

Biodynamics

Biodynamics Corp.
3511 NE 45th St. #2
Seattle, WA
(800) 869-6987
www.biodyncorp.com

Omron

OMRON Healthcare, Inc.
300 Lakeview Pkwy.
Vernon Hills, IL 60061
(847) 680-6200
www.omronhealthcare.com

RJL

RJL Systems
33955 Harper Ave.
Clinton TWP, MI 48035
(800) 528-4513
www.rjlsystems.com

Tanita

Tanita Corp.
2625 S. Clearbrook Dr.
Arlington Heights, IL 60005
(800) TANITA-8
www.tanita.com

Tri-frequency

Daninger Medical Technology
140 Fisher Rd.
Columbus, OH 43228
Phone: (614) 276-8267

Valhalla

Valhalla Scientific Inc.
9955 Mesa Rim Rd.
San Diego, CA 92121
(858) 457-5576
www.valhallascientific.com

Xitron Hydra ECF/ICF

Xitron Technologies
8 Claremont
Trabuco Canyon, CA 92679
(949) 766-4495
www.xitron-tech.com

Product	Manufacturer's Address
Calibration instruments/supplies	
Skinfold calibration blocks (15 mm)	Creative Health Products 7621 East Joy Rd. Ann Arbor, MI 48105 (800) 742-4478 www.chponline.com
Standard calibration weights	Ohaus Scale Corp. 29 Hanover Rd. Florham, NJ 07932 (800) 672-7722 www.ohaus.com
Vernier caliper	L.S. Starrett Co. Athol, MA (978) 249-3551 www.lsstarrett.com
Dual-energy X-ray absorptiometers	
Hologic	Hologic, Inc. 35 Crosby Dr. Bedford, MA 01730 (781) 999-7300 www.hologic.com
Norland	Norland Medical Systems, Inc. W6340 Hackbarth Rd. Fort Atkinson, WI 53538 (800) 563-9504 www.norland.com
Lunar	GE Lunar Medical Systems P.O. Box 414 Milwaukee, WI 53201 (608) 274-2663 www.gemedicalsystems.com
Scales	
Chatillon underwater weighing scale Detecto balance beam scale Health-O-Meter balance beam scale Health-O-Meter digital scale Seca digital scale	Creative Health Products 7621 East Joy Rd. Ann Arbor, MI 48105 (800) 742-4478 www.chponline.com
Skinfold calipers	
Adipometer (plastic)	Ross Products Division Abbott Laboratories 625 Cleveland Ave. Columbus, OH 43216 (800) 344-9739 www.ross.com
Body Caliper	The Caliper Company 7 Millside Lane Mill Valley, CA 94941 (800) 655-4960 www.bodycaliper.com

Fat-Control (plastic)	Creative Health Products
Fat-o-meter	7621 East Joy Rd.
Lafayette	Ann Arbor, MI 48105
Skyndex	(800) 742-4478
Slim-Guide	www.chponline.com
Harpenden	Quinton Instruments
	3303 Monte Villa Pkwy.
	Bothell, WA 98021
	(800) 426-0347
	www.quinton.com
Holtain	Pfister Import-Export, Inc.
	450 Barell Ave.
	Carlstadt, NJ 07072
	(201) 939-4606
Lange	Cambridge Scientific Products
	26 New St.
	Cambridge, MA 21613
	(888) 354-8908
	www.cambridgescientific.com
McGaw (plastic)	McGaw, Inc.
	P.O. Box 19791
	Irvine, CA 92713
	(714) 660-2055
	www.mcgaw.com

Stadiometers

Harpenden stadiometer	Pfister Import-Export, Inc.
Holtain stadiometer	450 Barell Ave.
	Carlstadt, NJ 07072
	Phone: (201) 939-4606

KEY POINTS

- Body composition is a key component of health and physical fitness; total body fat and fat distribution are related to disease risk.

- Standards for percent body fat can be used to classify body composition.

- Average %BF and standards for obesity vary according to age, gender, and physical activity levels.

- Hydrostatic weighing is a valid and reliable reference method for assessing body composition.

- Population-specific conversion formulas, based on multicomponent models of body composition, should be used to convert Db into percent body fat.

- The SKF method is widely used in field and clinical settings.

- Generalized SKF equations for the prediction of Db are reliable and valid for a wide range of individuals.

- Bioelectrical impedance analysis is a viable alternative for assessing body composition of diverse population subgroups.

- Circumferences and skeletal diameters can be used to estimate body composition.

- Body mass index is a crude index of total body fatness.

- Waist-to-hip ratio is an acceptable index of body fat distribution.

KEY TERMS

Learn the definition for each of the following key terms. Definitions of terms can be found in "Glossary of Terms," page 349.

air displacement plethysmography

anthropometry

Archimedes' principle

bioelectrical impedance analysis

body density

body volume

densitometry

dual-energy X-ray absorptiometry

fat-free body

fat-free mass

fat mass

hydrodensitometry

hydrostatic weighing

impedance

multicomponent model

near-infrared interactance

percent body fat (%BF)

reactance

relative body fat

residual volume

resistance

resistance index

skinfold

two-component model

underwater weighing

waist-to-hip ratio (WHR)

REVIEW QUESTIONS

In addition to being able to define each of the key terms, test your knowledge and understanding of the material by answering the following review questions.

1. Why is it important to assess the body composition of your clients?

2. What are the standards for classifying obesity and minimal levels of body fat for men and women?

3. What are the assumptions of the two-component model of body composition? Identify two commonly used two-component model equations for converting Db into %BF.

4. Explain how gender, ethnicity, and age affect FFB density and therefore two-component model estimates of %BF.

5. Name three methods that can be used to obtain reference measures of body composition. Which method is best? Explain your choice.

6. Identify two ways to measure (not estimate) your client's Db.

7. Distinguish between total Db and FFB density.

8. Describe how the HW method could be modified to test clients who are unable to be weighed underwater at RV.

9. Identify potential sources of measurement error for the SKF method.

10. In lay terms, explain the basic theory underlying the use of BIA.

11. To obtain accurate estimates of body composition using the BIA method, your client must adhere to pretesting guidelines. Identify these client guidelines.

12. Explain how BMI, WHR, and waist circumference may be used to identify clients at risk due to obesity.

13. Identify suitable field methods and prediction equations (i.e., SKF, BIA, or other anthropometric methods) to estimate body composition for each of the following subgroups of the population: older adults, children, obese individuals, and athletes.

REFERENCES

Adams, J., Mottola, M., Bagnall, K.M., and McFadden, K.D. 1982. Total body fat content in a group of professional football players. *Canadian Journal of Applied Sport Sciences* 7: 36-44.

American College of Sports Medicine (ACSM). 2000. *ACSM's guidelines for exercise testing and prescription,* 6th ed. Philadelphia: Lippincott Williams & Wilkins.

Ashley, C., and Tonery, J. 2000. Validity of commercially-available bioelectrical impedance measures of body composition. *Medicine & Science in Sports & Exercise* 32(Suppl.): S354 [abstract].

Baumgartner, R.N., Heymsfield, S.B., Lichtman, S., Wang, J., and Pierson, R.N. 1991. Body composition in elderly people: Effect of criterion estimates on predictive equations. *American Journal of Clinical Nutrition* 53: 1–9.

Baun, W.B., and Baun, M.R. 1981. A nomogram for the estimate of percent body fat from generalized equations. *Research Quarterly for Exercise and Sport* 52: 380–384.

Behnke, A.R. 1961. Quantitative assessment of body build. *Journal of Applied Physiology* 16: 960–968.

Behnke, A.R., and Wilmore, J.H. 1974. *Evaluation and regulation of body build and composition.* Englewood Cliffs, NJ: Prentice Hall.

Biaggi, R., Vollman, M., Nies, M., Brener, C., Flakoll, P., Levenhagen, D., Sun, M., Karabulut, Z., and Chen, K. 1999. Comparison of air-displacement plethysmography with hydrostatic weighing and bioelectrical impedance analysis for the assessment of body composition in healthy adults. *American Journal of Clinical Nutrition* 69: 898–903.

Bray, G.A. 1978. Definitions, measurements and classifications of the syndromes of obesity. *International Journal of Obesity* 2: 99–113.

Bray, G.A., and Gray, D.S. 1988a. Anthropometric measurements in the obese. In *Anthropometric standardization reference manual,* ed. T.G. Lohman, A.F. Roche, and R. Martorell, 131–136. Champaign, IL: Human Kinetics.

Bray, G.A., and Gray, D.S. 1988b. Obesity. Part I—Pathogenesis. *Western Journal of Medicine* 149: 429–441.

Brozek, J., Grande, F., Anderson, J.T., and Keys, A. 1963. Densitometric analysis of body composition: Revision of some quantitative assumptions. *Annals of the New York Academy of Sciences* 110: 113–140.

Bunt, J.C., Lohman, T.G., and Boileau, R.A. 1989. Impact of total body water fluctuations on estimation of body fat from body density. *Medicine & Science in Sports & Exercise* 21: 96–100.

Burgert, S.L., and Anderson, C.F. 1979. A comparison of triceps skinfold values as measured by the plastic McGaw caliper and the Lange caliper. *American Journal of Clinical Nutrition* 32: 1531–1533.

Callaway, C.W., Chumlea, W.C., Bouchard, C., Himes, J.H., Lohman, T.G., Martin, A.D., Mitchell, C.D., Mueller, W.H., Roche, A.F., and Seefeldt, V.D. 1988. Circumferences. In *Anthropometric standardization reference manual,* ed. T.G. Lohman, A.F. Roche, and R. Martorell, 39–54. Champaign, IL: Human Kinetics.

Cataldo, D., and Heyward, V. 2000. Pinch an inch: A comparison of several high-quality and plastic skinfold calipers. *ACSM's Health & Fitness Journal* 4(3): 12–16.

Caton, J.R., Mole, P.A., Adams, W.C., and Heustis, D.S. 1988. Body composition analysis by bioelectrical impedance: Effect of skin temperature. *Medicine & Science in Sports & Exercise* 20: 489–491.

Clarys, J.P., Martin, A.D., Drinkwater, D.T., and Marfell-Jones, M.J. 1987. The skinfold: Myth and reality. *Journal of Sports Sciences* 5: 3–33.

Collins, M., Millard-Stafford, M., Sparling, P., Snow, T., Rosskopf, L., Webb, S., and Omer, J. 1999. Evaluation of the Bod Pod for assessing body fat in collegiate football players. *Medicine & Science in Sports & Exercise* 31: 1350–1356.

Cote, D.K., and Adams, W.C. 1993. Effect of bone density on body composition estimates in young adult black and white women. *Medicine & Science in Sports & Exercise* 25: 290–296.

Dempster, P., and Aitkens, S. 1995. A new air displacement method for the determination of human body composition. *Medicine & Science in Sports & Exercise* 27: 1692–1697.

Despres, J.P., Prud'homme, D., Pouliot, M.C., Tremblay, A., and Bouchard, C. 1991. Estimation of deep adipose-tissue accumulation from simple anthropometric measurements in men. *American Journal of Clinical Nutrition* 54: 471–477.

Deurenberg, P., van der Kooy, K., Evers, P., and Hulshof, T. 1990. Assessment of body composition by bioelectrical impedance in a population aged >60 y. *American Journal of Clinical Nutrition* 51: 3–6.

Deurenberg, P., Weststrate, J.A., Paymans, I., and van der Kooy, K. 1988. Factors affecting bioelectrical impedance measurements in humans. *European Journal of Clinical Nutrition* 42: 1017–1022.

Deurenberg. P., Westrate, J.A., and Seidell, J.C. 1991. Body mass index as a measure of body fatness: Age- and sex-specific prediction formulas. *British Journal of Nutrition* 65: 105–114.

Donnelly, J.R., Brown, T.E., Israel, R.G., Smith-Sintek, S., O'Brien, K.F., and Caslavka, B. 1988. Hydrostatic weighing without head submersion: Description of a method. *Medicine & Science in Sports & Exercise* 20: 66–69.

Eaton, A.W., Israel, R.G., O'Brien, K.F., Hortobagyi, T., and McCammon, M.R. 1993. Comparison of four methods to assess body composition in women. *European Journal of Clinical Nutrition* 47: 353–360.

Edwards, D.A., Hammond, W.H., Healy, M.J., Tanner, J.M., and Whitehouse, R.H. 1955. Design and accuracy of calipers for measuring subcutaneous tissue thickness. *British Journal of Nutrition* 9: 133–143.

Elia, M., Parkinson, S.A., and Diaz, E. 1990. Evaluation of near infra-red interactance as a method for predicting body composition. *European Journal of Clinical Nutrition* 44: 113–121.

Elsen, R., Siu, M.L., Pineda, O., and Solomons, N.W. 1987. Sources of variability in bioelectrical impedance determinations in adults. In *In vivo body composition studies*, ed. K.J. Ellis, S. Yasamura, and W.D. Morgan, 184–188. London: Institute of Physical Sciences in Medicine.

Frisancho, A.R. 1984. New standard of weight and body composition by frame size and height for assessment of nutritional status of adults and the elderly. *American Journal of Clinical Nutrition* 40: 808–819.

Gibson, A., Heyward, V., and Mermier, C. 2000. Predictive accuracy of Omron Body Logic Analyzer in estimating relative body fat of adults. *International Journal of Sport Nutrition and Exercise Metabolism* 10: 216–227.

Gleichauf, C.N., and Rose, D.A. 1989. The menstrual cycle's effect on the reliability of bioimpedance measurements for assessing body composition. *American Journal of Clinical Nutrition* 50: 903–907.

Going, S.B., Massett, M.P., Hall, M.C., Bare, L.A., Root, P.A., Williams, D.P., and Lohman, T.G. 1993. Detection of small changes in body composition by dual-energy X-ray absorptiometry. *American Journal of Clinical Nutrition* 57: 845–850.

Graves, J.E., Pollock, M.L., Colvin, A.B., Van Loan, M., and Lohman, T.G. 1989. Comparison of different bioelectrical impedance analyzers in the prediction of body composition. *American Journal of Human Biology* 1: 603–611.

Gray, D.S., Bray, G.A., Gemayel, N., and Kaplan, K. 1989. Effect of obesity on bioelectrical impedance. *American Journal of Clinical Nutrition* 50: 255–260.

Gruber, J.J., Pollock, M.L., Graves, J.E., Colvin, A.B., and Braith, R.W. 1990. Comparison of Harpenden and Lange calipers in predicting body composition. *Research Quarterly for Exercise and Sport* 61: 184–190.

Harrison, G.G., Buskirk, E.R., Carter, L.J.E., Johnston, F.E., Lohman, T.G., Pollock, M.L., Roche, A.F., and Wilmore, J.H. 1988. Skinfold thicknesses and measurement technique. In *Anthropometric standardization reference manual*, ed. T.G. Lohman, A.F. Roche, and R. Martorell, 55–70. Champaign, IL: Human Kinetics.

Hawkins, J.D. 1983. An analysis of selected skinfold measuring instruments. *Journal of Health, Physical Education, Recreation and Dance* 54(1): 25–27.

Hayes, P.A., Sowood, P.J., Belyavin, A., Cohen, J.B., and Smith, F.W. 1988. Sub-cutaneous fat thickness measured by magnetic resonance imaging, ultrasound, and calipers. *Medicine & Science in Sports & Exercise* 20: 303–309.

Heymsfield, S.B., Wang, J., Lichtman, S., Kamen, Y., Kehayias, J., and Pierson, R.N. 1989. Body composition in elderly subjects: A critical appraisal of clinical methodology. *American Journal of Clinical Nutrition* 50: 1167–1175.

Heyward, V.H., Cook, K.L., Hicks, V.L., Jenkins, K.A., Quatrochi, J.A., and Wilson, W. 1992. Predictive accuracy of three field methods for estimating relative body fatness of nonobese and obese women. *International Journal of Sport Nutrition* 2: 75–86.

Heyward, V.H., Jenkins, K.A., Cook, K.L., Hicks, V.L., Quatrochi, J.A., Wilson, W., and Going, S. 1992. Validity of single-site and multi-site models of estimating body composition of women using near-infrared interactance. *American Journal of Human Biology* 4: 579–593.

Heyward, V.H., and Stolarczyk, L.M. 1996. *Applied body composition assessment*. Champaign, IL: Human Kinetics.

Houtkooper, L.B., Going, S.B., Westfall, C.H., Lohman, T.G. 1989. Prediction of fat-free body corrected for bone mass from impedance and anthropometry in adult females. *Medicine & Science in Sports & Exercise* 21: 539 [abstract].

Houtkooper, L.B., Lohman, T.G., Going, S.B., and Hall, M.C. 1989. Validity of bioelectric impedance for body composition assessment in children. *Journal of Applied Physiology* 66: 814–821.

Israel, R.G., Houmard, J.A., O'Brien, K.F., McCammon, M.R., Zamora, B.S., and Eaton, A.W. 1989. Validity of near-infrared spectrophotometry device for estimating human body composition. *Research Quarterly for Exercise and Sport* 60: 379–383.

Jackson, A. 1984. Research design and analysis of data procedures for predicting body density. *Medicine & Science in Sports & Exercise* 16: 616–620.

Jackson, A.S., and Pollock, M.L. 1976. Factor analysis and multivariate scaling of anthropometric variables for the assessment of body composition. *Medicine & Science in Sports & Exercise* 8: 196–203.

Jackson, A.S., and Pollock, M.L. 1978. Generalized equations for predicting body density of men. *British Journal of Nutrition* 40: 497–504.

Jackson, A.S., and Pollock, M.L. 1985. Practical assessment of body composition. *The Physician and Sportsmedicine* 13: 76–90.

Jackson, A.S., Pollock, M.L., Graves, J.E., and Mahar, M.T. 1988. Reliability and validity of bioelectrical impedance in determining body composition. *Journal of Applied Physiology* 64: 529–534.

Jackson, A.S., Pollock, M.L., and Ward, A. 1980. Generalized equations for predicting body density of women. *Medicine & Science in Sports & Exercise* 12: 175–182.

Janot, J., Gibson, A., Faria, E., Mermier, C., Wilmerding, V., and Heyward, V. 2001. Body composition assessment of physically active adults: Hydrodensitometry vs. air displacement plethysmography (Bod Pod). *Medicine & Science in Sports & Exercise* 33: S16 [abstract].

Keys, A., and Brozek, J. 1953. Body fat in adult man. *Physiological Reviews* 33: 245–325.

Khaled, M.A., McCutcheon, M.J., Reddy, S., Pearman, P.L., Hunter, G.R., and Weinsier, R.L. 1988. Electrical impedance in assessing human body composition: The BIA method. *American Journal of Clinical Nutrition* 47: 789–792.

Kohrt, W. 1995. Body composition by DXA: Tried and true? *Medicine & Science in Sports & Exercise* 27: 1349–1353.

Kushner, R.F. 1992. Bioelectrical impedance analysis: A review of principles and applications. *Journal of the American College of Nutrition* 11: 199–209.

Kushner, R.F., and Schoeller, D.A. 1986. Estimation of total body water in bioelectrical impedance analysis. *American Journal of Clinical Nutrition* 44: 417–424.

Leger, L.A., Lambert, J., and Martin, P. 1982. Validity of plastic skinfold caliper measurements. *Human Biology* 54: 667–675.

Lockner, D., Heyward, V., Baumgartner, R., and Jenkins, K. 2000. Comparison of air-displacement plethysmography, hydrodensitometry, and dual X-ray absorptiometry for assessing body composition of children 10 to 18 years of age. *Annals of the New York Academy of Sciences* 904: 72–78.

Lohman, T.G. 1981. Skinfolds and body density and their relation to body fatness: A review. *Human Biology* 53: 181–115.

Lohman, T.G. 1987. *Measuring body fat using skinfolds* [videotape]. Champaign, IL: Human Kinetics.

Lohman, T.G. 1989. Bioelectrical impedance. In *Applying new technology to nutrition: Report of the ninth roundtable on medical issues,* 22–25. Columbus, OH: Ross Laboratories.

Lohman, T.G. 1992. *Advances in body composition assessment. Current issues in exercise science series.* Monograph no. 3. Champaign, IL: Human Kinetics.

Lohman, T.G., Boileau, R.A., and Slaughter, M.H. 1984. Body composition in children and youth. In *Advances in pediatric sport sciences,* ed. R.A. Boileau, 29–57. Champaign, IL: Human Kinetics.

Lohman, T.G., Houtkooper, L., and Going, S. 1997. Body fat measurement goes high-tech: Not all are created equal. *ACSM's Health & Fitness Journal* 7: 30–35.

Lohman, T.G., Pollock, M.L., Slaughter, M.H., Brandon, L.J., and Boileau, R.A. 1984. Methodological factors and the prediction of body fat in female athletes. *Medicine & Science in Sports & Exercise* 16: 92–96.

Lohman, T.G., Roche, A.F., and Martorell, R., eds. 1988. *Anthropometric standardization reference manual.* Champaign, IL: Human Kinetics.

Loy, S., Likes, E., Andrews, P., Vincent, W., Holland, G.J., Kawai, H., Cen, S., Swenberger, J., VanLoan, M., Tanaka, K., Heyward, V., Stolarczyk, L., Lohman, T.G., and Going, S.B. 1998. Easy grip on body composition measurements. *ACSM's Health & Fitness Journal* 2(5): 16–19.

Lukaski, H.C. 1986. Use of the tetrapolar bioelectrical impedance method to assess human body composition. In *Human body composition and fat patterning,* ed. N.G. Norgan, 143–158. Wageningen, Netherlands: Euronut.

Martin, A.D., Drinkwater, D.T., and Clarys, J.P. 1992. Effects of skin thickness and skinfold compressibility on skinfold thickness measurements. *American Journal of Human Biology* 4: 453–460.

Martin, A.D., Ross, W.D., Drinkwater, D.T., and Clarys, J.P. 1985. Prediction of body fat by skinfold caliper: Assumptions and cadaver evidence. *International Journal of Obesity* 9 (Suppl. 1): 31–39.

McCrory, M.A., Gomez, T.D., Bernauer, E.M., and Mole, P.A. 1995. Evaluation of a new displacement plethysmograph for measuring human body composition. *Medicine & Science in Sports & Exercise* 27: 1686–1691.

McLean, K.P., and Skinner, J.S. 1992. Validity of Futrex-5000 for body composition determination. *Medicine & Science in Sports & Exercise* 24: 253–258.

Micozzi, M.S., Albanes, D., Jones, Y., and Chumlea, W.C. 1986. Correlations of body mass indices with weight, stature, and body composition in men and women in NHANES I and II. *American Journal of Clinical Nutrition* 44: 725–731.

Mitchell, C.O., Rose, J.F., Mitchell, C.O., Familoni, B., Winders, S.E., and Lancaster, E. 1993. The use of multifrequency bioelectrical impedance analysis to estimate fluid volume changes as a function of the menstrual cycle. In *Human body composition: In vivo methods, models and assessment,* ed. K.J. Ellis and J.D. Eastman, 189–191. New York: Plenum Press.

Morrow, J.R., Jackson, A.S., Bradley, P.W., and Hartung, G.H. 1986. Accuracy of measured and predicted residual lung volume on body density measurement. *Medicine & Science in Sport & Exercise* 18: 647–652.

National Cholesterol Education Program (NCEP). 2001. Executive summary of the third report of the National Cholesterol Education Program (NCEP) expert panel on detection, evaluation, and treatment of high blood cholesterol in adults (adult treatment panel III). *Journal of the American Medical Association* 285: 2486–2497.

Ng, N. 1997. *Comprehensive body composition software.* Champaign, IL: Human Kinetics.

Nielsen, D.H., Cassady, S.L., Wacker, L.M., Wessels, A.K., Wheelock, B.J., and Oppliger, R.A. 1992. Validation of the Futrex-5000 near-infrared spectrophotometer analyzer for assessment of body composition. *Journal of Orthopaedic and Sports Physical Therapy* 16: 281–287.

Norton, K., Marfell-Jones, M., Whittingham, N., Kerr, D., Carter, L., Saddington, K., and Gore, C. 2000. Anthropometric assessment protocols. In *Physiological tests for elite athletes,* ed. C. Gore, 66–85. Champaign, IL: Human Kinetics.

Nunez, C., Kovera, A., Pietrobelli, A., Heshka, S., Horlick, M., Kehayias, J., Wang, Z., and Heymsfield, S. 1999. Body composition in children and adults by air displacement plethysmography. *European Journal of Clinical Nutrition* 53: 382–387.

Oppliger, R.A., Nielsen, D.H., and Vance, C.G. 1991. Wrestlers' minimal weight: Anthropometry, bioimpedance, and hydrostatic weighing compared. *Medicine & Science in Sports & Exercise* 23: 247–253.

Ortiz, O., Russell, M., Daley, T.L., Baumgartner, R.N., Waki, M., Lichtman, S., Wang, S., Pierson, R.N., and Heymsfield, S.B. 1992. Differences in skeletal muscle and bone mineral mass between black and white females and their relevance to estimates of body composition. *American Journal of Clinical Nutrition* 55: 8–13.

Peters, D., Fox, K., Armstrong, N., Sharpe, P., and Bell, M. 1992. Assessment of children's abdominal fat distribution by magnetic resonance imaging and anthropometry. *International Journal of Obesity* 16(Suppl. 2): S35 [abstract].

Pollock, M., and Jackson, A.S. 1984. Research progress in validation of clinical methods of assessing body composition. *Medicine & Science in Sports & Exercise* 16: 606–613.

Quatrochi, J.A., Hicks, V.L., Heyward, V.H., Colville, B.C., Cook, K.L., Jenkins, K.A., and Wilson, W. 1992. Relationship of optical density and skinfold measurements: Effects of age and level of body fatness. *Research Quarterly for Exercise and Sport* 63: 402–409.

Rodd, D., Ho, L., and Enzler, D. 1999. Validity of Tanita TBF-515 bioelectrical impedance scale for estimating body fat in young adults. *Medicine & Science in Sports & Exercise* 31(Suppl.): S201 [abstract].

Ross, W.D., and Marfell-Jones, M.J. 1991. Kinanthropometry. In *Physiological testing of the high-performance athlete,* ed. J.D. MacDougall, H.A. Wenger, and H.J. Green, 75–115, Champaign, IL: Human Kinetics.

Ross, W.D., Crawford, S.M., Kerr, D.A., Ward, R., Bailey, D.A., and Mirwald, R.M. 1988. Relationship of the body mass index with skinfolds, girths, and bone breadths in Canadian men and women aged 20-79 years. *American Journal of Physical Anthropology* 77: 169–173.

Roubenoff, R., Kehayias, J.J., Dawson-Hughes, B., and Heymsfield, S.B. 1993. Use of dual-energy X-ray absorptiometry in body-composition studies: Not yet a "gold standard." *American Journal of Clinical Nutrition* 58: 589–591.

Segal, K.R., Van Loan, M., Fitzgerald, P.I., Hodgdon, J.A., and Van Itallie, T.B. 1988. Lean body mass estimation by bioelectrical impedance analysis: A four-site cross-validation study. *American Journal of Clinical Nutrition* 47: 7–14.

Seidell, J.C., Oosterlee, A., Thijssen, M., Burema, J., Deurenberg, P., Hautvast, J., and Ruijs, J. 1987. Assessment of intra-abdominal and subcutaneous abdominal fat: Relation between anthropometry and computed tomography. *American Journal of Clinical Nutrition* 45: 7–13.

Seip, R., and Weltman, A. 1991. Validity of skinfold and girth based regression equations for the prediction of body composition in obese adults. *American Journal of Human Biology* 3: 91–95.

Siri, W.E. 1961. Body composition from fluid space and density. In *Techniques for measuring body composition,* ed. J. Brozek and A. Henschel, 223–224. Washington, D.C.: National Academy of Sciences.

Slaughter, M.H., Lohman, T.G., Boileau, R.A., Horswill, C.A., Stillman, R.J., Van Loan, M.D., and Bemben, D.A. 1988. Skinfold equations for estimation of body fatness in children and youth. *Human Biology* 60: 709–723.

Thomas, T.R., and Etheridge, G.L. 1980. Hydrostatic weighing at residual volume and functional residual capacity. *Journal of Applied Physiology* 49: 157–159.

Timson, B.F., and Coffman, J.L. 1984. Body composition by hydrostatic weighing at total lung capacity and residual volume. *Medicine & Science in Sports & Exercise* 16: 411–414.

Tran, Z.V., and Weltman, A. 1988. Predicting body composition of men from girth measurements. *Human Biology* 60: 167–175.

Tran, Z.V., and Weltman, A. 1989. Generalized equation for predicting body density of women from girth measurements. *Medicine & Science in Sports & Exercise* 21: 101–104.

Van Loan, M.D., and Mayclin, P.L. 1987. Bioelectrical impedance analysis: Is it a reliable estimator of lean body mass and total body water? *Human Biology* 59: 299–309.

Van Loan, M.D., and Mayclin, P.L. 1992. Body composition assessment: Dual-energy X-ray absorptiometry (DEXA) compared to reference methods. *European Journal of Clinical Nutrition* 46: 125–130.

Wagner, D., and Heyward, V. 2000. Validity of two-component models for estimating body fat of black men. *Journal of Applied Physiology* 90:649–656.

Wagner, D., Heyward, V., and Gibson, A. 2000. Validation of air displacement plethysmography for assessing body composition. *Medicine & Science in Sports & Exercise* 32: 1339–1344.

Wagner, D., Heyward, V., and Stolarczyk, L. 1997. Body mass index as a measure of body fatness: Influence of gender, age, and ethnicity. Presented at Southwest ACSM annual meeting, Las Vegas, NV.

Ward, R., Rempel, R., and Anderson, G.S. 1999. Modeling dynamic skinfold compression. *American Journal of Human Biology* 11: 521–537.

Ward, R., and Anderson, G.S. 1998. Resilience of anthropometric data assembly strategies to imposed error. *Journal of Sports Sciences* 16: 755-759.

Weltman, A., Levine, S., Seip, R.L., and Tran, Z.V. 1988. Accurate assessment of body composition in obese females. *American Journal of Clinical Nutrition* 48: 1179–1183.

Weltman, A., Seip, R.L., and Tran, Z.V. 1987. Practical assessment of body composition in adult obese males. *Human Biology* 59: 523–535.

Whatley, S., Florence, M., Ransdell, L., Yates, J., and Clasey, J. 1999. Validity of five bioelectrical impedance analyzers used to estimate body composition in young adults. *Medicine & Science in Sports & Exercise* 31(Suppl.): S203 [abstract].

WHO Report. 1998. Obesity: preventing and managing a global epidemic. *Report of a WHO Consultation on Obesity.* Geneva: World Health Organization.

Williams, D.P., Going, S.B., Massett, M.P., Lohman, T.G., Bare, L.A., and Hewitt, M.J. 1993. Aqueous and mineral fractions of the fat-free body and their relation to body fat estimates in men and women aged 49-82 years. In *Human body composition: In vivo methods, models and assessment,* ed. K.J. Ellis and J.D. Eastman, 109–113. New York: Plenum Press.

Wilmore, J.H., and Behnke, A.R. 1969. An anthropometric estimation of body density and lean body weight in young men. *Journal of Applied Physiology* 27: 25–31.

Wilmore, J.H., and Behnke, A.R. 1970. An anthropometric estimation of body density and lean body weight in young women. *American Journal of Clinical Nutrition* 23: 267–274.

Wilmore, J.H., Frisancho, R.A., Gordon, C.C., Himes, J.H., Martin, A.D., Martorell, R., and Seefeldt, R.D. 1988. Body breadth equipment and measurement techniques. In *Anthropometric standardization reference manual,* ed. T.G. Lohman, A.F. Roche, and R. Martorell, 27–38. Champaign, IL: Human Kinetics.

Wilmore, K.M., McBride, P.J., and Wilmore, J.H. 1994. Comparison of bioelectric impedance and near-infrared interactance for human body composition assessment in a population of self-perceived overweight adults. *International Journal of Obesity* 18: 375–381.

Zando, K.A., and Robertson, R.J. 1987. The validity and reliability of the Cramer skyndex caliper in the estimation of percent body fat. *Athletic Training* 22: 23–25, 79.

chapter 9

Designing Weight Management and Body Composition Programs

KEY QUESTIONS

- What is obesity and how prevalent is it worldwide?
- What are the health risks associated with having high or low levels of body fat?
- What are the primary causes of overweight and obesity?
- How is healthy body weight determined?
- What are the guidelines for a well-balanced diet? Are vitamin and mineral supplements necessary for most clients?

- What steps should I follow in planning a weight management program?
- What are the recommended guidelines for weight loss and weight gain programs?
- Why is exercise important for weight management?
- What types of exercise are best for weight loss?
- Does exercising without dieting improve body composition?

"Aim for a healthy body weight." This is the very first guideline statement in the most recent *Dietary Guidelines for Americans* (U.S. Department of Health and Human Services 2000a). Health and longevity are threatened when a person is either overweight or underweight. Overweight and obesity increase one's risk of developing serious cardiovascular, pulmonary, and metabolic diseases and disorders. Likewise, individuals who are underweight may have a higher risk than others of cardiac, musculoskeletal, and reproductive disorders. Thus, healthy weight is key to a healthy and longer life.

As a health/fitness professional, you have an enormous challenge and responsibility to help determine a healthy body weight for your clients and to provide scientifically sound weight management programs for them. This chapter presents guidelines and techniques for determining healthy body weight. You will learn about weight control principles and practices, as well as guidelines for designing exercise programs for weight loss, weight gain, and body composition change.

OBESITY, OVERWEIGHT, AND UNDERWEIGHT: DEFINITIONS AND TRENDS

Individuals with body fat levels falling at or near the extremes of the body fat continuum are likely to have serious health problems that reduce life expectancy and threaten their quality of life. Obese individuals have a higher risk of cardiovascular disease, dyslipidemia, hypertension, glucose intolerance, insulin resistance, diabetes mellitus, obstructive pulmonary disease, gallbladder disease, osteoarthritis, and certain types of cancer (U.S. Department of Health and Human Services 2000a). The prevalences of hypercholesterolemia, hypertension, and type 2 diabetes are, respectively, 2.9, 2.1, and 2.9 times greater in overweight than non-overweight persons (National Institutes of Health Consensus Development Panel 1985). Obesity is independently associated with coronary heart disease (CHD), heart failure, cardiac arrhythmia, stroke, and menstrual irregularities (Pi-Sunyer 1999).

At the opposite extreme, underweight individuals with too little body fat tend to be malnourished. These people have a relatively higher risk of fluid-electrolyte imbalances, osteoporosis and osteopenia, bone fractures, muscle wasting, cardiac arrhythmias and sudden death, peripheral edema, and renal and reproductive disorders (Fohlin 1977; Mazess, Barden, and Ohlrich 1990; Vaisman, Corey, Rossi, Goldberg, and Pencharz 1988). One disease associated with extremely low body fat levels is anorexia nervosa. **Anorexia nervosa**, an eating disorder found primarily in females, is characterized by excessive weight loss. Anorexia nervosa is estimated to afflict 1% of the female population (American Psychiatric Association 1994). Compared to normal women, those with anorexia have extremely low body fat (8% to 13% body fat), signs of muscle wasting, and less bone mineral content and bone density (Mazess et al. 1990; Vaisman, Rossi et al. 1988).

Definitions of Obesity, Overweight, and Underweight

Obesity is an excessive amount of body fat relative to body weight and is not synonymous with overweight. In many epidemiological studies, overweight is defined as a body mass index (BMI) between 25 and 29.9 kg/m^2; obesity is defined as a BMI of 30 kg/m^2 or more; and **underweight** is defined by a BMI of less than 18.5 kg/m^2 (U.S. Department of Health and Human Services 2000a). Because these criteria do not take into account the composition of the individual's body weight, they are limited as indexes of obesity and may result in misclassifications of underweight, overweight, and obesity. There is considerable variability in body composition for any given BMI. Some individuals with low BMIs may have as much relative body fat as those with higher BMIs. Older

people have more relative body fat at any given BMI than younger people (Baumgartner, Heymsfield, and Roche 1995). Thus, the prevalence of obesity could be worse than currently thought.

Trends in Overweight and Obesity

Trends in overweight and obesity among adults vary internationally (Flegal 1999). The prevalence of obesity is highest in Western Samoa (57% of men and 74% of women are obese) and pacific island populations. In some European countries (i.e., Germany and United Kingdom), the United States, and Israel, the prevalence of obesity ranges from 15% to 20% for adult men and 17% to 32% for adult women. The prevalence of obesity is lower, ranging between 3% and 5% for men and between 4% and 13% for women, in less developed countries (Brazil and Australia), Asian countries (China and Japan), and a few Scandinavian countries (Denmark and Sweden).

Obesity is on the rise worldwide, reaching epidemic proportions in some countries. Canada, Finland, New Zealand, the United Kingdom, Western Samoa, and the United States all reported large recent increases (i.e., >5%) in overweight and obesity among adults (Flegal 1999). Since 1960, overweight and obesity in the United States have increased across all age, gender, and ethnic groups (Grundy et al. 1999). Approximately 55% of American adults are overweight or obese; more than 20% of children and adolescents are overweight (Kuczmarski, Flegal, Campbell, and Johnson 1994; Troiano, Flegal, Kuczmarski, Campbell, and Johnson 1995). Because of the health risk and medical costs associated with obesity, the U.S. Surgeon General has recently established a goal of reducing the prevalence of obesity in adults to no more than 15% by the year 2010 (U.S. Department of Health and Human Services 2000b).

OBESITY: TYPES AND CAUSES

Combating obesity is not an easy task. Many overweight and obese individuals have incorporated patterns of overeating and physical inactivity into their lifestyles, while others have developed eating disorders, exercise addictions, or both. In an effort to lose weight quickly and to prevent weight gain, many are lured by fad diets and exercise gimmicks; and some resort to extreme behaviors, such as avoiding food, bingeing and purging, and exercising compulsively. In a survey of weight control practices of adults in the United States, Serdula et al. (1994) reported that 38% of women and 24% of men were trying to lose weight by counting calories, participating in organized weight loss programs, taking special supplements or diet pills, or fasting. Only 50% of those trying to lose weight reported using the recommended method of restricting caloric intake and increasing physical activity.

In a more recent report of leisure-time physical activity among overweight adults in the United States ("Prevalence of Leisure-Time Physical Activity" 2000), two-thirds of overweight adults reported that they engaged in physical activity to try to lose weight; however, only 20% met the national recommendation for physical activity (at least 30 min of moderate-intensity activity, most days of the week, preferably daily). Most of these individuals exercised 30 min or longer per session; but only a minority exercised at least five times per week. Therefore, low frequency of physical activity was the main reason that the physical activity recommendation was not met.

Types of Obesity

The way in which fat is distributed in the body may be more important than total body fat for determining one's risk of disease. The waist-to-hip ratio (WHR) is strongly associated with visceral fat, and the impact of regional fat distribution on health is related to the amount of visceral fat located in the abdominal cavity. Abdominal fat is strongly associated with diseases such as CHD, diabetes, hypertension, and hyperlipidemia (Bjorntorp 1988; Blair, Habricht, Sims, Sylwester, and Abraham 1984; Ducimetier, Richard, and Cambien 1989).

The terms **android obesity** and **gynoid obesity** refer to the localization of excess body fat mainly in the upper body (android) or lower body (gynoid). Android obesity (apple shaped) is more typical of males; gynoid obesity (pear shaped) is more characteristic of females. However, some men may have gynoid obesity, and some women have android obesity. Other terms are also used to describe types of obesity and regional fat distribution. Android obesity is frequently simply called **upper-body obesity,** and gynoid obesity is often described as **lower-body obesity.**

In field settings, you can assess regional fat distribution using the WHR. Chapter 8 presents measurement procedures (see pp. 185-186 and WHR norms (see table 8.7, p. 183). Generally, young adults with WHR values in excess of 0.94 for men and 0.82 for women are at very high risk for adverse health consequences (Bray and Gray 1988).

Causes of Overweight and Obesity

Many questions may arise in regard to overweight and obesity. This section addresses common questions relating to the causes of overweight and obesity.

■ *Why do people gain or lose weight?*

An energy imbalance in the body results in a weight gain or loss. There is an energy balance when the caloric intake equals the caloric expenditure. A **positive energy balance** is created when the input (food intake) exceeds the expenditure (resting metabolism plus activity level). For every 3500 kcal of excess energy accumulated, 1 lb (0.45 kg) of fat is stored in the body. A **negative energy balance** is produced when the energy expenditure exceeds the energy input. This can be accomplished by reducing the food intake or increasing the physical activity level. A caloric deficit of approximately 3500 kcal produces a loss of 1 lb of fat.

■ *How are energy needs and energy expenditure measured?*

Energy need and expenditure are measured in kilocalories (kcal). A **kilocalorie** is defined as the amount of heat needed to raise the temperature of 1 kg (2.2 lb) of water 1° C. Direct calorimetry is used to measure the energy yield and caloric equivalent of various foods. These foods are burned in a closed chamber in the presence of oxygen, and the amount of heat liberated is measured precisely in kilocalories. Table 9.1 gives the energy yield and caloric equivalents for carbohydrate, protein, and fat.

Table 9.1 Energy Yield and Caloric Equivalents for Macronutrients		
Nutrient	**Energy yield (kcal/g)**	**Caloric equivalents (kcal/L O_2)**
Carbohydrate	4.1	5.1
Protein	4.3	4.4
Fat	9.3	4.7

The energy or caloric need is a function of an individual's metabolic rate and physical activity level. The **basal metabolic rate (BMR)** is a measure of the minimal amount of energy (kcal) needed to maintain basic and essential physiological functions. Basal metabolic rate varies according to age, gender, body size, and body composition. For assessment of BMR, the individual needs to be rested and fasted and should be in a controlled environment. Since this is not always practical, we use the term **resting metabolic rate (RMR)** to indicate the energy required to maintain essential physiological processes in a relaxed, awake, and reclined state.

You can measure energy expenditure during basal, resting, or activity states using indirect calorimetry. In this case, the body's energy expenditure is estimated from the oxygen utilization. Every liter of oxygen consumed per minute yields approximately 5 kcal (see table 9.1). Intense physical activity can increase the rate of energy expenditure more than 10 times above the resting level.

■ *How is RMR regulated?*

Thyroxine is extremely important in regulating RMR. Inadequate levels of this hormone can be produced by thyroid tumors or lack of iodine in the diet. Underproduction of thyroxine can reduce RMR 30% to 50%. If energy input and expenditure are not adjusted accordingly, the positive energy balance that is created results in a weight gain.

Growth hormone, epinephrine, norepinephrine, and various sex hormones may elevate RMR as much as 15% to 20%. These hormones increase during exercise and may be responsible for the elevation in RMR after cessation of exercise.

■ *Does weight gain increase both the number and size of fat cells?*

Obesity is associated with increases in the both the number and size of fat cells. A normal-weight individual has 25 to 30 billion fat cells, whereas an obese person may have as many as 42 to 106 billion fat cells. Also, the adipose cell size of obese individuals is on the average 40% larger than that of non-obese persons (Hirsh 1971). An increase in fat cell number **(hyperplasia)** occurs rapidly during the first year of life and again during adolescence but remains fairly stable in adulthood, except in cases of morbid obesity. Fat cells increase in size **(hypertrophy)** during the adolescent growth spurt and continue to grow when excess fat is stored in the cells as triglycerides. Weight gain in adults is typically characterized by the enlargement of existing fat cells, rather than the creation of new fat cells. Also, caloric restriction and exercise are effective in reducing fat cell size but not the number of fat cells in adults (Hirsh 1971). Perhaps the key to preventing obesity is to closely monitor the dietary intake and energy expenditure, especially during the adolescent growth spurt and puberty. This could potentially retard the development of new fat cells and control the size of existing fat cells.

■ *What is the relative importance of genetics and environment in developing obesity?*

Scientists have debated the relative contributions of genetics and environment to obesity. Mayer (1968) observed that only 10% of children who had normal-weight parents were obese. The probability of being obese is increased to 40% and 80%, respectively, if one parent or both parents are obese. Although these data suggest a strong genetic influence, they do not rule out environmental influences such as eating and exercise habits.

In a controlled study of long-term (100 days) overfeeding in identical twins, Bouchard et al. (1990) observed large individual differences in the tendency toward obesity and distribution of body fat, even within each pair of twins. Changes in body weight due to overfeeding of twins were moderately correlated ($r = 0.55$). Overall, increases in body weight, fat mass, trunk fat, and visceral fat were three times greater in high-weight gainers compared to low-weight gainers. These data suggest that genotype explains some, but not all, of a person's adaptation to a sustained energy surplus. Approximately 25% of the variability among individuals in absolute and relative body fat is attributed to genetic factors and 30% is associated with cultural (environmental) factors (Bouchard, Perusse, Leblanc, and Theriault 1988).

Hill and Melanson (1999) suggested that the major cause of obesity in the United States is our environment. Over the past 30 years, the U.S. population has been exposed to an environment that strongly promotes the consumption of high-fat, energy-dense foods (increased energy intake) and reliance on technology that discourages physical activity and reduces the amount of physical activity (decreased energy expenditure) needed for daily living.

WEIGHT MANAGEMENT PRINCIPLES AND PRACTICES

Proper nutrition (eating a well-balanced diet) and daily physical activity are key components of a weight management program. In weight management programs, most clients are interested in losing body weight and body fat, but some need to gain body weight. The basic principle underlying safe and effective weight loss programs is that weight can be lost only through a negative energy balance, which is produced when the caloric expenditure exceeds the caloric intake. The most effective way of creating a caloric deficit is through a combination of diet (restricting caloric intake) and exercise (increasing caloric expenditure). On the other hand, for weight gain programs, the caloric intake must exceed the caloric expenditure in order to create a positive energy balance. "Weight Management Principles" summarizes principles and practices underlying the design of weight management programs.

Weight Management Principles

Weight loss

- A well-balanced diet for good nutrition contains carbohydrate, protein, fat, vitamin, minerals, and water.

- The weight loss should be gradual—no more than 2 lb a week.

- The caloric intake should be at least 1200 kcal/day, and the caloric deficit should not exceed 1000 kcal/day.

- A caloric deficit of 3500 kcal is needed to lose 1 lb of fat.

- Weight loss should be due to loss of fat rather than lean body tissue.

- On the same diet, a taller, heavier person will lose weight at a faster rate than a shorter, lighter person due to a higher RMR.

- Weight loss rate decreases over time, because the difference between the caloric intake and caloric needs gets smaller as one loses weight.

- Men lose weight faster than women due to a higher RMR.

- The individual should eat at least 3 meals a day.

- Quick weight loss diets, diet pills, and appetite suppressants should be avoided.

- Carnitine supplementation does not promote body fat loss.

- Compulsive eating behaviors should be identified and modified.

Weight gain

- The dietary protein intake should be increased to 1.2–1.6 $g \cdot kg^{-1}$ body weight.

- The weight gain should be gradual—no more than 2 lb a week.

- The daily caloric intake should exceed caloric needs by 400 to 500 kcal/day.

- A positive energy balance of 2800 to 3500 is needed to gain 1 lb of muscle tissue.

- Weight gain should be due to increased FFM rather than fat mass.

- The individual should eat 3 meals and 2 to 3 healthy snacks per day, e.g., dried fruits, nuts, seeds, and some liquid meals.

- Protein powders are no more effective than natural protein sources (e.g., lean meats, skim milk, and egg whites).

- Protein and amino acid supplements do not promote muscle growth.

- Vitamin B12, boron, and chromium supplementation does not increase FFM.

Exercise

- The major cause of obesity is lack of physical activity, not overeating.

- For fat-weight loss, aerobic exercise should be performed daily or twice daily.

- Resistance exercise training is excellent for maintaining FFM (for weight loss) and increasing FFM (for weight gain).

- For weight loss, exercise helps create a caloric deficit by increasing caloric expenditure.

- Exercise is better than dieting for maximizing fat loss and minimizing lean tissue loss.

- Compared to fat, muscle tissue is more metabolically active and uses more calories at rest.

- Low-intensity, longer-duration exercise maximizes total energy expenditure better than high-intensity, shorter-duration exercise.

- RMR remains elevated 30 min or longer after vigorous exercise.

- At a given heart rate, the more physically fit individual expends calories at a faster rate than the less fit individual.

- Exercise does not increase appetite.

- Passive exercise devices (e.g., vibrators and sauna belts) do not massage away excess fat.

- Spot-reduction exercises do not preferentially mobilize subcutaneous fat stored near the exercising muscles.

- To increase caloric expenditure, avoid using labor-saving devices at home and work.

People can win the battle of controlling body weight and obesity by not only understanding why they eat and monitoring their food intake closely, but also by incorporating more physical activity into their lifestyles. The physically active lifestyle is characterized by

- daily aerobic exercise;
- strength and flexibility exercises;
- increased participation in recreational activities such as bowling, golf, tennis, and dancing; and
- increased physical activity in the daily routine at home and work through restricting use of labor-saving devices such as escalators, power tools, automobiles, and home and garden appliances.

In addition to these suggestions, you should encourage your clients to follow the *Dietary Guidelines for Americans* (U.S. Department of Health and Human Services 2000a):

- Aim for fitness:
  - Aim for a healthy weight.
  - Be physically active each day.
- Build a healthy base:
  - Let the pyramid guide your food choices (see figure 9.4, p. 213).
  - Choose a variety of grains daily, especially whole grains.
  - Keep food safe to eat.
- Choose sensibly:
  - Choose a diet that is low in saturated fat and cholesterol and moderate in total fat.
  - Choose beverages and foods to moderate your intake of sugars.
  - Choose and prepare foods with less salt.
  - If you drink alcoholic beverages, do so in moderation.

WELL-BALANCED NUTRITION

Before you can help your clients with their weight management, you must understand good nutrition. A well-balanced diet should contain adequate amounts of protein, fat, carbohydrate, vitamins, minerals, and water. A 1985 survey of food intakes of 658 men and 1459 women between the ages of 19 and 50 years indicated that the average percentage of total energy intake from carbohydrate (46%), fat (37%), and protein (16%) did not comply with U.S. dietary goals (i.e., 58% carbohydrate,

30% fat, and 12% protein). Also, the average dietary cholesterol (435 mg·dl^{-1}) and sodium intake of men exceeded the recommended levels. Women, on the average, took in 78% of the estimated safe and adequate daily dietary intake for calcium, 61% of that for iron, 60% of that for zinc, and 72% of that for magnesium (U.S. Department of Health and Human Services 1988).

Carbohydrates

Three kinds of carbohydrates are sugars, starches, and cellulose. Carbohydrates are classified as either complex (e.g., fruits, vegetables, whole grains, and legumes) or simple (e.g., processed foods or foods high in sugar). In the past, this classification was used to describe the body's glycemic response (i.e., increase in blood glucose and insulin after consumption of food) to various types of foods; however, the glycemic response to simple and complex carbohydrates varies greatly. Some complex carbohydrates are metabolized as rapidly as simple sugars. Thus, foods are now categorized based on the body's glycemic response to them (high, moderate, or low) through use of the **glycemic index (GI).** The GI is a rating of the immediate effect of a given food on blood glucose levels and is obtained by comparing the glycemic response to that food with the glycemic response to glucose or white bread (GI = 100). High glycemic index carbohydrates (GI > 60) enter the bloodstream quickly and are recommended to replenish blood glucose levels during and after exercise, whereas carbohydrates with a low (GI < 40) to moderate (GI = 40 to 60) glycemic response are best for sustaining blood glucose levels during long-term exercise (Clark 1997). Lists of GI values for various foods may be found in nutrition books and journals and on Web sites (see Clark 1997; Foster-Powell and Miller 1995; Miller 2001).

The largest proportion (58% to 65%) of the daily caloric intake should be in the form of carbohydrates. The ingestion of refined and processed sugars should be limited to 10% of the daily caloric intake. Complex carbohydrates (i.e., starches and fiber) and naturally occurring sugars should be consumed to meet the carbohydrate requirements of a well-balanced diet. Diets with a high fiber content (cellulose) are less likely to produce colon cancer and hemorrhoids compared to low-fiber diets.

Carbohydrates are stored in the liver and muscle as glycogen. However, the amount of glucose that can be stored in the body as muscle and liver glycogen is limited. If the glycogen storage capability of the body is exceeded, a positive energy balance is created. These excess calories in the form of carbohydrate provide the building blocks for the synthesis of trigyclerides, which are eventually stored in adipose tissue and in the muscles as intramuscular fat.

Protein

Approximately 12% to 15% of the daily caloric intake should be protein. The diet should include sources of the essential amino acids needed for protein synthesis. Lack of these essential amino acids may produce a loss of muscle tissue or prevent the synthesis of hormones, enzymes, and cellular structures. The amount of protein that the average individual needs to meet the daily protein requirements of the body is 0.8 $g \cdot kg^{-1}$ of body weight. Protein supplementation beyond the average level is usually not necessary unless the individual is participating in a strenuous training program. In such cases, the person's daily protein intake may be increased to 1.2 to 2.0 $g \cdot kg^{-1}$ of body weight in the early stages of training. This amount represents about 150% to 250% of the current RDA for adults (Lemon 1998).

Excess protein cannot be stored in the body and is broken down into amino acids. Amino acids also cannot be stored and therefore will be used as fuel for energy. Too much protein in the diet causes dehydration due to excessive production of urea, which must be eliminated in the urine.

Fats

In the typical American diet, approximately 34% of the daily caloric intake is in the form of fats (Lenfant and Ernst 1994; U.S. Department of Agriculture 1998). In the United States, adults lowered the percent of caloric intake from total fat from 45% in 1965 to 34% in 1995. However, this decrease in relative (%) fat intake is a result of increased total caloric intake. A higher number of calories consumed reduces the calculated percentage of calories from fat even when there is no decrease in total fat consumption (U.S. Department of Agriculture 1998).

Some dietary fat is needed to supply essential fatty acids and to absorb fat-soluble vitamins. In addition, free fatty acids are an important energy source during aerobic exercise. However, because of a possible link between serum triglyceride and cholesterol levels with atherosclerosis, hypertension, and CHD, individuals should restrict dietary fat intake, especially their intake of saturated fats, trans fatty acids, and cholesterol (U.S. Department of Health and Human Services 2000a). In the *Dietary Guidelines for Americans* (U.S. Department of Health and Human Services 2000a), the recommendation is that total fat intake not exceed 30% of the daily caloric intake. Saturated fat and trans fatty acid intake should not be greater than one-third of the total fat intake or 10% of the total daily caloric intake. The remaining fat intake should be evenly divided between polyunsaturated fats (10% of total daily kilocalories) and monounsaturated fats (10% of total daily kilocalories). Excess fat in the diet cannot be used to synthesize glucose; instead, the free fatty acids are resynthesized and stored as triglyceride in the muscle and adipose tissue.

The National Cholesterol Education Program (2001) recommends a "Therapeutic Lifestyle Changes Diet" (table 9.2) to promote weight loss in those who are overweight and to reduce serum cholesterol levels. This diet limits dietary intakes of saturated fat and trans fatty acids (<7% of total calories), total fat (25% to 35% of total calories), and cholesterol (<200 mg per day).

Vitamins, Minerals, and Water

A well-balanced diet usually does not need to be supplemented to meet the minimum daily vitamin and mineral requirements of the body. Table 9.3 gives recommended dietary allowances (RDA), adequate intakes (AI), and upper intake levels (UL) for vitamins and minerals.

Vitamins

Eating a well-balanced diet typically provides an individual's vitamin requirements. The body does not store the water-soluble vitamins (B complex and C); and in the case of most of these vitamins, an excess amount is excreted in the urine. The excess accumulation of fat-soluble vitamins (A, D, E, and K) may produce decalcification of bones, headaches, nausea, diarrhea, and other toxic effects (Williams 1992).

Antioxidant vitamins (C, E, and beta-carotene) may protect against muscle damage following intense, eccentric exercise by counteracting the negative effects of free radicals and lipid peroxidation on muscle tissue (Singh 1992). However, additional research is needed before one can recommend antioxidant vitamin supplementation as a means to prevent exercise-induced muscle damage (Goldfarb 1993).

Table 9.2   Nutrient Composition of the Therapeutic Lifestyle Changes Diet

Nutrient	Recommended intake
Saturated fat[a]	<7% of total calories
Polyunsaturated fat	Up to 10% of total calories
Monounsaturated fat	Up to 20% of total calories
Total fat	25-35% of total calories
Carbohydrate[b]	50-60% of total calories
Fiber	20-30 g/day
Protein	Approximately 15% of total calories
Cholesterol	<200 mg/day
Total calories[c]	Balance energy intake and expenditure to maintain desirable body weight/prevent weight gain

[a]Trans fatty acids are another low-density lipoprotein-raising fat that should be kept to a low intake.

[b]Carbohydrates should be derived predominantly from foods rich in complex carbohydrates including grains, especially whole grains, fruits, and vegetables.

[c]Daily energy expenditure should include at least moderate physical activity (contributing approximately 200 kcal/day).

Data from National Cholesterol Education Program (2001), "Executive Summary of the Third Report of the National Cholesterol Education Program Expert Panel on Detection, Evaluation and Treatment of High Blood Cholesterol in Adults (Adult Treatment Panel III)," *Journal of the American Medical Association* 285 (19): 2490.

Minerals

The most common mineral deficiencies are of iron, zinc, and calcium. Physically active individuals, particularly those who choose to exclude meat from their diets, need to plan their diets carefully so that adequate amounts of iron and zinc are available. In some cases, it may be appropriate for you to recommend daily supplementation of iron, zinc, and calcium at 100% RDA in order to ensure adequate intake of these nutrients.

Iron is found in hemoglobin (in the red blood cells), which transports oxygen to exercising muscles. Iron deficiency has been frequently reported for both male and female athletes, but is more common among women (Clarkson 1990). Thus, iron supplementation may be warranted for some exercising individuals (Rajaram et al. 1995).

Zinc plays an important role in energy metabolism (as a cofactor for enzymes), hormonal function, and the immune system. The average zinc intake of sedentary and athletic women in the United States is below the RDA (12 mg per day); for men, it typically exceeds the RDA (Clarkson and Haymes 1994). Zinc deficiency may result in

decreased strength and endurance (Krotkiewski, Gudmundsson, Backstrom, and Mandroukas 1982).

The recommended adequate intake (AI) for calcium is 1000 mg per day for men and women less than 51 years of age and 1200 mg per day for older (51-70+ yr) adults. Most individuals can meet their calcium requirements by eating a well-balanced diet that contains milk products. When this is not possible, they should use calcium supplements.

Adequate dietary calcium intake and exercise are essential for bone mineralization and skeletal growth. Inadequate bone mineralization or excessive bone resorption results in bone loss and osteoporosis (Sanborn 1990). In early-menopausal women, a high calcium intake (1500 mg per day), in combination with estrogen therapy, deterred bone loss. Calcium supplementation alone did not prevent bone loss in this group (Ettinger, Genault, and Cann 1987).

The typical American diet contains more sodium than the recommended daily amount. The *Dietary Guidelines for Americans* (U.S. Department of Health and Human Services 2000a) recommends limiting salt intake to less than 2400 mg per day

Table 9.3 Guidelines for Vitamin and Mineral Intakes: RDAs, AIs, and ULs* for Adults

	Men Age (years)				Women Age (years)				ULs Both sexes
	19-30	31-50	51-70	70+	19-30	31-50	51-70	70+	19-70+
Vitamins									
A (μg RE)[a]	1000	1000	1000	1000	800	800	800	800	NA[c]
D (μg/d)	**5**	**5**	**10**	**15**	**5**	**5**	**10**	**15**	50
E (mg/d)	15	15	15	15	15	15	15	15	1000
K (μg)	70	80	80	80	60	65	65	65	NA
C (mg/d)	90	90	90	90	75	75	75	75	NA
Thiamin (mg/d)	1.2	1.2	1.2	1.2	1.1	1.1	1.1	1.1	NA
Riboflavin (mg/d)	1.3	1.3	1.3	1.3	1.1	1.1	1.1	1.1	NA
Niacin (mg/d)	1.6	1.6	1.6	1.6	1.4	1.4	1.4	1.4	35
B6 (mg/d)	1.3	1.3	1.7	1.7	1.3	1.3	1.5	1.5	100
Folate (μg/d)	400	400	400	400	400	400	400	400	1000
B12 (μg/d)	2.4	2.4	2.4	2.4	2.4	2.4	2.4	2.4	NA
Pantothenic acid (mg/d)	**5**	**5**	**5**	**5**	**5**	**5**	**5**	**5**	NA
Biotin (μg/d)	**30**	**30**	**30**	**30**	**30**	**30**	**30**	**30**	NA
Choline (mg/d)	**550**	**550**	**550**	**550**	**425**	**425**	**425**	**425**	3500
Minerals									
Calcium (mg/d)	**1000**	**1000**	**1200**	**1200**	**1000**	**1000**	**1200**	**1200**	2500
Phosphorous (mg/d)[b]	700	700	700	700	700	700	700	700	3000-4000
Magnesium (mg/d)	400	420	420	420	310	320	320	320	350[d]
Fluoride (mg/d)	**4**	**4**	**4**	**4**	**3**	**3**	**3**	**3**	10
Iron (mg)	10	10	10	10	15	15	10	10	NA
Zinc (mg)	15	15	15	15	12	12	12	12	NA
Iodine (μg)	150	150	150	150	150	150	150	150	NA
Selenium (μg/d)	55	55	55	55	55	55	55	55	400

[a]Retinol equivalents: 1 RE = 1 μg retinol or 6 μg beta-carotene.

[b]3000 mg/d for >70 years; 4000 mg/d for 19-70 years.

[c]Not available.

[d]UL is for supplemental magnesium only.

*Recommended dietary allowances (RDAs) are in ordinary type, and adequate intakes (AIs) are in bold type. The RDA is the intake that meets the needs of almost all (97-98%) individuals in a group. The AI is believed to cover needs of all individuals in the group; however, sufficient scientific evidence is not available to estimate the RDA for this nutrient. The AI can be used to set goals for individuals. The tolerable upper intake level (UL) is the maximum amount of the nutrient that is unlikely to have adverse health effects in most healthy individuals.

Based on data from the National Academy of Sciences. National Academy Press, Washington, D.C., 2000.

(approximately 1 level teaspoon of salt). Excess salt (sodium chloride) intake may disrupt the electrolyte balance of the body and lead to increased fluid retention, hypertension, and calcium excretion. Thus, the amount of sodium in the diet should be restricted, especially for hypertensive or coronary-prone individuals.

Fraudulent claims sway many physically active individuals, particularly bodybuilders and strength-trained athletes, into believing that multivitamin and mineral supplements enhance muscle growth and exercise performance. Research suggests that long-term use of vitamin-mineral supplements does not increase strength or sport performance (Telford, Catchpole, Deakin, Hahn, and Plank 1992). Scientific studies (Williams 1993) demonstrate that

- vitamin B12 supplementation does not increase muscle growth or strength;
- carnitine (a vitamin-like compound) supplementation does not facilitate loss of body fat;
- chromium supplementation does not increase fat-free mass or decrease body fat;
- boron supplementation does not increase serum testosterone or fat-free mass; and
- magnesium supplementation does not improve muscle strength.

Water

The major sources of water for the body are fluid intake, food intake, and oxidation of foodstuffs by the body. Water is lost in urine, feces, perspiration, and expired air. During strenuous exercise, as much as 3 L of water may be lost through sweating. This water loss should be replenished immediately to prevent dehydration and electrolyte imbalances. Fluid replacement should not be restricted during exercise. Although plain water is effective for this purpose much of the time, carbohydrate sport drinks may also be used to maintain blood glucose levels and replace fluids lost during exercise. These beverages are effective in replenishing muscle glycogen stores after exercise. The ideal fluid replacement beverage contains some sodium and glucose or sucrose. These guidelines for fluid replacement are for everyone, but especially for individuals who are competing or engaging in intense, long-duration (>1 hr) activities (Nadel 1988):

- Drink 2 1/2 cups 2 hr prior to exercise.
- Drink 1 1/2 cups 15 min before competition.

- Do not restrict fluids during exercise; drink at least 1 cup every 15 to 20 min during exercise.
- When you are exercising in the heat, the beverage should contain small amounts of sodium.
- During intense training, the beverage should contain 6% to 8% carbohydrate (glucose or sucrose).

DESIGNING WEIGHT MANAGEMENT PROGRAMS: PRELIMINARY STEPS

In designing weight management programs for weight loss or weight gain, you need to set body weight goals and assess the caloric intake and expenditure for your clients.

Setting Body Weight Goals

To set healthy body weight goals for your clients, you must first assess their present body weight, BMI, or body fat levels. You can easily measure the client's body weight by using a calibrated bathroom or doctor's scale. Clients should wear indoor clothing but not shoes.

When you are evaluating your client's body weight, you should not use height-weight tables established by the Metropolitan Life Insurance Company (Society of Actuaries and Association of Life Insurance Medical Directors of America 1980). These tables are limited for two reasons:

- The values represent height and weight with shoes and clothing. Whether individuals were measured with shoes and clothing was not standardized.
- Data were obtained from individuals who could afford life insurance; the data represent predominantly young to middle-aged white males and females and therefore are not representative of other population groups.

The *Dietary Guidelines for Americans* (U.S. Department of Health and Human Services 2000a) recommends using BMI to determine a healthy body weight range. Calculate your client's BMI and refer to table 8.6 (page 183) to determine if the client's BMI value falls within the healthy range. Individuals with a BMI from 18.5 up to 25 are considered to be at a **healthy body weight.**

Determining a healthy body weight from either BMI or any height-weight table alone may lead to invalid conclusions regarding your client's level of body fatness and health risk. These methods do not take into account the body composition of the individual. For example, with the use of BMI or height-weight tables, many mesomorphs having a large fat-free mass are classified as overweight, yet their body fat content may be lower than average. Similarly, individuals may be overfat or obese even though they are underweight according to the BMI and height-weight tables. Therefore, you should use the body composition technique to estimate a healthy body weight and body fat level for your clients.

When you use the body composition technique for estimating healthy body weight and body fat levels, assess the fat-free mass (FFM) and percent fat (%BF) using one of the methods described in chapter 8. A healthy body weight is based on the client's present FFM and %BF goal. Because some fat is needed for good health and nutrition, individuals should attempt to achieve a %BF somewhere between the low and upper values recommended in table 8.1 (see p. 162). Remember, minimal %BF depends on age and is estimated to be 5% to 10% for males and 12% to 15% for females. Cutoff values for obesity are also age dependent, ranging from >22% to >31% BF for males and >35% to >38% BF for females. Figure 9.1 illustrates a sample calculation of healthy body weight using the body composition technique.

With aging, there is a tendency to accumulate body weight and excess fat. Typically, adults may expect to gain 15 lb (9 kg) of fat weight and lose 5 lb (2.3 kg) of lean body mass per decade of life (Evans and Rosenberg 1992; Forbes 1976; Paffenbarger and Olsen 1996). This weight gain is primarily characterized by an increase in body fat and a decrease in muscle mass and is associated with declining physical activity levels with age. Each individual should attempt to maintain body weight and fatness at healthy levels.

Assessing Caloric Intake and Expenditure

The second step in planning weight management programs is to assess the client's energy (calorie) intake and expenditure. You will use these baseline data to estimate the rate of weight loss or weight gain and the amount of time needed to achieve long-term goals of body composition and body weight.

Energy Intake

A food record (see appendix E.1, "Food Record and RDA Profile," p. 322) is used to determine an

---

Demographic Data

Client: 31-year-old male

Current body composition:

    Body weight = 185 lb (84.1 kg)
    Body fat = 20% BF
    Fat-free mass (FFM) = 148 lb (67.3 kg)

Goals: 12% BF and 88% FFM

Steps:

1. Determine the client's present % BF using one of the body composition methods (see chapter 8).

2. Calculate the client's present FFM (in lb): 185 lb $\times$ 0.80 (current % FFM) = 148 lb.

3. Set reasonable body composition goals for client: 12% BF and 88% FFM.

4. Divide the present FFM (in lb) by the % FFM goal to obtain target body weight: 148 lb/0.88 = 168 lb (76.4 kg).

5. Calculate weight loss by subtracting target body weight from present body weight: 185 − 168 = 17 lb (7.7 kg). Assuming that FFM is maintained, this client must lose 17 lb of fat to achieve his target body weight and body fat level.

Figure 9.1 Sample calculation of healthy body weight using body composition method.

individual's daily caloric intake. The client keeps a record of the type and quantity of foods eaten each day for three to seven days. Use computer software to assess the average daily caloric intake and to compare average nutrient intakes to recommended amounts for each nutrient (see appendix E.2, "Sample Computerized Analysis of Food Intake," p. 324, for sample output). The food record also can help you analyze dietary patterns such as types of foods consumed, frequency of eating, and the caloric content of each meal.

Energy Expenditure

Assess the calorie needs of an individual by estimating RMR and the additional calories expended during work, household chores, personal daily activities, and exercise. Various methods used to estimate RMR are summarized below.

Estimation of Resting Metabolic Rate

The RMR is the minimum amount of calories needed to sustain the vital functions of the body during a relaxed, reclined, and waking state. Since RMR is proportional to the body size and surface area of the individual, taller, heavier persons have a higher RMR than shorter, lighter persons. You can estimate body surface area (BSA) from height and weight using the nomogram in figure 9.2.

The average male or female between 20 and 40 years of age burns 38 kcal/hr and 35 kcal/hr, respectively, for each square meter of BSA. For example, according to method I for estimating RMR, a 5 ft 2 in. (157.5 cm), 120-lb (54.5 kg) female has a body surface area of 1.54 m^2 and a daily resting metabolic need of 1294 kcal (1.54 m^2 × 35 kcal·hr^{-1} × 24 hr).

You can obtain a simpler but less accurate estimate of RMR by multiplying the body weight in pounds by a factor of 10 or 11 for women or men, respectively (see method IV). With this method, the resting metabolic need for the woman in our example is 1200 kcal (120 lb × 10).

Resting metabolic rate gradually decreases with age because the number of metabolically active cells is reduced. The RMR declines 2% to 5% during each decade of life after age 25 (Sharkey 1990). To prevent gradual weight gain with aging, people must reduce caloric intake or increase physical activity level. The Harris-Benedict (1919) equations (method II) are widely used to estimate RMR. These equations are gender specific and take into account not only the height and weight, but also age. In 1984, Roza and Shizgal cross-validated

Methods of Estimating Resting Metabolic Rate (RMR)

Method	Equation
I. Body surface area (BSA)[a]	
Men	RMR = BSA × 38 kcal·hr^{-1} × 24 hr
Women	RMR = BSA × 35 kcal·hr^{-1} × 24 hr
II. Harris-Benedict equations[b]	
Men	RMR = 66.473 + 13.751(BM) + 5.0033(ht) − 6.755(age)
Women	RMR = 655.0955 + 9.463(BM) + 1.8496(ht) − 4.6756(age)
III. Fat-free mass (FFM)	
Men and women	RMR = 500 + 22(FFM in kg)
IV. Quick estimate: lb BM	
Men	RMR = BM (in lb) × 11 kcal·lb^{-1}
Women	RMR = BM (in lb) × 10 kcal·lb^{-1}
V. Quick estimate: kg BM	
Men	RMR = BM (in kg) × 24.2 kcal·kg^{-1}
Women	RMR = BM (in kg) × 22.0 kcal·kg^{-1}

[a]Adjust RMR for age. RMR decreases 2% to 5% per decade after age 40.

[b]BM (body mass) in kilograms; ht in centimeters; age in years.

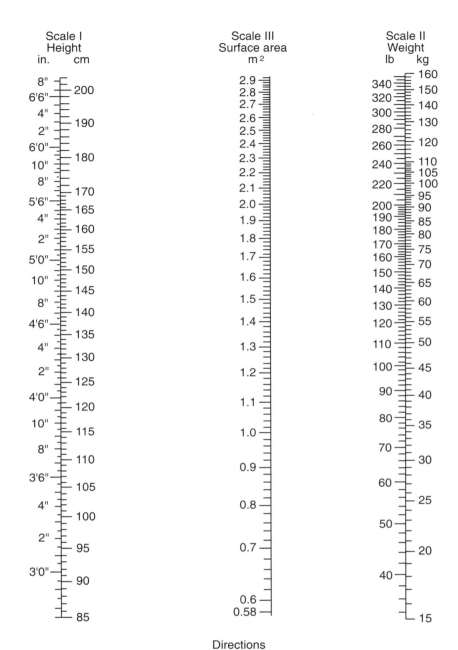

Scale I
Height
in.   cm

Scale III
Surface area
m²

Scale II
Weight
lb   kg

Directions
To find body surface of a client, locate the height in inches (or centimeters) on Scale I and the weight in pounds (or kilograms) on Scale II. Place a straight edge (ruler) between these two points which will intersect Scale III at the client's surface area.

Figure 9.2 Nomogram to predict body surface area.

Reprinted, by permission, from W.E. Collins, 1967, *Clinical Spirometry,* Braintree, MA: Warren E. Collins. Copyright 1967 by Warren E. Collins, 33.

these original equations and developed new equations using data from a large number of subjects and concluded that the original equations published in 1919 yielded identical estimates of resting energy expenditure. Compared to more technologically sophisticated methods, the Harris-Benedict equations are more practical in terms of effort and expense, and their level of accuracy is sufficient for purposes of planning weight management programs.

In addition to body size and age, RMR is influenced by body composition. Muscular individuals have a higher RMR than fatter individuals of the same body weight because fat tissue is less metabolically active than muscle tissue. The RMRs of women are 5% to 10% lower than those of men (McArdle, Katch, and Katch 1996). This lower rate may be attributable to a greater relative fat content and lower FFM for women. To use method III (p. 208), you must measure the fat-free mass of your client using one of the body composition methods suggested in chapter 8.

Estimation of Additional Caloric Requirements

Resting metabolic rate accounts for 50% to 70% of total daily caloric needs, but this value depends on the activity level and occupation of the person. The percentage is greater for less active individuals, who require fewer calories above the resting level. For example, if a sedentary male office worker has a resting metabolic need of 1680 kcal, the additional caloric need as a consequence of the nature of his work is approximately 40% above resting level, or 672 kcal. Provided he performs no additional physical activities, his total daily caloric need is 2352 kcal. In this case, RMR accounts for 71% of his total daily caloric requirements. Table 9.4 presents additional caloric requirements for selected occupational activity levels.

After determining the daily caloric needs of your clients from their RMR and occupation, you can estimate their additional caloric expenditure due to physical activity and exercise by using a physical activity log (appendix E.3, "Physical Activity Log," p. 329). The individual records every activity performed and the total amount of time spent in each activity. The estimated energy expenditure for a variety of activities is listed in appendix E.4, "Gross Energy Expenditure for Conditioning Exercises, Sports, and Recreational Activities," page 330. You can calculate the total caloric expenditure for each activity by converting the METs to $kcal \cdot kg^{-1} \cdot hr^{-1}$ (1 MET = 1 $kcal \cdot kg^{-1} \cdot hr^{-1}$) and multiplying this value by the client's body weight (kg). This yields the total amount of kilocalories that the client expends per hour of that activity. You can determine the $kcal \cdot min^{-1}$ expenditure by dividing the $kcal \cdot hr^{-1}$ by 60 min. Calculate the total energy expenditure by multiplying the $kcal \cdot min^{-1}$ by the duration of the activity.

Keeping a physical activity log is a very time-consuming process for both you and your client; and it may not increase the accuracy of your estimate of additional caloric expenditure because many clients tend to overestimate the actual du-

Table 9.4 Additional Energy Requirements for Selected Activity Levels

Occupational activity level*	Percentage above basal metabolism	
	Men	Women
Sedentary	15	15
Lightly active	40	35
Moderately active	50	45
Very active	85	70
Exceptionally active	110	100

*Examples for each occupational activity levels are as follows:

Sedentary = inactive.

Lightly active = most professionals, office workers, shop workers, teachers, homemakers.

Moderately active = workers in light industry, most farm workers, active students, department store workers, soldiers not in active service, commercial fishing workers.

Very active = full-time athletes and dancers, unskilled laborers, forestry workers, military recruits and soldiers in active service, mine workers, steel workers.

Exceptionally active = lumberjacks, blacksmiths, female construction workers.

ration of their physical activity. It may be best to just ask your clients to list the frequency, intensity, and average time for the physical activities and sports that they perform on a regular basis; you can then determine their caloric expenditure for each activity as just described. Add these values to the daily caloric need estimated for the individual's RMR and occupation, and advise clients that on days they are active they can increase their caloric intake accordingly.

DESIGNING WEIGHT LOSS PROGRAMS

When the caloric expenditure exceeds the caloric intake, a negative energy balance or caloric deficit is created. The most effective way of producing this deficit is to use a combination of caloric restriction and exercise. Because a deficit of 3500 kcal is needed to lose 1 lb (0.45 kg) of fat, you can easily calculate the daily caloric deficit that is needed to result in the target weekly weight loss you set for your client. An average deficit of 500 kcal will produce a weekly weight loss of approximately 1 lb (0.45 kg), given that 500 kcal × 7 days = 3500 calories. An average deficit of 1000 will produce a weight loss of 2 lb (0.90 kg) a week (1000 kcal × 7 days, or 2 lb). The daily caloric deficit should not exceed 1000 kcal per day.

To ensure that the weight loss is a result of the loss of body fat rather than lean body tissue, you should

- use the body composition method to estimate the client's healthy body weight and fat loss;

- encourage daily participation in aerobic exercise and resistance training programs to enhance the loss of fat and to conserve FFM; and

- prescribe a high-carbohydrate, low-fat diet to prevent the depletion of muscle glycogen stores and to maximize the protein-sparing effect of carbohydrate.

When you design the weight loss program of diet and exercise, use descriptive data to help you set reasonable goals for your clients. These data include age, gender, height, body weight, relative body fat (%BF), %BF goal, average caloric intake, cardiorespiratory fitness level, and occupation. Figure 9.3 illustrates the steps to follow in designing a weight loss program.

Weight Loss Diets

It is strongly recommended that you consult and work closely with a licensed nutritionist or registered dietitian when modifying and planning diets for your clients. For suggestions and advice that you can give to your clients to promote successful weight reduction or weight maintenance, see Clark (1997). When comparing your client's typical nutrient intakes to recommended dietary intakes, you should focus on the following questions:

- How does the average caloric intake compare with the caloric needs and expenditure of the individual?

- What is the relative percentage of carbohydrate, protein, and fat in the diet?

- How much of the total fat intake is saturated fat?

- Is the minimum daily protein requirement being met?

- What is the dietary cholesterol level?

- What is the sodium intake?

- Are the vitamin and mineral requirements being met through the food intake?

- How many meals per day does the person eat? What is the average caloric content of each meal? At what meal are most of the kilocalories consumed?

- What types of snack foods does the person eat? (If the diet contains a lot of junk food, suggest more nutritious snack foods.)

- At what time of day does eating appear to be a problem?

Prescribing a Safe Weight Loss Diet

A high-carbohydrate, low-fat diet provides an excellent source of energy and typically contains as much as 58% to 70% carbohydrate, 12% to 15% protein, and 20% to 30% fat. In planning a well-balanced diet with these relative amounts of macronutrients, refer to the Food Guide Pyramid (see figure 9.4) to determine the number of servings from each of the food groups. Table 9.5 lists common sources for protein, carbohydrate (starches and sugars), and fat. Be sure to consult with your clients when selecting food choices within each group for their diets. Computerized software programs are available to help you plan nutritious and well-balanced meals for your clients.

Educating Your Clients About Quick Weight Loss Diets

The desire to lose weight quickly and easily makes clients vulnerable to fad diets that may be unsafe and nutritionally unsound. Teach them that the safest way to lose weight is to limit caloric intake while eating a well-balanced diet and increasing physical activity and exercise. Some diets ignore the importance of well-balanced meals for adequate nutrition by excluding or restricting the carbohydrate, fat, or protein intake. Recently, the American Institute for Cancer Research (2000) analyzed and summarized the potential effectiveness and possible health risks associated with four popular fad diets promoted in the following books: *Dr. Atkins' New Diet Revolution, The New Beverly Hills Diet, Protein Power,* and *Suzanne Somers' Get Skinny on Fabulous Food.* All four of these plans recommend a daily caloric intake that is well below average requirements. These diets typically omit certain foods and sometimes even entire food groups. The following questions deal with the dangers of quick weight loss diets.

<u>Summary of Client's Demographic Data</u>
1. Client's age and gender (35 yr female)
2. Height (62 in. or 157.5 cm)
3. Body weight (131 lb or 59.55 kg)
4. Percent fat (26% BF); relative FFM (74%)
5. Percent fat goal (20% BF); relative FFM goal (80%)
6. Average daily caloric intake (2000 kcal)
7. Cardiorespiratory fitness level (below average)
8. Occupation (secretary)

<u>Steps:</u>
1. Assess the body weight and body composition of the client.
2. Assess the daily caloric intake of the subject (use 3- or 7-day food records).
3. Estimate a healthy target body weight based on the client's percent fat goal.
   Present FFM = 96.9 lb (131 lb × 0.74) (relative FFM)
   Target body weight = 121 lb (96.9 lb/0.80) (relative FFM goal)
4. Calculate the weight loss and total caloric deficit needed to achieve that weight loss.
   a. Weight loss = 10 lb (131 lb − 121 lb)
   b. Caloric deficit = 35,000 kcal (10 lb × 3,500 kcal · lb^{-1})
5. Estimate the daily energy expenditure of the client from the equation: Energy expenditure = RMR + daily activity level.
   a. RMR = 655.0955 + 9.463 (59.55 kg) + 1.8496 (157.5 cm) − 4.6756 (35 yr) = 1346 kcal
   b. Daily occupational activity level: lightly active 35% above basal level (see table 9.4).
      Additional kcal = 1346 × 0.35 = 471 kcal
   c. Total energy expenditure = 1346 + 471 = 1817 kcal
6. Plan to produce a caloric deficit of 700 to 800 kcal per day by reducing the caloric intake by 500 kcal per day and increasing the caloric expenditure by 200 to 300 kcal per day through exercise. To calculate caloric expenditure during exercise refer to appendix E.4. Multiply the calories burned per minute per kilogram of body weight by the duration of the activity and the client's body weight. Continue this program until the total caloric deficit of 35,000 kcal is reached.

Week 1	exercise = 100 kcal · day^{-1} × 7 days	=	700 kcal
	diet = 500 kcal · day^{-1} × 7 days	=	3,500 kcal
	Total	=	4,200 kcal
Week 2	exercise = 150 kcal · day^{-1} × 7 days	=	1,050 kcal
	diet = 500 kcal · day^{-1} × 7 days	=	3,500 kcal
	Total	=	4,550 kcal
Week 3-4	exercise = 200 kcal · day^{-1} × 14 days	=	2,800 kcal
	diet = 500 kcal · day^{-1} × 14 days	=	7,000 kcal
	Total	=	9,800 kcal
Week 5-6	exercise = 250 kcal · day^{-1} × 14 days	=	3,500 kcal
	diet = 500 kcal · day^{-1} × 14 days	=	7,000 kcal
	Total	=	10,500 kcal
Week 7	exercise = 300 kcal · day^{-1} × 7 days	=	2,100 kcal
	diet = 500 kcal · day^{-1} × 7 days	=	3,500 kcal
	Total	=	5,600 kcal
	Total Weeks 1-7	=	34,650 kcal

In a little over 7 weeks the client will lose approximately 10 lb. This is a gradual average weight loss of 1 1/2 lb per week. Reassess the body composition to see if the percent fat goal was reached.
7. Put the client on a maintenance diet and exercise program.
   a. Calculate the total energy expenditure using an estimate of RMR based on the new body weight.
      RMR + activity level + exercise = total energy expenditure where:
      RMR = 1303 kcal (use Harris-Benedict formula substituting a body weight of 55 kg)
      Occupational activity level = 456 kcal (1303 × 0.35)
      Exercise = 300 kcal
      Total energy expenditure = 1303 + 456 + 300 = 2059 kcal
   b. Advise the client that if she continues to exercise daily, expending approximately 300 kcal per workout, she may increase her caloric intake to 2060 kcal per day. However, for days in which she cannot exercise, the caloric intake must be restricted to 1760 kcal.

Figure 9.3 Steps for designing a weight loss program. FFM = fat-free mass; BF = body fat; RMR = resting metabolic rate.

Table 9.5	Common Sources of Carbohydrate, Protein, and Fat
Macronutrient	**Food sources**
Carbohydrate	
Starches	Pasta, rice, grains, breads, cereals, potatoes, dried beans and peas
Sugars	Fruits, candy, cookies, cakes, jelly, sugar, honey, syrup, molasses, soda pop
Protein	Meats, fish, poultry, eggs, milk, yogurt, cheese, nuts, dried beans
Fat	
Saturated	Animal fats, butter, cheese, whole milk, mayonnaise, egg yolks, ice cream, chocolate, lard, hydrogenated oils, coconut and palm oils
Polyunsaturated	Some margarines, nuts, and oils (i.e., corn, safflower, soybean, cottonseed, sesame, and sunflower oils)
Monounsaturated	Olive, canola, and peanut oils and avocado

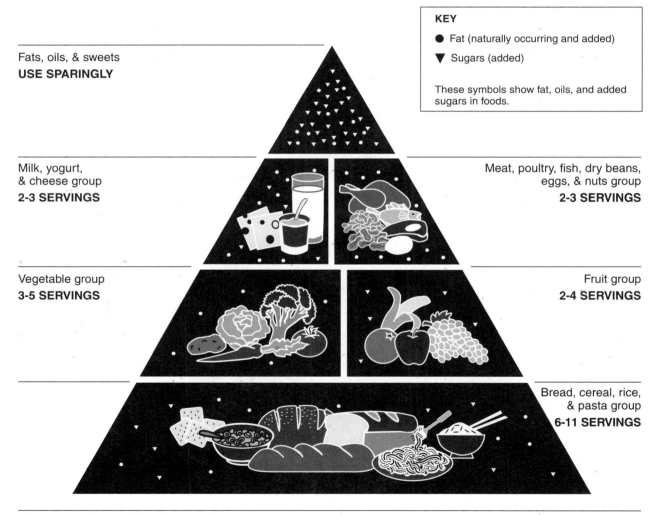

KEY

● Fat (naturally occurring and added)

▼ Sugars (added)

These symbols show fat, oils, and added sugars in foods.

Fats, oils, & sweets
USE SPARINGLY

Milk, yogurt, & cheese group
2-3 SERVINGS

Meat, poultry, fish, dry beans, eggs, & nuts group
2-3 SERVINGS

Vegetable group
3-5 SERVINGS

Fruit group
2-4 SERVINGS

Bread, cereal, rice, & pasta group
6-11 SERVINGS

Figure 9.4 The Food Guide Pyramid.

From "The Food Guide Pyramid" by U.S. Department of Agriculture, Human Nutrition Information Service, 1992, Leaflet No. 572, U.S. Government Printing Office, Washington, D.C.

■ *Why should a weight loss diet include at least 58% to 70% carbohydrate?*

Carbohydrate, in the form of glucose, helps maintain normal function of the nervous system, because nerve tissue relies solely on glucose as a fuel for energy. Consuming adequate amounts of carbohydrate on a daily basis prevents the depletion of glycogen stores and synthesis of glucose from the body's protein (protein-sparing effect). When glycogen stores are depleted, the glucose needs of the body are met through the breakdown of muscle protein. This produces a loss of lean tissue rather than fat. Carbohydrate is also essential for fat metabolism. When carbohydrates are restricted or carbohydrate stores are depleted, more free fatty acids are mobilized from adipose tissue than can be metabolized by the body. This results in the incomplete breakdown of lipids and the formation of ketone bodies that may cause ketosis.

In addition, muscle glycogen and glucose are the primary fuels used during intense short-term exercise and prolonged submaximal exercise. Inclusion of adequate amounts of carbohydrate in the diet prevents muscle glycogen depletion and the consequent reduction in endurance performance. Carbohydrates with a high GI are also recommended for replacing muscle glycogen immediately after exercise (Manore and Thompson 2000).

■ *Why do low-carbohydrate diets produce such rapid weight loss?*

Diets that limit or totally exclude carbohydrate intake produce a rapid weight loss. When the carbohydrate intake is low, muscle glycogen stores are depleted rapidly. For every gram of carbohydrate, 3 g of water is stored in the body. Thus, when glycogen stores are depleted, the loss of water leads to a dramatic weight loss because each liter of water weighs approximately 2 lb (0.90 kg). The weight is regained rapidly, however, when carbohydrate intake returns to normal.

■ *Why are low-carbohydrate diets unsafe?*

Low carbohydrate intake may lead to undue fatigue, hypoglycemia, and ketosis. As mentioned earlier, in the body's attempt to remedy low blood glucose levels, more free fatty acids are mobilized from adipose tissue than can be metabolized, resulting in an incomplete breakdown of fat and the formation of ketone bodies by the liver. The production of ketone bodies may exceed the body's ability to metabolize them (ketosis). The excess ketone bodies normally are excreted in the urine and expired air. In this condition, however, the blood pH may be lowered to dangerous levels. Examples of popular diets that are low in carbohydrates or that totally eliminate intake of carbohydrates are Dr. Atkins' New Diet Revolution and the Yudkin, Stillman, Cooper, Mayo Clinic, and Scarsdale diets.

■ *Are high-protein diets safe?*

High-protein diets that limit carbohydrate intake promote muscle tissue loss. When carbohydrate intake is restricted, the body meets its glucose needs by breaking down muscle proteins. The average exercising individual needs no more than 1.2 to 1.6 g of protein per kilogram of body weight each day to meet the additional protein requirements of the body (Lemon 1998; Lemon, Tarnopolsky, MacDougall, and Atkinson 1992; Tarnopolsky et al. 1992). Protein intake beyond this level does not promote protein synthesis. Instead, the excess protein is metabolized. The amino acids are deaminated, the excess nitrogen is excreted in the urine as urea, and the remaining carbon skeleton is converted to glucose or used as an energy fuel.

Some high-protein diets require drinking large quantities of water to prevent dehydration caused by excess urea production and to wash away ketone bodies. Dehydration and the additional stress placed on the kidneys may be potentially dangerous, especially for individuals with kidney problems or gout. Examples of popular diets that are high in protein are the Protein Power, Pennington, Stillman, Cooper, Mayo Clinic, and Scarsdale diets.

■ *Why are high-fat diets unsafe?*

Diets that allow unlimited consumption of fats produce high levels of serum cholesterol and triglycerides. This is potentially unhealthy because cholesterol in the form of low-density lipoproteins is associated with atherosclerosis and CHD. Typically, high-fat diets are high in calories. Each gram of fat yields 9.3 kcal, while protein and carbohydrate yield 4.3 and 4.1 $kcal \cdot g^{-1}$, respectively (see table 9.1). Thus, the total quantity of food that a person can consume on a high-fat diet is less than on a high-carbohydrate or high-protein diet when the calorie intake is the same. Because there are no metabolic pathways in the body for converting fatty acids to glucose, excess fat is stored in adipose tissue. The Atkins diet is an example of a high-fat diet that restricts carbohydrate intake and allows unlimited consumption of meat and fat.

■ *Are diets with a low GI safe and effective for weight loss?*

Monitoring the GI of various foods is important for individuals with diabetes and endurance athletes (food intake before, during, and after exercise). Diets composed primarily of foods with a low GI also have been promoted for weight loss (e.g., Sugar Busters). Foods that are slowly converted into blood glucose (i.e., low GI) have a high satiety index and therefore satisfy the appetite without making it necessary to consume excess calories. However, the American Diabetes Association warns that several foods with a low GI also have a high fat content (e.g., chocolate and peanuts). Thus, basing a diet primarily on the GI may put some individuals at higher risk for heart attacks and strokes (American Institute for Cancer Research 2000). Since there have been only a few clinical weight loss trials using the GI exclusively, the usefulness of this index as a weight management tool remains questionable (American Institute for Cancer Research 2000).

■ *What is the danger of fasting or skipping meals to promote weight loss?*

For some people, abstaining from food completely may be easier than limiting the amount of food eaten. Fasting, however, may produce serious problems such as kidney malfunction, hyperuricemia, loss of hair, dizziness, fainting, and muscle cramping. When the body is deprived of food, it responds by increasing the fat-depositing enzymes and storing more fat. Also, because carbohydrate and fat are not readily available as a source of energy, the body metabolizes protein to meet its energy needs.

Skipping meals to restrict caloric intake also leads to an increase in the deposition and storage of fat. When we eat just one meal per day, the body is subjected to a fasting condition (23-hr fast) that increases the fat-depositing enzymes. The body quickly adapts to this condition by increasing the percentage of food absorbed by the small intestine. For this reason, nutrition experts advise eating at least three meals a day, or as many as six small meals a day.

Exercise Prescription for Weight Loss

Exercise alone—without dieting—has only a modest effect on weight loss. The most successful weight loss programs, therefore, use a combination of dieting and exercising to optimize the energy deficit and to maintain weight loss (ACSM 1998). The exercise portion of the weight loss regimen is designed to produce a weight loss by increasing the caloric expenditure. Select an aerobic activity of sufficient intensity and duration to expend approximately 250 to 300 kcal or 4 kcal·kg⁻¹ of body weight per exercise session (ACSM 1998). See the following guidelines for developing an exercise prescription for weight loss.

GUIDELINES FOR EXERCISE PRESCRIPTION FOR WEIGHT LOSS

- **Mode:** Group I or II aerobic activities (see p. 89)
- **Intensity and duration:** An intensity that can be sustained for at least 30 to 45 min
- **Kcal expenditure:** 250 to 300 kcal or 4 kcal·kg⁻¹ of body weight per exercise session
- **Frequency:** At least three days per week
- **Length of program:** Dependent on desired weight loss

Benefits of Exercise

This section highlights some common questions about the benefits of exercise in a weight loss program.

■ *Why is exercise an essential part of weight loss programs?*

In addition to increasing energy expenditure and helping to create a negative energy balance for weight loss, adding exercise to dieting increases the amount of fat lost. Exercise also maintains or slows down the loss of FFM that occurs with dieting only and is important for maintaining weight loss after dieting (Manore and Thompson 2000).

Pavlou, Steffee, Lerman, and Burrows (1985) studied the contribution of exercise to the preservation of FFM in mildly obese males on a rapid weight loss diet. The exercise group dieted and participated in an eight-week walking-jogging program, three days a week. The nonexercising group dieted only. Although the total weight loss of the exercise (–11.8 kg) and nonexercise (–9.2 kg) groups was similar, the composition of the weight loss differed significantly. The exercise group maintained FFM (–0.6 kg) while the nonexercise group lost a significant amount of FFM (–3.3 kg). Also, the exercise group lost more fat (11.2 kg) than the nonexercise group (5.9 kg). In other words, for the nonexercising subjects, only 64% of the total weight loss was fat weight compared to 95% for the exercising subjects. The researchers concluded that the addition of aerobic exercise to the dietary regimen preserves existing FFM, increases fat utilization for energy production, and is more effective in reducing fat stores than diet alone.

Similarly, Kraemer, Volek, et al. (1999) compared the effects of a weight loss dietary regimen with and without exercise in overweight men. The diet-only group did not exercise; the exercise groups participated in either an aerobic exercise program or a combined aerobic and resistance training exercise program, three days per week for 12 weeks. By the end of the program, all three groups lost a similar amount of body weight (~9 to 10 kg), but the composition of the weight loss differed significantly. For the diet-only group, only 69% of the total weight loss was fat weight compared to 78% for the diet plus aerobic exercise group and 97% for the diet and exercise (aerobic + resistance training) group. These results suggest that using a combination of aerobic and resistance training exercises in conjunction with dieting is more effective than dieting alone for preserving FFM and maximizing fat loss.

■ How does exercise promote fat loss and the preservation of lean body mass?

In response to aerobic and resistance training exercise, levels of growth hormone, epinephrine, and norepinephrine increase. These hormones stimulate the mobilization of fat from storage and activate the enzyme lipase, which breaks down triglycerides into free fatty acids. Free fatty acids are then metabolized and serve as an important energy source, especially during aerobic exercise. Heavy resistance training exercise also stimulates the release of anabolic hormones such as testosterone and growth hormone, resulting in increased protein synthesis, muscle growth, and FFM (Kraemer et al. 1991).

■ How does improved cardiorespiratory fitness help control body weight?

As the individual's cardiorespiratory fitness level increases through training, the amount of work that the person can accomplish at a given submaximal heart rate increases. Thus, the more fit individual expends calories at a faster rate than the less fit individual at a given exercise heart rate. For example, at a heart rate of 150 bpm, the rate of energy expenditure is approximately 10 and 15 kcal·min^{-1} for fair and superior fitness levels, respectively (Sharkey 1990).

During high-intensity aerobic exercise, lactate production increases and inhibits fatty acid metabolism. However, endurance training increases the lactate threshold (point at which lactate accumulates significantly in the blood). In aerobically trained individuals, the percentage of the energy derived from the oxidation of free fatty acids during submaximal exercise is greater than that derived from glucose oxidation (Coyle 1995; Mole, Oscai, and Holloszy 1971). The reduction in muscle glycogen utilization is also associated with a greater rate of oxidation of intramuscular tri-glyceride (Coyle 1995).

■ What effect does exercise have on the RMR?

Another reason for including exercise in the weight loss program is its positive effect on RMR. Research indicates that exercise may counter the reduction in RMR that usually occurs as a result of dieting (Thompson, Manore, and Thomas 1996). It is well known that the rate of weight loss declines in the later stages of dieting due to a decrease in RMR. The lowered RMR is an energy-conserving metabolic adaptation to prolonged periods of caloric restriction (Donahue, Lin, Kirschenbaum, and Keesey 1984). In a study of 12 overweight females, Donahue et al. (1984) reported that diet alone caused a 4.4% reduction in the relative RMR (RMR/BW). After the addition of eight weeks of aerobic exercise to the program, the relative RMR increased by 5%. The net effect of exercise was to offset the diet-induced metabolic adaptation and return the RMR to the normal, pre-diet level.

Exercise may also facilitate weight loss by causing an increase in postexercise RMR. Moderate-to high-intensity aerobic exercise increases the postexercise RMR by 5% to 16%, and the elevated RMR may persist for 12 to 39 hr postexercise (Bahr, Ingnes, Vaage, Sjersted, and Newsholme 1987; Bielinski, Schultz, and Jequier 1985; Sjodin et al. 1996). The postexercise elevation in RMR appears to be related to the exercise intensity and duration (Brehm 1988). Cycling at 70% $\dot{V}O_2$max for 20 min produced a 5% to 14% elevation in RMR for 12 hr in young, healthy men (Bahr, Ingnes, Vaage, Sjersted, and Newsholme 1987). Although it is tempting to apply these findings to clients who are elderly or obese, it is not known whether the postexercise metabolic response of these individuals is similar to that of young men.

Types of Exercise

This section addresses common concerns regarding the types of exercise suitable for weight loss programs.

■ Is aerobic exercise better than resistance exercise for weight loss?

One study evaluated the effects of aerobic and/or resistance training, in combination with dieting (i.e., moderate caloric restriction), in moderately overweight women (Marks, Ward, Morris, Castellani, and Rippe 1995). All the exercise intervention groups (cycling only, resistance training only, and combination of cycling and resistance training) maintained FFM. The diet-only group lost only a minimal amount of FFM; this result suggests that FFM can be maintained provided that the daily caloric intake is at least 1200 kcal a day. Compared to a control group, all diet and exercise intervention groups lost greater amounts of body weight (–3.7 to –5.4 kg) and fat mass, but there were no differences in weight loss and fat loss among the intervention groups. These data suggest that resistance training may be as effective as aerobic training in weight loss programs.

A recent study (Bryner et al. 1999) compared the effects of 12 weeks of resistance or aerobic training on the FFM and RMR of individuals on a very low calorie diet (800 kcal per day liquid diet). One group exercised aerobically (walking, biking, or stair climbing) for 1 hr, four days per week; the other group performed resistance training exercises (two to four sets, 8- to 15-RM for 10 exercises). The body weight of the aerobic exercise group decreased more than that of the resistance-trained group; however, the FFM and RMR of the aerobic exercise group also decreased significantly. The resistance-trained group, on the other hand, maintained FFM and significantly increased RMR. These findings suggest that resistance training may be superior to aerobic training in preserving FFM and RMR of individuals on a very low calorie diet.

■ Is high-intensity exercise better than light-to moderate-intensity exercise for weight loss?

An important reason for including exercise as part of a weight loss program is to maximize energy expenditure, thereby creating a larger negative energy balance. Close examination of energy expenditure during selected physical activities (appendix E.4, "Gross Energy Expenditure for Conditioning Exercises, Sports, and Recreational Activities," p. 330) reveals that increases in speed (intensity) of exercise produce only small increases in the rate of energy expenditure (METs). For example, if a 123-lb woman increases the speed of running from a slow (5.0 mph or 12 min/mile) to a faster speed (7.0 mph or 8.5 min/mile), the rate of expenditure increases only 3.2 kcal·min^{-1}. At the 8.5 min/mile pace, the woman expends 11.5 METs (11.5 kcal·kg^{-1}·min^{-1} or 10.7 kcal·min^{-1}) and is able to run a maximum distance of 3 miles (4.8 km). The duration of the workout is 25.5 min (8.5 min·mile^{-1} × 3 miles), and the total caloric expenditure is 274 kcal (25.5 min × 10.7 kcal·min^{-1}). When she reduces the exercise intensity by decreasing her speed to a 12 min/mile pace, her relative energy expenditure decreases (8 METs or 8 kcal·kg^{-1}·min^{-1} or 7.5 kcal·min^{-1}), but she is able to run a distance of 4 miles (6.4 km). The duration of the workout increases to 48 min (12 min·mile^{-1} × 4 miles), and the total caloric expenditure is increased (48 min × 7.5 kcal·min^{-1} = 360 kcal). Thus, the duration of the exercise and total distance may be somewhat more important than the speed (intensity) of exercise for maximizing the energy expenditure.

■ Are spot reduction exercises effective for decreasing body fat in localized regions of the body?

Specific spot reduction exercises are no more effective than general aerobic exercise for changing limb and body girth measurements or for altering total body composition (Carns, Schade, Liba, Hellebrandt, and Harris 1960; Noland and Kearney 1978; Roby 1962; Schade, Hellebrandt, Waterland, and Carns 1962). Katch, Clarkson, Kroll, McBride, and Wilcox (1984) assessed changes in the diameter of adipose cells from the abdomen, gluteal, and subscapular sites resulting from a 27-day training program in which each subject performed 5004 sit-ups. Although the training significantly reduced fat cell diameter, the effect was similar at all three sites: abdomen, –6.4%; gluteal, –5.0%; and subscapular, –3.7%. It appears that a sit-up exercise program does not preferentially reduce the fat in the abdominal region.

Despres, Bouchard, Tremblay, Savard, and Marcotte (1985) reported that a 20-week cycling program significantly reduced %BF and body weight. Cycling affected trunk skinfolds (SKFs) (–22%) more than extremity SKFs (–12.5%). If fat was mobilized preferentially from subcutaneous stores near the exercising muscle mass, one would expect the lower-extremity SKFs to be more affected by cycling than the trunk SKFs. Yet Despres et al. noted an 18% reduction in the suprailiac SKF compared to a 13% reduction in the thigh SKF. This suggests that subcutaneous fat cells in the abdomen are more sensitive to the lipolytic effect of catecholamines than subcutaneous fat cells in the thighs (Smith, Hammerstein, Bjorntorp, and Kral 1979).

The enzyme lipoprotein-lipase is responsible for lipid accumulation. In women, lipoprotein-lipase activity is higher in the gluteofemoral region than in the abdominal region (Litchell and Boberg 1978). Estrogen and progesterone appear to enhance lipoprotein-lipase activity in women. Also, the lipolytic response to catecholamines is lower in the femoral than in the abdominal depots for both men and women (Rebuffe-Scrive 1985).

Thus, the regional distribution and mobilization of adipose tissue appear to follow a biologically selective pattern regardless of type of exercise. Even with weight reduction, the relative fat distribution remains stable as measured by the WHR; however, the waist-to-thigh ratio decreases, suggesting that the thigh region is slightly more resistant to fat mobilization in women (Ashwell, McCall, Cole, and Dixon 1985).

DESIGNING WEIGHT GAIN PROGRAMS

Because genetics plays an important role in weight gain, some clients may have difficulty gaining weight, especially if they have inherited a high RMR. Before prescribing weight gain programs, you should rule out the possibility that diseases and psychological disorders associated with malnutrition (e.g., anorexia nervosa) are not causing your client to be underweight.

The number of additional calories needed in order for a person to gain 1 lb (0.45 kg) of muscle tissue has not yet been firmly established. However, research suggests that an excess of 2800 to 3500 kcal is required. Thus, adding 400 to 500 kcal to the estimated daily caloric needs (RMR + occupational activity level) of the individual should produce a gradual weight gain of 1 lb per week (Williams 1992). The caloric intake must also be adjusted for additional calories expended during exercise.

Weight Gain Diets

Again, it is highly recommended that you consult with a trained nutrition professional when planning weight gain diets. When comparing your client's typical nutrient intakes to recommended dietary intakes, you should focus on the same questions as outlined for weight loss programs (see "Weight Loss Diets," p. 211).

To ensure that your client's weight gain is due to increases in lean tissues rather than body fat, you should

- use the body composition method to estimate a healthy target body weight and gain in FFM;
- plan a high-calorie, well-balanced diet in which 60% to 65% of the total kilocalorie intake is derived from carbohydrate, 12% to 15% from protein, and 23% to 25% from fat;
- increase daily protein intake to 1.2 to 1.6 g per kilogram of body weight to increase muscle size; and
- monitor body composition regularly throughout the weight gain program using methods described in chapter 8.

Exercise Prescription for Weight Gain

As part of the weight gain program, you should prescribe resistance training to increase muscle size. A high-volume resistance training program is the best approach to maximize the development of muscle size (see table 7.3). Because some clients may not be able to tolerate this volume of training at first, novice weight lifters should start slowly by performing only three sets of each exercise at the prescribed intensity and by reducing the number of exercises for each muscle group. Depending on your client's goal, this may be sufficient to increase FFM. For some clients, however, you may need to progressively increase the training volume in order to elicit further improvements in muscle size and FFM. Recommended guidelines for developing an exercise prescription for weight gain are as follows:

GUIDELINES FOR EXERCISE PRESCRIPTION FOR WEIGHT GAIN

- **Mode:** Resistance training
- **Intensity:** 70% to 75% 1-RM or 10- to 12-RM
- **Sets:** Three for novices; more than three for advanced weight lifters
- **Number of exercises:** One to two per muscle group for novices; three to four per muscle group for advanced weight lifters
- **Duration:** 60 min or longer
- **Frequency:** Three days a week for novices; five to six days a week for advanced weight lifters
- **Length of program:** Dependent on desired weight gain

DESIGNING PROGRAMS TO IMPROVE BODY COMPOSITION

Some clients may wish to improve their body composition without changing their body weight. For these individuals, you can design exercise programs to either decrease body fat, increase FFM, or both. Research has shown that regular participation in an exercise program may alter an individual's body composition. Aerobic exercise and resistance training are effective modes for decreasing SKF thicknesses, fat weight, and %BF of both women and men.

Questions About Exercise and Body Composition Changes

- *What is the effect of aerobic exercise training on body fat?*

Numerous studies have been conducted to determine the effect of aerobic exercise training on body composition. The modes of exercise include cycling, walking, jogging, running, and swimming. Wilmore, Royce, Girandola, Katch, and Katch (1970) reported that a 10-week jogging program (three times per week) produced a significant increase in body density of sedentary men. Because total body weight decreased and FFM remained stable, the increase in body density was attributed almost entirely to fat loss. Pollock et al. (1971) also noted that a 20-week (four times a week) walking program produced a decrease in %BF and total body weight of men.

- *Which aerobic exercise mode is best for maximizing fat loss?*

One study compared cycling, running, and walking of equal frequency, duration, and intensity (Pollock, Dimmick, Miller, Kendrick, and Linnerud 1975). All three programs produced significant reductions in %BF and body weight. Also, Despres, Bouchard, Tremblay, Savard, and Marcotte (1985) reported that a 20-week cycling program (four to five times a week) resulted in significant reductions in body weight, %BF, and fat cell weight in a group of sedentary men. On the basis of these studies it appears that aerobic exercise modes are equally effective in altering body composition.

- *How many times a week should I exercise to maximize the loss of body fat?*

The frequency of the training program may affect the magnitude of the changes in body composition. Pollock, Miller, Linnerud, and Cooper (1975) compared aerobic exercise programs consisting of two, three, or four days a week. Even though the total mileage and caloric expenditure were the same, exercising two days a week was not sufficient to produce significant alterations in body composition. The authors concluded that a three or four day a week program produces significant body composition changes, with four days a week being superior to three.

- *What effect does resistance training have on body fat and FFM?*

Dynamic resistance training is effective for decreasing %BF and increasing FFM of men and women (Brown and Wilmore 1974; Cullinen and Caldwell 1998; Mayhew and Gross 1974; Wilmore 1974). Cullinen and Caldwell (1998) found that normal-weight women (19 to 44 years) participating in a moderate-intensity resistance training program (2 days per week for 12 weeks) significantly increased FFM (~4.5%) and decreased %BF (~8.7%). In Wilmore's study (1974), subjects trained two days a week for 10 weeks. At each training session, they performed two sets of 7- to 9-RM for eight different weight training exercises. Men and women exhibited similar alterations in body composition. Although the total body weight remained stable, the FFM increased significantly for both sexes. As a result of resistance training, the relative body fat decreased 9.6% and 10.0% for women and men, respectively.

- *How does exercise promote body composition changes?*

The significant loss of fat weight and %BF with aerobic exercise and resistance training is a function of hormonal responses to the exercise. Exercise increases the circulatory levels of growth hormone (GH), and the levels remain elevated for 1 to 2 hr after exercise (Hartley et al. 1972; Hartley 1975). Exercise also stimulates the release of catecholamines from the adrenal medulla. Both GH and catecholamines increase the mobilization of free fatty acids from storage (Hartley 1975). Eventually, the muscle may metabolize these free fatty acids during rest and low-intensity exercise.

The increase in FFM with resistance training may be due to muscle hypertrophy, increased protein content in the muscle, or increased bone density. Muscle hypertrophy and increased protein are mediated by changes in serum testosterone and GH levels in response to weightlifting. Immediately following heavy resistance weightlifting, serum testosterone levels are significantly elevated for men but not for women (Fahey, Rolph, Moungmee,

Nagel, and Mortara 1976; Weiss, Cureton, and Thompson 1983). Growth hormone levels in men are increased significantly for 15 min following a 21-min bout of high-intensity (85% of 1-RM) leg press exercises. However, low-intensity, high-repetition (28% of 1-RM, 21 reps per set) leg presses produced no significant change in GH even though the total amount of work and duration of exercise were equal. Thus, the intensity and number of repetitions play a role in GH release in response to weightlifting exercise (Vanhelder, Radomski, and Goode 1984).

In addition, resistance training has an effect on the hormonal profiles of younger (30 years) and older (62 years) men (Kraemer, Hakkinen, et al. 1999). Following a 10-week, periodized strength-power training program, young men had significant increases in free testosterone at rest and in response to weightlifting exercise. Younger men also showed increases in resting levels of insulin-like growth factor-binding protein-3 after training. For the older men, training produced a significant increase in total testosterone in response to weightlifting exercise, as well as a significant reduction in resting cortisol levels.

Exercise Prescription for Body Composition Change

While light- to moderate-intensity aerobic exercise may be more beneficial for fat loss, high-intensity resistance training is better for FFM gain. Thus, combining aerobic and resistance training exercises may be the most effective way to alter body composition of non-dieting individuals (Dolezal and Potteiger 1998). When designing exercise programs to promote changes in body composition, adhere to the following guidelines. Prescribe aerobic exercise to reduce body fat and resistance training exercise to increase FFM.

GUIDELINES FOR EXERCISE PRESCRIPTION FOR FAT LOSS

- **Goal:** Fat loss
- **Mode:** Type I or II aerobic activities (see p. 89)
- **Intensity:** Light to moderate (50% to 75% $\dot{V}O_2$reserve)
- **Duration:** 30 to 45 min
- **Frequency:** Minimum of three days a week
- **Length:** Minimum of eight weeks

GUIDELINES FOR EXERCISE PRESCRIPTION FOR FAT-FREE MASS GAIN

- **Goal:** Increase FFM and reduce body fat
- **Mode:** Dynamic resistance training
- **Intensity:** 70% to 85% 1-RM
- **Repetitions:** 6 to 12 reps
- **Sets:** Three sets
- **Frequency:** Minimum of three days per week
- **Length:** Minimum of eight weeks

KEY POINTS

- Obesity is an excess of body fat that increases health risks.
- Two types of obesity are upper-body (android) and lower-body (gynoid) obesity.
- The number of fat cells in the body is determined primarily during childhood and adolescence.
- Weight gain in adults is associated with an increase in the size of existing fat cells (hypertrophy), rather than an increase in the number of fat cells (hyperplasia).
- Physical inactivity is a more common cause of obesity than overeating.

- The body composition method provides a useful estimate of a healthy body weight.
- Well-balanced nutrition includes adequate amounts of carbohydrate, protein, fat, minerals, vitamins, and water.
- A high-carbohydrate, low-fat diet provides an excellent source of energy and complies with the recommendations in *Dietary Guidelines for Americans*.
- Effective weight loss programs create a negative energy balance by restricting caloric intake and increasing physical activity and exercise; weight gain programs create a positive energy balance by increasing caloric intake.

- For weight loss programs, the combined daily caloric deficit due to calorie restriction and extra exercise should not exceed 1000 kcal; for weight gain programs, the daily caloric intake should exceed the energy need by no more than 400 to 500 kcal.

- Adding a combination of aerobic and resistance training exercises to the dieting regimen is an effective way to maximize fat loss and preserve FFM during weight loss.

- For weight gain programs, resistance training will ensure that most of the weight gain is due to increases in lean body tissues.

- Aerobic exercise and resistance training are effective ways to improve body composition without changing body weight.

KEY TERMS

Learn the definition for each of the following key terms. Definitions of terms can be found in "Glossary of Terms," page 349.

android obesity
anorexia nervosa
basal metabolic rate (BMR)
glycemic index (GI)
gynoid obesity
healthy body weight
hyperplasia
hypertrophy

kilocalorie
lower-body obesity
negative energy balance
obesity
positive energy balance
resting metabolic rate (RMR)
underweight
upper-body obesity

REVIEW QUESTIONS

In addition to being able to define each of the key terms, test your knowledge and understanding of the material by answering the following review questions.

1. Using BMI, what are the cutoff values for classification of obesity, overweight, healthy body weight, and underweight?

2. Describe how you can determine a healthy body weight for your client.

3. For typical weight loss programs, identify the minimal caloric intake per day and maximal caloric deficit (i.e., negative energy balance) per day. What is the best way to create this daily caloric deficit?

4. Explain why a taller, heavier person will lose weight at a faster rate than a shorter, lighter person when both individuals are on the same diet.

5. For well-balanced nutrition, what are the recommended proportions of carbohydrate, fat, and protein in the diet?

6. Explain why exercise is an important component of weight loss and weight gain programs.

7. Estimate the daily caloric intake for a 50-year-old, 150-lb (68-kg) female professor who is 5 ft 5 in. and who bikes a total of 60 min, five days per week, to and from the university.

8. Why are low-carbohydrate, high-protein diets not recommended for weight loss?

9. Describe the basic exercise prescriptions for weight loss and weight gain programs.

REFERENCES

American College of Sports Medicine (ACSM). 1988. The recommended quantity and quality of exercise for developing and maintaining cardiorespiratory and muscular fitness, and flexibility in healthy adults. *Medicine & Science in Sports & Exercise* 30: 975–991.

American Institute for Cancer Research. 2000. Fad diets versus dietary guidelines. **http://www.aicr.org**.

American Psychiatric Association. 1994. *Diagnostic and statistical manual of mental disorders:* IV, 4th ed. Washington, D.C.: Author.

Ashwell, M., McCall, S.A., Cole, T.J., and Dixon, A.K. 1985. Fat distribution and its metabolic complications: Interpretations. In *Human body composition and fat distribution,* ed. N.G. Norgan, 227–242. Wageningen, Netherlands: Euronut.

Bahr, R., Ingnes, I., Vaage, O., Sjersted, O.M., and Newsholme, E.A. 1987. Effect of duration of exercise on excess post-exercise O_2 consumption. *Journal of Applied Physiology* 62: 485–490.

Baumgartner, R.N., Heymsfield, S.B., and Roche, A.F. 1995. Human body composition and the epidemiology of chronic disease. *Obesity Research* 3: 73–95.

Bielinski, R., Schultz, Y., and Jequier, E. 1985. Energy metabolism during the postexercise recovery in man. *American Journal of Clinical Nutrition* 42: 69–82.

Bjorntorp, P. 1988. Abdominal obesity and the development of non-insulin diabetes mellitus. *Diabetes and Metabolism Reviews* 4: 615–622.

Blair, D., Habricht, J.P., Sims, E.A., Sylwester, D., and Abraham, S. 1984. Evidence of an increased risk for hypertension with centrally located body fat, and the effect of race and sex on this risk. *American Journal of Epidemiology* 119: 526–540.

Bouchard, C., Perusse, L., Leblanc, C., Tremblay, A., and Theriault, G. 1988. Inheritance of the amount and distribution of human body fat. *International Journal of Obesity* 12: 205–215.

Bouchard, C., Tremblay, A., Despres, J.P., Nadeau, A., Lupien, P.J., Theriault, G., Dussault, J., Moorjani, S., Pinault, S., and Fournier, G. 1990. The response of long-term overfeeding in identical twins. *New England Journal of Medicine* 322: 1477–1482.

Bray, G.A., and Gray, D.S. 1988. Obesity. Part I—Pathogenesis. *Western Journal of Medicine* 149: 429–441.

Brehm, B.A. 1988. Elevation of metabolic rate following exercise—implications for weight loss. *Sports Medicine* 6: 72–78.

Brown, C.H., and Wilmore, J.H. 1974. The effects of maximal resistance training on the strength and body composition of women athletes. *Medicine and Science in Sports* 6: 174–177.

Bryner, R.W., Ullrich, I.H., Sauers, J., Donley, D., Hornsby, G., Kolar, M., and Yeater, R. 1999. Effects of resistance vs. aerobic training combined with an 800 calorie liquid diet on lean body mass and resting metabolic rate. *Journal of the American College of Nutrition* 18(2): 115–121.

Carns, M.L., Schade, M.L., Liba, M.R., Hellebrandt, F.A., and Harris, C.W. 1960. Segmental volume reduction by localized and generalized exercise. *Human Biology* 32: 370–376.

Clark, N. 1997. *Sports nutrition guidebook.* Champaign, IL: Human Kinetics.

Clarkson, P.M. 1990. Tired blood: Iron deficiency in athletes and effects of iron supplementation. *Sports Science Exchange* 3(28). Gatorade Sports Science Institute, Quaker Oats Co.

Clarkson, P.M., and Haymes, E.M. 1994. Trace mineral requirements for athletes. *International Journal of Sport Nutrition* 4: 104–119.

Collins, W.E. 1967. *Clinical spirometry.* Braintree, MA: Author.

Coyle, E.F. 1995. Fat metabolism during exercise. *Sports Science Exchange* 8(6). Gatorade Sports Science Institute, Quaker Oats Co.

Cullinen, K., and Caldwell, M. 1998. Weight training increases fat-free mass and strength in untrained young women. *Journal of the American Dietetic Association* 98(4): 414–418.

Despres, J.P., Bouchard, C., Tremblay, A., Savard, R., and Marcotte, M. 1985. Effects of aerobic training on fat distribution in male subjects. *Medicine & Science in Sports & Exercise* 17: 113–118.

Dolezal, B.A., and Potteiger, J.A. 1998. Concurrent resistance and endurance training influence basal metabolic rate in nondieting individuals. *Journal of Applied Physiology* 85: 695–700.

Donahue, C.P., Lin, D.H., Kirschenbaum, D.S., and Keesey, R.E. 1984. Metabolic consequence of dieting and exercise in the treatment of obesity. *Journal of Counseling and Clinical Psychology* 52: 827–836.

Ducimetier, P., Richard, J., and Cambien, F. 1989. The pattern of subcutaneous fat distribution in middle-aged men and the risk of coronary heart disease: The Paris prospective study. *International Journal of Obesity* 10: 229–240.

Ettinger, B., Genault, H.K., and Cann, C.E. 1987. Postmenopausal bone loss is prevented by treatment with low-dosage estrogen with calcium. *Annals of Internal Medicine* 106: 40–45.

Evans, W., and Rosenberg, I. 1992. *Biomarkers.* New York: Simon & Schuster.

Fahey, T.D., Rolph, R., Moungmee, P., Nagel, J., and Mortara, S. 1976. Serum testosterone, body composition, and strength of young adults. *Medicine and Science in Sports* 8: 31–34.

Flegal, K.M. 1999. The obesity epidemic in children and adults: Current evidence and research issues. *Medicine & Science in Sports & Exercise* 31: S509–S514.

Fohlin, L. 1977. Body composition, cardiovascular and renal function in adolescent patients with anorexia nervosa. *Acta Paediatrica Scandinavica* 268(Suppl.): 7–20.

Forbes, G.B. 1976. Adult decline in the lean body mass. *Human Biology* 48: 151–173.

Foster-Powell, K., and Miller, J. 1995. International tables of glycemic index. *American Journal of Clinical Nutrition* 62: 871S–893S.

Goldfarb, A. 1993. Antioxidants: Role of supplementation to prevent exercise-induced oxidative stress. *Medicine & Science in Sports & Exercise* 25: 232–236.

Grundy, S.M., Blackburn, G., Higgins, M., Lauer, R., Perri, M.G., and Ryan, D. 1999. Physical activity in the prevention and treatment of obesity and its comorbidities: Evidence report of independent panel to assess the role of physical activity in the treatment of obesity and its comorbidities. *Medicine & Science in Sports & Exercise* 31: S502–S508.

Harris, J.A., and Benedict, F.G. 1919. *A biometric study of basal metabolism in man* (publication no. 279). Washington, D.C.: Carnegie Institute.

Hartley, L.H. 1975. Growth hormone and catecholamine response to exercise in relation to physical training. *Medicine and Science in Sports* 7: 34–36.

Hartley, L.H., Mason, J.W., Hogan, R.P., Jones, L.G., Kotchen, T.A., Mougey, E.H., Wherry, R., Pennington, L., and Ricketts, P. 1972. Multiple hormonal responses to graded exercise in relation to physical conditioning. *Journal of Applied Physiology* 33: 602–606.

Hill, J.O., and Melanson, E.L. 1999. Overview of the determinants of overweight and obesity: Current evidence and research issues. *Medicine & Science in Sports & Exercise* 31: S515–S521.

Hirsh, J. 1971. Adipose cellularity in relation to human obesity. *Advances in Internal Medicine* 17: 289–300.

Katch F.I., Clarkson, P.M., Kroll, W., McBride, T., and Wilcox, A. 1984. Effects of sit-up exercise training on adipose cell size and adiposity. *Research Quarterly for Exercise and Sport* 55: 242–247.

Kraemer, W.J., Gordon, S.J., Fleck, S.J., Marchitelli, L.J., Mello, R., Dziados, J.E., Friedl, K., Harman, E., Maresh, C., and Fry, A.C. 1991. Endogenous anabolic hormonal and growth factor responses to heavy resistance exercise in males and female. *International Journal of Sports Medicine* 12: 228–235.

Kraemer, W.J., Häkkinen, K., Newton, R.U., Nindl, B.C., Volek, J.S., McCormick, M., Gotshalk, L.A., Gordon, S.E., Fleck, S.J., Campbell, W.W., Putukian, M., and Evans, W.J. 1999. Effects of heavy-resistance training on hormonal response patterns in younger vs. older men. *Journal of Applied Physiology* 87: 982–992.

Kraemer, W.J., Volek, J.S., Clark, K.L., Gordon, S.E., Puhl, S.M., Koziris, L.P., McBride, J.M., Triplett-McBride, N.T., Putukian, M., Newton, R.U., Häkkinen, K., Bush, J.A., and Sabastianelli, W.J. 1999. Influence of exercise training on physiological and performance changes with weight loss in men. *Medicine & Science in Sports & Exercise* 31: 1320–1329.

Krotkiewski, M., Gudmundsson, M., Backstrom, P., and Mandroukas, K. 1982. Zinc and muscle strength and endurance. *Acta Physiologica Scandinavica* 116: 309–311.

Kuczmarski, R.J., Flegal, K.M., Campbell, S.M., and Johnson, C.L. 1994. Increasing prevalence of overweight among U.S. adults: The National Health and Nutrition Examination Surveys, 1960 to 1991. *Journal of the American Medical Association* 272: 205–211.

Lemon, P.W. 1998. Effects of exercise on dietary protein requirements. *International Journal of Sport Nutrition* 8: 426–447.

Lemon, P.W., Tarnopolsky, M.A., MacDougall, J.D., and Atkinson, S.A. 1992. Protein requirements and muscle mass/strength changes during intensive training in novice bodybuilders. *Journal of Applied Physiology* 73: 767–775.

Lenfant, C., and Ernst, N. 1994. Daily dietary fat and total food-energy intakes: Third National Health and Nutrition Examination Survey, Phase I, 1988-91. *Morbidity and Mortality Weekly Report* 43: 116–117.

Litchell, H., and Boberg, J. 1978. The lipoprotein lipase activity of adipose tissue from different sites in obese women and relationship to cell size. *International Journal of Obesity* 2: 47–52.

Manore, M., and Thompson, J. 2000. *Sport nutrition for health and performance.* Champaign, IL: Human Kinetics.

Marks, B.L., Ward, A., Morris, D.H., Castellani, J., and Rippe, J.M. 1995. Fat-free mass is maintained in women following a moderate diet and exercise program. *Medicine & Science in Sports & Exercise* 27: 1243–1251.

Mayer, J. 1968. *Overweight: Causes, costs and control.* Englewood Cliffs, NJ: Prentice Hall.

Mayhew, J.L., and Gross, P.M. 1974. Body composition changes in young women with high resistance weight training. *Research Quarterly* 45: 433–440.

Mazess, R.B., Barden, H.S., and Ohlrich, E.S. 1990. Skeletal and body-composition effects of anorexia nervosa. *American Journal of Clinical Nutrition* 52: 438–441.

McArdle, W.D., Katch, F.I., and Katch, V.L. 1996. *Exercise physiology.* Baltimore: Williams & Wilkins.

Miller, J.B. 2001. GI research. **http://www.glycemicindex.com**.

Mole, P.A., Oscai, L.B., and Holloszy, J.O. 1971. Adaptation of muscle to exercise: Increase in levels of palmityl CoA synthetase, carnitine palmityl-transferase, and palmityl CoA dehydrogenase and the capacity to oxidize fatty acids. *Journal of Clinical Investigation* 50: 2323–2329.

Nadel, E.R. 1988. New ideas for rehydration during and after exercise in hot weather. *Sports Science Exchange* 1(3). Gatorade Sports Science Institute, Quaker Oats Co.

National Academy of Sciences. 2000. *Dietary reference intakes.* Washington, D.C.: National Academy Press.

National Cholesterol Education Program. 2001. Executive summary of the third report of the National Cholesterol Education Program (NCEP) Expert Panel on detection, evaluation, and treatment of high blood cholesterol in adults (Adult Treatment Panel III). *Journal of the American Medical Association* 285(19): 2486–2497.

National Institutes of Health Consensus Development Panel. 1985. Health implications of obesity: National Institutes of Health Consensus development statement. *Annals of Internal Medicine* 103: 1073–1079.

Noland, M., and Kearney, J.T. 1978. Anthropometric and densitometric responses of women to specific and general exercise. *Research Quarterly* 49: 322–328.

Paffenbarger, R.S., and Olsen, E. 1996. *LifeFit: An effective exercise program for optimal health and a longer life.* Champaign, IL: Human Kinetics.

Pavlou, K.N., Steffee, W.P., Lerman, R.H., and Burrows, B.A. 1985. Effects of dieting and exercise on lean body mass, oxygen uptake, and strength. *Medicine & Science in Sports & Exercise* 17: 466–471.

Pi-Sunyer, F.X. 1999. Comorbidities of overweight and obesity: Current evidence and research issues. *Medicine & Science in Sports & Exercise* 31: S602–S608.

Pollock, M.L., Dimmick, J., Miller, H.S., Kendrick, Z., and Linnerud, A.C. 1975. Effects of mode of training on cardiovascular function and body composition of middle-aged men. *Medicine and Science in Sports* 7: 139–145.

Pollock, M.L., Miller, H.S., Janeway, R., Linnerud, A.C., Robertson, B., and Valentino, R. 1971. Effects of walking on body composition and cardiovascular function of middle-aged men. *Journal of Applied Physiology* 30: 126–130.

Pollock, M.L., Miller, H.S., Linnerud, A.C., and Cooper, K.H. 1975. Frequency of training as a determinant for improvement in cardiovascular function and body composition of middle-aged men. *Archives of Physical Medicine and Rehabilitation* 56: 141–145.

Prevalence of leisure-time physical activity among overweight adults—United States, 1998. 2000. *Morbidity and Mortality Weekly Report* 49(15), April 21.

Rajaram, S., Weaver, C.M., Lyle, R.M., Sedlock, D.A., Martin, B., Templin, T.J., Beard, J.L., and Percival, S.S. 1995. Effects of long-term moderate exercise on iron status in young women. *Medicine & Science in Sports & Exercise* 27: 1105–1110.

Rebuffe-Scrive, M. 1985. Adipose tissue metabolism and fat distribution. In *Human body composition and fat distribution,* ed. N.G. Norgan, 212–217. Wageningen, Netherlands: Euronut.

Roby, R.B. 1962. Effect of exercise on regional subcutaneous fat accumulations. *Research Quarterly* 33: 273–278.

Roza, A.M., and Shizgal, H.M. 1984. The Harris Benedict equation reevaluated: Resting energy requirements and the body cell mass. *American Journal of Clinical Nutrition.* 40: 168–182.

Sanborn, C.F. 1990. Exercise, calcium, and bone density. *Sports Science Exchange* 2(24). Gatorade Sports Science Institute, Quaker Oats Co.

Schade, M., Hellebrandt, F.A., Waterland, J.C., and Carns, M.L. 1962. Spot reducing in overweight college women: Its influence on fat distribution as determined by photography. *Research Quarterly* 33: 461–471.

Serdula, M.K., Williamson, D.F., Anda, R.F., Levy, A., Heaton, A., and Byers, T. 1994. Weight control practices in adults: Results of a multistate telephone survey. *American Journal of Public Health* 84: 1821–1824.

Sharkey, B.J. 1990. *Physiology of fitness,* 3rd ed. Champaign, IL: Human Kinetics.

Singh, V. 1992. A current perspective on nutrition and exercise. *Journal of Nutrition* 122: 760–765.

Sjodin, A.M., Forslund, A.H., Westerterp, K.R., Andersson, A.B., Forslund, J.M., and Hambraeus, L.M. 1996. The influence of physical activity on BMR. *Medicine & Science in Sports & Exercise* 28: 85–91.

Smith, U., Hammerstein, J., Bjorntorp, P., and Kral, J.G. 1979. Regional differences and effect of weight reduction on human fat cell metabolism. *European Journal of Clinical Investigation* 9: 327–332.

Society of Actuaries and Association of Life Insurance Medical Directors of America. 1980. *1979 build study.* New York: Metropolitan Life Insurance.

Tarnopolsky, M.A., Atkinson, S.A., MacDougall, J.D., Chesley, A., Phillips, S., and Schwarcz, H.P. 1992. Evaluation of protein requirements for trained strength athletes. *Journal of Applied Physiology* 73: 1986–1995.

Telford, R., Catchpole, E., Deakin, V., Hahn, A., and Plank, A. 1992. The effect of 7 to 8 months of vitamin/mineral supplementation on athletic performance. *International Journal of Sport Nutrition* 2: 135–153.

Thompson, J., Manore, M., and Thomas, J. 1996. Effects of diet and diet-plus-exercise programs on resting metabolic rate: A meta-analysis. *International Journal of Sport Nutrition* 6: 41–61.

Troiano, R.P., Flegal, K.M., Kuczmarski, R.J., Campbell, S.M., and Johnson, C.L. 1995. Overweight prevalence and trends for children and adolescents. The National Health and Nutrition Examination Surveys 1963-1991. *Archives of Pediatric and Adolescent Medicine* 149: 1085–1091.

U.S. Department of Agriculture. 1992. *The food guide pyramid.* Hyattsville, MD: Human Nutrition Information Service.

U.S. Department of Agriculture, Center for Nutrition Policy and Promotion. 1998. Is total fat consumption really decreasing? *Nutrition Insights,* no. 5 (April). Washington, D.C.: U.S. Government Printing Office.

U.S. Department of Health and Human Services. 1988. *The Surgeon General's report on nutrition and health* (DHHS [PHS] publication no. 88-50210). Washington, D.C.: U.S. Government Printing Office.

U.S. Department of Health and Human Services. 2000a. *Dietary guidelines for Americans.* Washington, D.C.: U.S. Government Printing Office.

U.S. Department of Health and Human Services. 2000b. *Healthy people 2010: Understanding and improving health—overweight and obesity,* 15. Washington, D.C.: U.S. Government Printing Office.

Vaisman, N., Corey, M., Rossi, M.F., Goldberg, E., and Pencharz, P. 1988. Changes in body composition during refeeding of patients with anorexia nervosa. *Journal of Pediatrics* 113: 925–929.

Vaisman, N., Rossi, M.F., Goldberg, E., Dibden, L.J., Wykes, L.J., and Pencharz, P.B. 1988. Energy expenditures and body composition in patients with anorexia nervosa. *Journal of Pediatrics* 113: 919–924.

Vanhelder, W.P., Radomski, M.W., and Goode, R.C. 1984. Growth hormone responses during intermittent weight lifting exercise in men. *European Journal of Applied Physiology* 53: 31–34.

Weiss, L.W., Cureton, K.J., and Thompson, F.N. 1983. Comparison of serum testosterone and androstenedione responses to weight lifting in men and women. *European Journal of Applied Physiology* 50: 413–419.

Williams, M.H. 1992. *Nutrition for fitness and sport.* Dubuque, IA: Brown & Benchmark.

Williams, M.H. 1993. Nutritional supplements for strength trained athletes. *Sports Science Exchange* 6(6). Gatorade Sports Science Institute, Quaker Oats Co.

Wilmore, J.H. 1974. Alterations in strength, body composition, and anthropometric measurements consequent to a 10-week weight training program. *Medicine and Science in Sports* 6: 133–138.

Wilmore, J.H., Royce, J., Girandola, R.N., Katch, F.I., and Katch, V.L. 1970. Body composition changes with a 10-week program of jogging. *Medicine and Science in Sports* 2: 113–119.

chapter 10

Assessing Flexibility and Designing Stretching Programs

KEY QUESTIONS

- What is the difference between static and dynamic flexibility?
- What factors affect flexibility?
- How is flexibility assessed?
- Are all types of stretching exercises safe and effective for improving flexibility?

- What are the recommended guidelines for designing a stretching program?
- Can low back syndrome be prevented?
- What exercises are specifically recommended for low back care programs?

Flexibility is an important, yet often neglected, component of health-related fitness. Adequate levels of flexibility are needed for maintenance of functional independence and performance of activities of daily living such as bending to pick up a newspaper or getting out of the back seat of a two-door car. Over the years, flexibility tests have been included in most health-related fitness test batteries, since it has been long thought that lack of flexibility is associated with musculoskeletal injuries and low back pain. However, compared to research on other physical fitness components, there are not many studies substantiating the importance of flexibility to health-related fitness.

Research suggests that individuals with too little (ankylosis) or too much (hypermobility) flexibility are at higher risk than others for musculoskeletal injuries (Jones and Knapik 1999), but there is limited evidence that a greater-than-normal amount of flexibility actually decreases injury risk (Knudson, Magnusson, and McHugh 2000). Also,

research fails to support an association between lumbar/hamstring flexibility and the occurrence of low back pain (Jackson et al. 1998; Plowman 1992). Still, flexibility should be included in health-related fitness test batteries to identify individuals at the extremes who may have a higher risk of musculotendinous injury.

This chapter describes direct and indirect methods for assessing flexibility. It presents guidelines for designing flexibility programs, as well as recommendations for prescribing exercises suitable for low back care programs.

BASICS OF FLEXIBILITY

Flexibility and joint stability are highly dependent on the joint structure, as well as the strength and number of ligaments and muscles spanning the joint. To fully appreciate the complexity of flexibility, you should review the anatomy of joints and muscles. This section deals with the definitions and nature of flexibility and also presents factors influencing joint mobility.

Definitions and Nature of Flexibility

Flexibility is the ability of a joint, or series of joints, to move through a full **range of motion** (ROM) without injury. **Static flexibility** is a measure of the total ROM at the joint and is limited by the extensibility of the musculotendinous unit. **Dynamic flexibility** is a measure of the rate of torque or resistance developed during stretching throughout the ROM. Although dynamic flexibility accounts for 44% to 66% of the variance in static flexibility (Magnusson et al. 1997; McHugh, Kremenic, Fox, and Gleim 1998), more research is needed to firmly establish the relationship between static and dynamic flexibility and to determine whether these two types of flexibility are distinct entities or two aspects of the same flexibility component (Knudson et al. 2000).

The ROM is highly specific to the joint (i.e., specificity principle) and depends on morphological factors such as the joint geometry and the joint capsule, ligaments, tendons, and muscles spanning the joint. The joint structure determines the planes of motion and may limit the ROM at a given joint. **Triaxial joints** (e.g., ball-and-socket joints of the hip and shoulder) afford a greater degree of movement in more directions than either the **uniaxial** or **biaxial joints** (see table 10.1).

The tightness of soft-tissue structures such as muscle, tendons, and ligaments is a major limitation to both static and dynamic flexibility. Johns and Wright (1962) determined the relative contribution of soft tissues to the total resistance encountered by the joint during movement:

- Joint capsule—47%
- Muscle and its fascia—41%
- Tendons and ligaments—10%
- Skin—2%

The joint capsule and ligaments consist predominantly of collagen, a nonelastic connective tissue. The muscle and its fascia, however, have elastic connective tissue; therefore, they are the most important structures in terms of reducing resistance to movement and increasing dynamic flexibility.

The tension within the muscle-tendon unit affects both static flexibility (ROM) and dynamic flexibility (stiffness or resistance to movement). The tension within this unit is attributed to the **viscoelastic properties** of connective tissues, as well as to the degree of muscular contraction resulting from the stretch reflex (McHugh, Magnusson, Gleim, and Nicholas 1992). Individuals with less flexibility and tighter muscles and tendons have a greater contractile response during stretching exercises and a greater resistance to stretching. The **elastic deformation** of the muscle-tendon unit during stretching is proportional to the load or tension applied, whereas the **viscous deformation** is proportional to the speed at which the tension is applied. When the muscle and tendon are stretched and held at a fixed length (e.g., during static stretching), the tension within the unit, or tensile stress, decreases over time (McHugh et al. 1992). This is called **stress relaxation**. A single static stretch sustained for 90 sec produces a 30% increase in viscoelastic stress relaxation and decreases muscle stiffness for up to 1 hr (Magnusson 1998). Thus, static stretching exercise is an excellent way to induce viscoelastic stress relaxation.

Table 10.1   Joint Classification by Structure and Function

Type of joint	Axes of rotation	Movements	Examples
Gliding	Nonaxial	Gliding, sliding, twisting	Intercarpal, intertarsal, tarsometatarsal
Hinge	Uniaxial	Flexion, extension	Knee, elbow, ankle, interphalangeal
Pivot	Uniaxial	Medial and lateral rotation	Proximal radioulnar, atlantoaxial
Condyloid and saddle	Biaxial	Flexion, extension, abduction, adduction, circumduction	Wrist, atlanto-occipital, metacarpophalangeal, first carpometacarpal
Ball and socket	Triaxial	Flexion, extension, abduction, adduction, circumduction, rotation	Hip, shoulder

Factors Affecting Flexibility

Flexibility is related to body type, age, gender, and physical activity level. This section addresses some commonly asked questions about flexibility.

■ *Does body type limit flexibility?*

Individuals with large hypertrophied muscles or excessive amounts of subcutaneous fat may score poorly on ROM tests because adjacent body segments in these people contact each other sooner than in those with smaller limb and trunk girths. However, this does not necessarily mean that all heavily muscled or obese individuals have poor flexibility. Many bodybuilders and obese individuals who routinely stretch their muscles have adequate levels of flexibility.

■ *Why do older individuals tend to be less flexible than younger people?*

Inflexible and older individuals have increased muscle stiffness and a lower stretch tolerance compared to younger individuals with normal flexibility (Magnusson 1998). As muscle stiffness increases, static flexibility progressively decreases with aging (Brown and Miller 1998; Gajdosik et al. 1999). A decline in physical activity and development of arthritic conditions, rather than a specific effect of aging, are the primary causes for the loss of flexibility as one grows older. Still, flexibility training can help to counteract age-related decreases in ROM. Girouard and Hurley (1995) reported significant improvements in shoulder and hip ROM of older men (50 to 69 years) following 10 weeks of flexibility training. Thus, older persons can benefit from flexibility training and should be encouraged to perform stretching exercises at least three times a week to counteract age-related decreases in ROM.

■ *Are females more flexible than males?*

Some evidence suggests that females generally are more flexible than males at all ages (Alter 1996; Payne, Gledhill, Katzmarzyk, Jamnik, and Keir 2000). The greater flexibility of women is usually attributed to gender differences in pelvic structure and hormones that may affect connective tissue laxity (Alter 1996). However, the effect of gender on ROM appears to be joint and motion specific. Females tend to have more hip flexion and spinal lateral flexion than males of the same age. On the other hand, males have greater ROM in hip extension and spinal flexion and extension in the thoracolumbar region (Norkin and White 1995).

■ *How do physical activity and inactivity affect flexibility?*

Habitual movement patterns and physical activity levels apparently are more important determinants of flexibility than gender, age, and body type (Harris 1969; Kirby, Simms, Symington, and Garner 1981). Lack of physical activity is a major cause of inflexibility. It is well documented that inactive persons tend to be less flexible than active persons (McCue 1953) and that exercise increases flexibility (deVries 1962; Chapman, deVries, and Swezey 1972; Hartley-O'Brien 1980). Disuse, due to lack of physical activity or immobilization, produces shortening of the muscles (i.e., **contracture**) and connective tissues, which in turn restricts joint mobility.

Moving the joints and muscles in a repetitive pattern or maintaining habitual body postures may restrict ROM because of the tightening and shortening of the muscle tissue. For example, joggers and people who sit behind a desk for long periods need to stretch the hamstrings and low back muscles to counteract the tautness developed in these muscle groups.

■ *Does warm-up affect flexibility?*

Wright and Johns (1960) reported that warming the joint (113 °F) produces a 20% increase in ROM, whereas cooling the joint (65 °F) results in a 10% to 20% decrease in flexibility. When you administer flexibility tests, make certain that (a) your client performs some type of warm-up activity to increase circulation and internal body temperature and (b) you administer multiple trials of each test item.

■ *Can you develop too much flexibility?*

It is important to recognize that excessive amounts of stretching and flexibility training may result in hypermobility, or an increased ROM of joints beyond normal, acceptable values. Hypermobility leads to **joint laxity** (looseness or instability) and may increase one's risk of musculoskeletal injuries. For example, it is not uncommon for gymnasts and swimmers to experience shoulder dislocations because of joint laxity and hypermobility. As an exercise specialist, you need to be able to accurately assess ROM and to design stretching programs that improve your clients' flexibility without compromising joint stability.

ASSESSMENT OF FLEXIBILITY

Field and clinical tests are available for assessing static flexibility. Although ROM data are important, measures of dynamic flexibility (i.e., joint stiffness and resistance to movement) may be more meaningful in terms of physical performance. Dynamic flexibility tests measure the increase in resistance during muscle elongation; several studies have shown that less stiff muscles are more effective in using the elastic energy during movements involving the stretch-shortening cycle (Kubo, Kawakami, and Fukunaga 1999; Kubo et al. 2000). However, dynamic flexibility testing is limited to the research setting because the equipment is expensive. Typically, static flexibility is assessed in field and clinical settings by direct or indirect measurement of the ROM.

GENERAL GUIDELINES FOR FLEXIBILITY TESTING

To assess a client's flexibility, you should select a number of test items because of the highly specific nature of flexibility (Dickinson 1968; Harris 1969). Direct tests that measure the range of joint rotation in degrees are usually more useful than indirect tests that measure static flexibility in linear units. When administering these tests,

- have the client perform a general warm-up prior to the test and avoid fast, jerky movements and stretching beyond the pain-free range of joint motion;
- administer three trials of each test item;
- compare the client's best score to norms in order to obtain a flexibility rating for each test item; and
- use the test results to identify joints and muscle groups in need of improvement.

Direct Methods of Measuring Static Flexibility

To assess static flexibility directly, measure the amount of joint rotation in degrees using a goniometer, flexometer, or inclinometer. The following sections describe the procedures for these tests.

Universal Goniometer Test Procedures

The universal **goniometer** is a protractor-like device with two steel or plastic arms that measure the joint angle at the extremes of the ROM (see figure 10.1). The stationary arm of the goniometer is attached at the zero line of the protractor, and the other arm is movable. To use the goniometer, place the center of the instrument so it coincides with the fulcrum, or axis of rotation, of the joint. Align the arms of the goniometer with bony landmarks along the longitudinal axis of each moving body segment. Measure the ROM as the difference between the joint angles (degrees) at the extremes of the movement.

Table 10.2 summarizes procedures for measuring ROM for various joints using a universal goniometer. For more detailed descriptions of these procedures, see Greene and Heckman (1994) and Norkin and White (1995). Table 10.3 presents average ROM values for healthy adults.

Flexometer Test Procedures

Another tool you can use to measure ROM is the Leighton **flexometer** (see figure 10.2). This device consists of a weighted 360° dial and weighted pointer. The ROM is measured in relation to the downward pull of gravity on the dial and pointer.

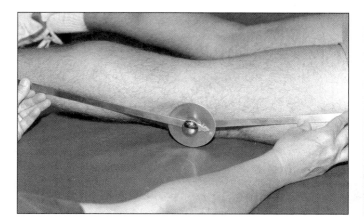
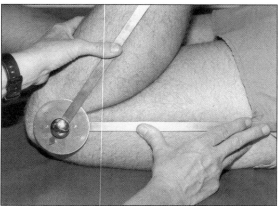

Figure 10.1   Measuring range of motion at knee joint using universal goniometer.

Table 10.2 Universal Goniometer Measurement Procedures

Joint	Body position	Axis of rotation	Goniometer position			Stabilization	Special considerations
			Stationary arm	Moving arm			
Shoulder							
Extension	Prone	Acromion process	Midaxillary line	Lateral epicondyle of humerus		Scapula and thorax	Elbow is slightly flexed and palm of hand faces body.
Flexion	Supine	Same as extension	Same as extension	Same as extension		Scapula and thorax	Palm of hand faces body.
Abduction	Supine	Anterior axis of acromion process	Midline of anterior aspect of sternum	Medial midline of humerus		Scapula and thorax	Palm of hand faces anteriorly; humerus is laterally rotated; elbow is extended.
Medial/lateral rotation	Supine	Olecranon process	Perpendicular to floor	Styloid process of ulna		Distal end of humerus and scapula	Arm is abducted 90°; forearm is perpendicular to supporting surface in mid-pronated-supinated position; humerus rests on pad so that it is level with acromion process.
Elbow							
Flexion	Supine	Lateral epicondyle of humerus	Lateral midline of humerus	Lateral midline of radial head and styloid process		Distal end of humerus	Arm is close to body; pad is placed under distal end of humerus; forearm is fully supinated.
Forearm							
Pronation	Sitting	Lateral to ulna styloid process	Parallel to anterior midline of humerus	Lies across dorsal aspect of forearm, just proximal to styloid processes of radius and ulna		Distal end of humerus	Arm is close to body, elbow flexed 90°; forearm is midway between supination and pronation (thumb toward ceiling).
Supination	Sitting	Medial to ulna styloid process	Parallel to anterior midline of humerus	Lies across ventral aspect of forearm, just proximal to styloid processes of radius and ulna		Distal end of humerus	Testing position is same as for pronation of forearm.

(continued)

Table 10.2 *(continued)*

Joint	Body position	Axis of rotation	Goniometer position			Stabilization	Special considerations
			Stationary arm	Moving arm			

Wrist

Joint	Body position	Axis of rotation	Stationary arm	Moving arm	Stabilization	Special considerations
Flexion and extension	Sitting	Lateral aspect of wrist over the triquetrum	Lateral midline of ulna, using olecranon and ulnar styloid processes for reference	Lateral midline of fifth metacarpal	Radius and ulna	Client sits next to supporting surface, abducts shoulder 90°, and flexes elbow 90°; forearm is in mid-supinated-pronated position; palm of hand faces ground; forearm rests on supporting surface; hand is free to move.
Radial or ulnar deviation	Sitting	Middle of dorsal aspect of wrist over capitate	Dorsal midline of forearm, using lateral humeral epicondyle as reference	Dorsal midline of third metacarpal	Distal ends of radius and ulna	Same as for wrist flexion.

Hip

Flexion and extension	Supine Prone	Lateral aspect of hip joint, using greater trochanter as reference	Lateral midline of pelvis	Lateral midline of femur, using lateral epicondyle for reference	Pelvis	Knee is allowed to flex as range of hip flexion is completed; knee is flexed during hip extension.
Abduction and adduction	Supine	Centered over anterior superior iliac spine	Horizontally align arm with imaginary line between anterior superior iliac spines	Anterior midline of femur, using midline of patella for reference	Pelvis	Knee is extended during abduction.
Medial/lateral rotation	Sitting	Centered over anterior aspect of patella	Perpendicular to floor	Anterior midline of lower leg, using crest of tibia and point midway between malleoli for reference	Distal end of femur; avoid rotation and lateral tilt of pelvis	Client sits on supporting surface, knees flexed 90°, place towel roll under distal end of femur; contralateral knee may need to be flexed so that hip being measured can complete full range of lateral rotation.

	Position	Axis	Stationary arm	Moving arm	Stabilization	Notes
Knee						
Flexion	Supine	Over the lateral epicondyle of femur	Lateral midline of femur, using greater trochanter for reference	Lateral midline of fibula, using lateral malleolus and fibular head for reference	Femur to prevent rotation, abduction, and adduction	As knee flexes, the hip also flexes.
Ankle						
Dorsiflexion and plantar flexion	Sitting	Over the lateral aspect of lateral malleolus	Lateral midline of fibula, using head of fibula for reference	Parallel to lateral aspect of fifth metatarsal	Tibia and fibula	Client sits on end of table with knee flexed and ankle positioned at 90°.
Subtalar						
Inversion and eversion	Sitting	Centered over anterior aspect of ankle midway between malleoli	Anterior midline of lower leg, using the tibial tuberosity for reference	Anterior midline of second metatarsal	Tibia and fibula	Client sits with knee flexed 90° and lower leg over edge of supporting surface.
Lumbar spine						
Lateral flexion	Standing	Centered over posterior aspect of spinous process of S1	Perpendicular to ground	Posterior aspect of spinous process of C7	Pelvis to prevent lateral tilt	Client stands erect with 0° of spinal flexion, extension, and rotation.
Rotation	Sitting	Centered over superior aspect of client's head	Parallel to imaginary line between tubercles of iliac crests	Imaginary line between two acromion processes	Pelvis to prevent rotation	Keep feet flat on floor to stabilize pelvis.

Table 10.3 Average Range of Motion (ROM) Values for Healthy Adults

Joint	ROM (degrees)	Joint	ROM
Shoulder		*Thoracic-lumbar spine*	
Flexion	150-180	Flexion	60-80
Extension	50-60	Extension	20-30
Abduction	180	Lateral flexion	25-35
Medial rotation	70-90	Rotation	30-45
Lateral rotation	90	*Hip*	
Elbow		Flexion	100-120
Flexion	140-150	Extension	30
Extension	0	Abduction	40-45
Radioulnar		Adduction	20-30
Pronation	80	Medial rotation	40-45
Supination	80	Lateral rotation	45-50
Wrist		*Knee*	
Flexion	60-80	Flexion	135-150
Extension	60-70	Extension	0-10
Radial deviation	20	*Ankle*	
Ulnar deviation	30	Dorsiflexion	20
Cervical spine		Plantar flexion	40-50
Flexion	45-60	*Subtalar*	
Extension	45-75	Inversion	30-35
Lateral flexion	45	Eversion	15-20
Rotation	60-80		

Data from the American Academy of Orthopaedic Surgeons (Greene and Heckman 1994) and the American Medical Association (1988).

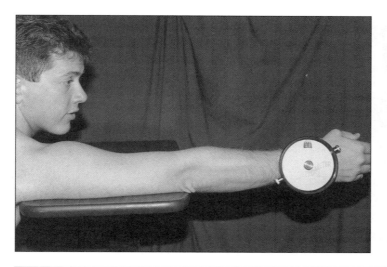 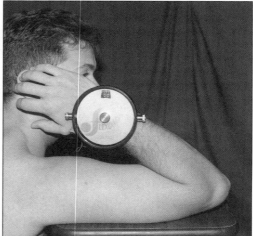

Figure 10.2 Measuring range of motion at elbow joint using Leighton flexometer.

To use this device, strap the instrument to the body segment, and lock the dial at 0° at one extreme of the ROM. After the client executes the movement, lock the pointer at the other extreme of the ROM. The degree of arc through which the movement takes place is read directly from the dial. Tests have been devised to measure the ROM at the neck, trunk, shoulder, elbow, radioulnar, wrist, hip, knee, and ankle joints using the Leighton flexometer (Leighton 1955; Hubley-Kozey 1991).

Inclinometer Test Procedures

The **inclinometer** is another type of gravity-dependent goniometer (see figure 10.3). To use this device, hold it on the distal end of the body segment. The inclinometer measures the angle between the long axis of the moving segment and the line of gravity. This device is easier to use than the flexometer and universal goniometer because it is held by hand on the moving body segment during the measurement and does not have to be aligned with specific bony landmarks. Also, the American Medical Association (1988) recommends the double-inclinometer technique, using two inclinometers, to measure spinal mobility (see figure 10.3).

Validity and Reliability of Direct Measures

The validity and reliability of these devices for directly measuring ROM are highly dependent on the joint being measured and technician skill. Radiography is considered to be the best reference method for establishing validity of goniometric measurements. Research shows high agreement between ROM measured by radiographs and universal goniometers for the hip and knee joints (Ahlback and Lindahl 1964; Enwemeka 1986). Mayer, Tencer, and Kristoferson (1984) reported no difference between radiography and the double-inclinometer technique for assessing spinal ROM of patients with low back pain.

The intratester and intertester reliability of goniometric measurements is affected by difficulty in identifying the axis of rotation and palpating bony landmarks. Measurements of upper-extremity joints are generally more reliable than ROM measurements of the lower-extremity joints (Norkin and White 1995). The intertester reliability of inclinometer measurements is variable and joint specific. Studies have presented reliability coefficients ranging from 0.48 for lumbar extension (Williams, Binkley, Bloch, Goldsmith, and Minuk 1993) to 0.96 for subtalar joint position (Sell, Verity, Worrell, Pease, and Wigglesworth 1994). In order to obtain accurate and reliable ROM measurements, you need a thorough knowledge of anatomy and of standardized testing procedures, as well training and practice to develop your measurement techniques.

Indirect Methods of Measuring Static Flexibility

Because of the belief that lack of flexibility is associated with low back pain and musculoskeletal injuries, most health-related fitness test batteries include a sit-and-reach test to evaluate the static flexibility of the lower back and hamstring muscles (Payne et al. 2000). The sit-and-reach test provides

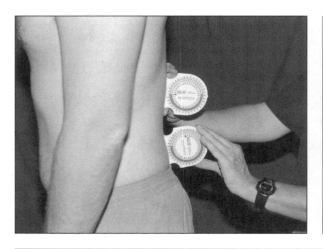
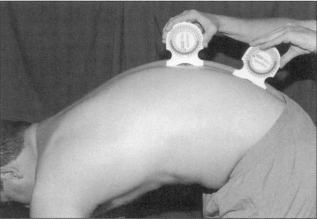

Figure 10.3 Measuring lumbosacral flexion using the double-inclinometer technique.

an indirect, linear measurement of the ROM. Several sit-and-reach protocols have been developed using either a yardstick (meter stick) or a box, or both, to measure flexibility in inches or centimeters.

Although some fitness professionals assume the sit-and-reach to be a valid measure of low back and hamstring flexibility, research has shown that these tests are moderately related to hamstring flexibility (r = 0.39 to 0.89), but poorly related to low back flexibility (r = 0.10 to 0.59) in children (Patterson et al. 1996), adults (Jackson and Langford 1989; Hui, Yuen, Morrow, and Jackson 1999; Hui and Yuen 2000; Martin, Jackson, Morrow, and Liemohn 1998; Minkler and Patterson 1994), and older adults (Jones, Rikli, Max, and Noffal 1998). Moreover, in a prospective study of adults, Jackson et al. (1998) reported that the sit-and-reach test has poor criterion-related validity and is unrelated to self-reported low back pain. Therefore, you should use these tests to identify individuals at the extremes who may have a higher risk of muscle injury because of hypermobility or lack of flexibility in the hamstring muscles. To assess low back flexibility, you may use the skin distraction test as an alternative to the sit-and-reach test.

The following sections describe the protocols for various types of sit-and-reach tests, as well as the skin distraction test. Before clients take any of these tests, have them perform a general warm-up to increase muscle temperature, as well as stretching exercises for the muscle groups to be tested. Unless otherwise stated, have your clients remove their shoes for all sit-and-reach test protocols. The ACSM (2000) recommends using either the standard or V sit-and-reach test.

Standard Sit-and-Reach Test

The standard sit-and-reach test uses a sit-and-reach box (12 in. [30.5 cm] high). Have the client sit on the floor with legs together, knees extended, and soles of the feet placed against the edge of the box (see figure 10.4). Most commercial sit-and-reach boxes have the zero point (front edge of box) set at 23 or 26 cm (Canadian Society of Exercise Physiology 1996). Instruct the client to reach forward slowly and as far as possible along the top of the box while keeping the two hands parallel (fingertips may overlap) and to hold this position momentarily (~2 sec). Make certain that the knees do not flex and that the client avoids leading with one hand. The score (in centimeters or inches) is the most distant point on the box contacted by the fingertips. Table 10.4 presents age-gender norms for this test.

Table 10.4 Percentile Ranks for the Standard Sit-and-Reach Test*

Rank	Age (years)									
	20-29		30-39		40-49		50-59		60-69	
	M	F	M	F	M	F	M	F	M	F
90	39	40	37	39	34	37	35	37	32	34
80	35	37	34	36	31	33	29	34	27	31
70	33	35	31	34	27	32	26	32	23	28
60	30	33	29	32	25	30	24	29	21	27
50	28	31	26	30	22	28	22	27	19	25
40	26	29	24	28	20	26	19	26	15	23
30	23	26	21	25	17	23	15	23	13	21
20	20	23	18	22	13	21	12	20	11	20
10	15	19	14	18	9	16	9	16	8	15

*Sit-and-reach scores measured in centimeters, using a box with the zero point set at 23 cm.

Adapted from the *Canadian Standardized Test of Fitness (CSTF) Operations Manual.* 3rd ed. 1986. Ottawa, Canada: Fitness Canada and Fitness and Amateur Sport Canada.

V Sit-and-Reach Test

The V sit-and-reach, also known as the YMCA sit-and-reach test, uses a yardstick instead of a box. Secure the yardstick to the floor by placing tape (12 in. long) at a right angle to the 15-in. (38 cm) mark on the yardstick. The client sits, straddling the yardstick, with the knees extended (but not locked) and legs spread 12 in. (30.5 cm) apart. The heels of the feet touch the tape at the 15-in. mark. Instruct the client to reach forward slowly and as far as possible along the yardstick while keeping the two hands parallel (fingertips may overlap) and to hold this position momentarily (~2 sec). Make certain that the knees do not flex and that the client avoids leading with one hand. The score (in centimeters or inches) is the most distant point on the yardstick contacted by the fingertips. Table 10.5 presents norms for the V sit-and-reach test.

Modified Sit-and-Reach Test

To account for a potential bias due to limb-length differences (i.e., individuals who have short legs relative to the trunk and arms may have an advantage when performing the standard sit-and-reach test), Hoeger (1989) developed a modified sit-and-reach test that takes into account the distance between the end of the fingers and the sit-and-reach box and uses the finger-to-box distance

as the relative zero point. This test uses a 12-in. (30.5 cm) sit-and-reach box (see figure 10.4). The client sits on the floor with buttocks, shoulders, and head in contact with the wall; extends the knees; and places the soles of the feet against the box. A yardstick is placed on top of the box with the zero end toward the client. Keeping the head and shoulders in contact with the wall, the client reaches forward with one hand on top of the other, and the yardstick is positioned so that it touches the fingertips. This procedure establishes the relative zero point for each client. As you firmly hold the yardstick in place, the client reaches forward slowly, sliding the fingers along the top of the yardstick. The score (in inches) is the most distant point on the yardstick contacted by the fingertips. Table 10.6 provides age-gender percentile norms for the modified sit-and-reach test.

Research comparing the standard and modified sit-and-reach test scores indicated that individuals with proportionally longer arms than legs (lower finger-to-box distance) had significantly better scores on the standard sit-and-reach test than those with moderate or high finger-to-box distances; in contrast, the modified sit-and-reach test scores did not differ significantly among the three groups (Hoeger, Hopkins, Button, and Palmer 1990; Hoeger and Hopkins 1992). However, Minkler and Patterson (1994) reported that the modified

Table 10.5 Percentile Ranks for the V Sit-and-Reach Test*

	Age (years)											
Rank	18-25		26-35		36-45		46-55		56-65		>65	
	M	F	M	F	M	F	M	F	M	F	M	F
90	22	24	21	23	21	22	19	21	17	20	17	20
80	20	22	19	21	19	21	17	20	15	19	15	18
70	19	21	17	20	17	19	15	18	13	17	13	17
60	18	20	29	32	25	30	24	29	13	16	12	17
50	17	19	26	30	22	28	22	27	11	15	10	15
40	15	18	24	28	20	26	19	26	9	14	9	14
30	14	17	21	25	17	23	15	23	9	13	8	13
20	13	16	18	22	13	21	12	20	7	11	7	11
10	11	14	14	18	9	16	9	16	5	9	4	9

*Sit-and-reach scores measured in inches.

Based on data from YMCA of the USA (2000). *YMCA Fitness Testing and Assessment Manual* 4th ed., Champaign, IL: Human Kinetics. Reprinted and adapted with permission of the YMCA of the USA, 101 N. Wacker Drive, Chicago, IL 60606.

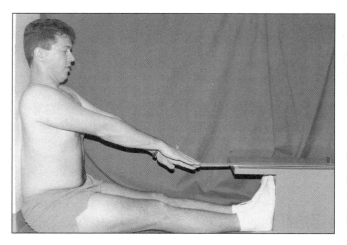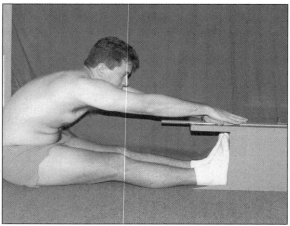

Figure 10.4   Modified sit-and-reach test.

sit-and-reach test was only moderately related to criterion measures of hamstring flexibility for women ($r = 0.66$) and men ($r = 0.75$) and poorly related to low back flexibility of women ($r = 0.25$) and men ($r = 0.40$). Similarly, Hui et al. (1999) compared the criterion-related validity of the standard and modified sit-and-reach tests and concluded that both tests were moderately valid measures of hamstring flexibility but poor measures of low back flexibility. Consequently, it appears that the validity of the modified sit-and-reach test is no better than that of the standard sit-and-reach test for assessing flexibility of the low back and hamstring muscle groups.

Table 10.6   Percentile Ranks for the Modified Sit-and-Reach Test*

Percentile rank	Women			Men		
	≤35 years	36-49 years	≥50 years	≤35 years	36-49 years	≥50 years
99	19.8	19.8	17.2	24.7	18.9	16.2
95	18.7	19.2	15.7	19.5	18.2	15.8
90	17.9	17.4	15.0	17.9	16.1	15.0
80	16.7	16.2	14.2	17.0	14.6	13.3
70	16.2	15.2	13.6	15.8	13.9	12.3
60	15.8	14.5	12.3	15.0	13.4	11.5
50	14.8	13.5	11.1	14.4	12.6	10.2
40	14.5	12.8	10.1	13.5	11.6	9.7
30	13.7	12.2	9.2	13.0	10.8	9.3
20	12.6	11.0	8.3	11.6	9.9	8.8
10	10.1	9.7	7.5	9.2	8.3	7.8
5	8.1	8.5	3.7	7.9	7.0	7.2
1	2.6	2.0	1.5	7.0	5.1	4.0

*Sit-and-reach scores measured to the nearest 0.25 in.

©Morton Publishing Company, *Lifetime Physical Fitness & Wellness* (1989) by Werner W.K. Hoeger.

Back-Saver Sit-and-Reach Test

The standard, modified, and V sit-and-reach tests require the client to stretch the hamstring muscles of both legs simultaneously, causing some discomfort when the anterior portions of the vertebrae are compressed during the stretch. The back-saver sit-and-reach test was devised to relieve some of this discomfort by measuring the flexibility of the hamstring muscles, one leg at a time. Instruct your client to place the sole of the foot of the extended (tested) leg against the edge of the sit-and-reach box and to flex the untested leg, placing the sole of that foot flat on the floor 2 to 3 in. to the side of the extended (tested) knee (see figure 10.5). Then follow the instructions for the standard sit-and-reach test to determine your client's flexibility score for each leg. Research suggests that the validity of this test (r = 0.39 to 0.71) is similar to that of the standard sit-and-reach test (r = 0.46 to 0.74) for assessing hamstring flexibility of men and women (Hui and Yuen 2000; Jones et al. 1998). Norms for this test are available elsewhere (see Cooper Institute for Aerobics Research 1992).

Modified Back-Saver Sit-and-Reach Test

While performing the back-saver sit-and-reach test, some participants may complain about the uncomfortable position of the untested leg. Hui and Yuen (2000), therefore, modified this test by having the client perform a single-leg sit-and-reach on a 12-in. (30.5 cm) bench (see figure 10.6). Instruct the client to place the untested leg on the floor with the knee flexed at a 90° angle. Align the sole of the foot of the tested leg with the 50-cm mark on the meter rule. Then follow the instructions for the standard sit-and-reach test to determine your client's hamstring flexibility for each leg. Hui and Yuen (2000) reported that the validity of this test (r = 0.50 to 0.67) for assessing hamstring flexibility was similar to that of the standard (r = 0.46 to 0.53) and V (r = 0.44 to 0.63) sit-and-reach tests. The modified back-saver test, however, was rated as the most comfortable compared to the other test protocols. Norms for this test have not yet been established.

Chair Sit-and-Reach Test

Many older individuals have difficulty performing sit-and-reach tests because functional limitations (e.g., obesity, low back pain, less flexibility) prevent them from getting down to and up from the floor. Therefore, Jones et al. (1998) devised a chair sit-and-reach protocol that is similar to the back-saver protocol in that only one leg at a time is tested, thereby reducing stress on the spine and lower back. Participants sit near the front edge of a folding chair (17-in. [43 cm] high seat) that is placed against a wall for stability. The tested leg is extended in front of the hip, with the heel on the floor and the ankle dorsiflexed approximately 90°. The untested leg is flexed so that the sole of the foot is flat on the floor about 6 to 12 in. (15 to 30.5 cm) to side of the body's midline. With the client's extended leg as straight as possible and hands on top of each other (palms down), instruct the client to slowly bend forward at the hip joint, keeping the spine as straight as possible and the head in normal alignment with the spine (client should not tuck head). The client reaches down the extended leg,

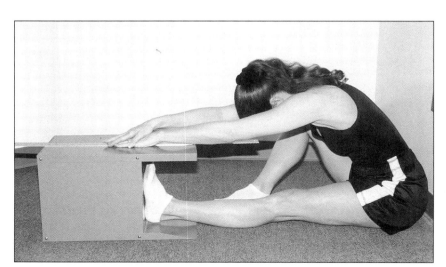

Figure 10.5 Back-saver sit-and-reach test.

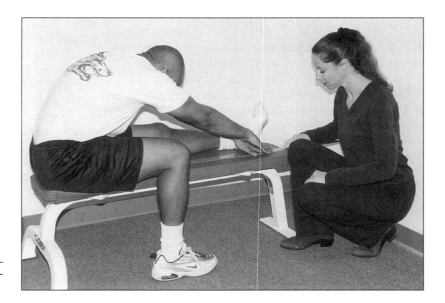

Figure 10.6 Modified back-saver sit-and-reach test.

trying to touch the toes, and holds this position for 2 sec (see figure 10.7). An 18-in. (45.7 cm) ruler is positioned parallel to the lower leg. The middle of the big toe (medial aspect) at the end of the shoe represents a "zero" score. Reaches short of the toes are recorded as minus scores; reaches beyond the toes are recorded as plus scores. Compared to the standard ($r = 0.71$ to 0.74) and back-saver ($r = 0.70$ to 0.71) sit-and-reach protocols, this test yielded similar criterion-related validity coefficients ($r = 0.76$ to 0.81) as a mea-

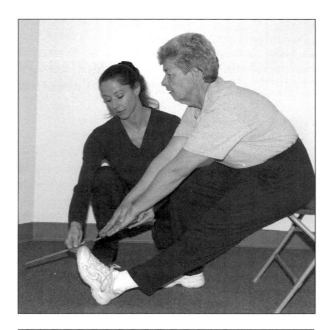

Figure 10.7 Chair sit-and-reach test.

sure of hamstring flexibility in older (>60 years) men and women. Norms for this test are available elsewhere (Rikli and Jones 2001).

Skin Distraction Test

The modified Schober test (Mcrae and Wright 1969) or the simplified skin distraction test (Van Adrichem and van der Korst 1973) is useful in assessing low back flexibility. These field tests are reliable and have good agreement with radiographic measurements of spinal flexion and extension (Williams, Binkley, Bloch, Glodsmith, and Minuk 1993). For the simplified skin distraction test, place a 0-cm mark on the midline of the lumbar spine at the intersection of a horizontal line connecting the left and right posterior superior iliac spines while the client is standing erect. Place a second mark 15 cm (5.9 in.) superior to the 0-cm mark (see figure 10.8). As the client flexes the lumbar spine, these marks move away from each other; use an anthropometric tape measure to measure the new distance between the two marks. The lumbar flexion score is the difference between this measurement and the initial length between the skin markings (15 cm). In a group of 15- to 18-year-old subjects, the simplified skin distraction scores averaged 6.7 ± 1.0 cm in males and 5.8 ± 0.9 cm in females. However, normal values for other age groups are not yet available. You can also use this technique to measure lumbar spinal extension (simplified skin attraction test) by having the client extend backward and measuring the difference between the initial length and the new distance between the superior and inferior skin markings.

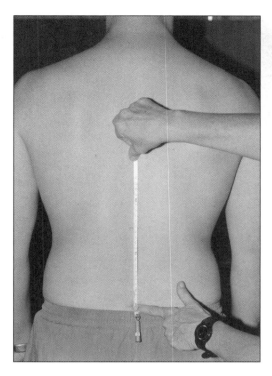

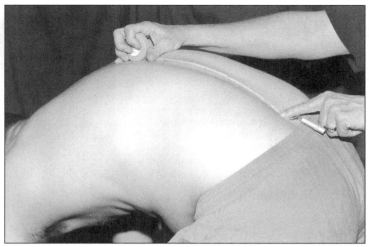

Figure 10.8 Measuring lumbosacral flexion using the simplified skin distraction test.

DESIGNING FLEXIBILITY PROGRAMS

After assessing your client's flexibility, you must identify those joints and muscle groups in need of improvement and select an appropriate exercise mode and specific exercises for the flexibility program. The specificity and progressive overload principles apply to the design of flexibility programs. As already mentioned, flexibility is highly joint specific (Cotten 1972; Harris 1969; Munroe and Romance 1975); therefore, to increase flexibility of a particular joint, select exercises that stretch the appropriate muscle groups. To improve ROM at the joint, your client must overload the muscle group by stretching the muscles beyond their normal resting length—but never beyond the pain-free ROM. Periodically your client will need to increase both the amount of time that the stretched position is maintained and the number of repetitions of the exercise to ensure the overload required for further improvement. The questions in this section address issues and concerns that you should consider when designing flexibility programs.

Modes of Stretching

Three types of stretching techniques are ballistic stretching, slow static stretching, and propriocep-

tive neuromuscular facilitation stretching. Table 10.7 summarizes the advantages and disadvantages of each of these stretching techniques.

■ *What mode of stretching is best for improving flexibility?*

All three types of stretching are effective in increasing the ROM (deVries 1962; Hartley-O'Brien 1980, Holt, Travis, and Okita 1970; Worrell, Smith, and Winegardner 1994). However, Wallin, Ekblom, Grahn, and Nordenborg (1985) reported significantly better improvement in the flexibility of the plantar flexors and hip adductors and extensors for subjects who trained using the PNF (11% to 25% increase) technique compared to ballistic stretching (3% to 7% increase).

■ *What is proprioceptive neuromuscular facilitation (PNF) and how is this technique used to improve flexibility?*

Proprioceptive neuromuscular facilitation stretching increases ROM by inducing muscle relaxation through spinal reflex mechanisms. Using the **contract-relax** technique, your client first performs an isometric contraction of the muscle group being stretched, and then proceeds with the slow static stretching (relaxation phase) of the muscle group. This technique is based on the concept of reciprocal inhibition. Theoretically, the isometric contraction of the antagonists (muscle group being stretched) induces a reflex facilitation and contraction of the agonist, which suppresses the contractile activity in the antagonist during the slow static stretching phase. The

Table 10.7   Comparison of Stretching Techniques

Factor	Ballistic	Slow static	PNF[a]
Risk of injury	High	Low	Medium
Degree of pain	Medium	Low	High
Resistance to stretch	High	Low	Medium
Practicality (time and assistance needed)	Good	Excellent	Poor
Efficiency (energy consumption)	Poor	Excellent	Poor
Effective for increasing ROM[b]	Good	Good	Good

[a]Proprioceptive neuromuscular facilitation.
[b]Range of motion.

isometric contraction of the antagonists also stimulates the Golgi tendon organs, resulting in a reflex relaxation of the same muscle group. However, the isometric contraction may promote a lingering discharge in the same muscle, which contributes to increased contractile activity in the muscle group during the relaxation (static stretching) phase of the contract-relax procedure (Moore and Hutton 1980).

Another type of PNF stretching is the **contract-relax with agonist contraction (CRAC)** technique. This method is identical to the contract-relax technique except that the stretching is assisted by a submaximal contraction of the opposing (agonist) muscle group. Theoretically, the voluntary contraction of the agonists induces additional inhibitory input to the antagonists (muscles being stretched) through reciprocal inhibition (Moore and Hutton 1980).

The neuromuscular mechanisms underlying muscle stretch are extremely complicated and not fully understood. Simple explanations concerning the role of reciprocal inhibition during muscle stretch are inadequate. For example, it as been shown that recurrent collateral pathways from motor neurons of agonists inhibit interneurons that normally reduce the excitation of alpha motor neurons of the antagonists during reciprocal inhibition. This results in an inhibition of inhibitory input to the antagonistic muscle groups (Hultborn, Illert, and Santini 1974).

■ *How are PNF stretches performed?*

The following steps are recommended for the use of PNF stretching techniques to increase static flexibility:

- Stretch the target muscle group by moving the joint to the end of its ROM.
- Isometrically contract the prestretched muscle group against an immovable resistance (such as a partner or wall) for 5 to 6 sec.
- Relax the contracted muscle group as you statically stretch the muscle (or your partner does) to a new point of limitation. With the contract-relax agonist contract technique, the opposing muscle group (agonist) contracts submaximally for 5 to 6 sec to facilitate relaxation and further stretching of the target muscle group.

For example, to stretch the pectoral muscles, the individual assumes a sitting position on the floor with the arms horizontally extended. The pectoral muscles are isometrically contracted as the partner offers resistance to horizontal flexion. Following the isometric contraction, the partner applies a slow static stretch as the horizontal extensors in the upper back are contracted submaximally.

■ *Why is slow static stretching safer than ballistic stretching?*

Many exercise specialists recommend using slow static stretching rather than ballistic stretching because there is less chance of injury and muscle soreness resulting from jerky, rapid movements. The **ballistic stretching** technique uses a relatively fast, bouncing motion to produce stretch. The momentum of the moving body segment, rather than external force, pushes the joint beyond its present ROM. This technique appears to be counterproductive for increasing muscle stretch. Muscle spindles signal changes in both muscle length and speed of contraction. The spindle responds more to the speed of movement than to the muscle's length or position. In fact, muscle spindle activity is directly proportional to the speed of movement. Thus, ballistic or dynamic stretching evokes the stretch reflex, producing more contraction and resistance to stretch in the muscle group being stretched. This places strain on the muscle-tendon unit and may cause microscopic tearing of muscle fibers and connective tissue.

In slow **static stretching,** your client stretches the muscle when the joint is positioned at the end of its ROM. While maintaining this lengthened position, the client slowly applies torque to the muscle to stretch it further. Because the dynamic portion of the muscle spindle rapidly adapts to the lengthened position, the spindle discharge is decreased. This lessens reflex contraction of the muscle and allows the muscle to relax (viscoelastic stress relaxation) and to be stretched even further.

▪ *Is PNF stretching better than slow static stretching?*

Moore and Hutton (1980) compared the relative level of muscle relaxation achieved during static stretching and PNF stretching procedures. They noted that the CRAC method produced larger gains in hip flexion than either the contract-relax or static stretching method. However, this technique produced greater electromyographic activity in the hamstring muscle group and was ranked as the most uncomfortable in terms of perceived pain ratings. It has also been reported that the CRAC technique is more effective for improving ROM than the contract-relax technique (Alter 1996).

A major disadvantage of the PNF technique is that the exercises, in some cases, cannot be performed alone. An assistant is needed to resist movement during the isometric contraction phase and to apply external force to the muscle during the stretching phase. Overstretching may cause injury, especially if the assistant has not been carefully trained in correct procedures. Assisted-stretching procedures, such as PNF, should be performed with care by trained clients or exercise professionals who understand the correct procedures and risks of incorrect stretching (Knudson et al. 2000).

The Exercise Prescription for Flexibility

When designing flexibility programs for your clients, follow the guidelines on page 244 and be sure to address the following questions regarding various aspects of their exercise prescriptions.

▪ *How many exercises should be included in a flexibility program?*

A well-rounded program includes at least one exercise for each of the major muscle groups of the body. It is important to select exercises for problem areas such as the lower back, hips, and posterior thighs and legs. Use the results of the flexibility tests to identify specific muscle groups with relatively poor flexibility, and include more than one exercise for these muscle groups. The workout should take 15 to 30 min depending on the number of exercises to be performed. Appendix F.1, "Selected Flexibility Exercises," page 336, illustrates flexibility exercises for various regions of the body. For additional flexibility exercises see Anderson (1980) and Alter (1996).

▪ *Are some stretching exercises safer than others?*

Some stretching exercises are not recommended for flexibility programs because they create excessive stress, thereby increasing your client's chance of musculoskeletal injuries—especially to the knee joints and low back region. Appendix F.2, "Exercise Do's and Don'ts," page 341, illustrates exercises that are contraindicated for flexibility programs and suggests alternative exercises that you can prescribe to increase the flexibility of specific muscle groups.

▪ *What is a safe intensity for stretching exercises?*

The intensity of the exercise for the slow static stretching and PNF stretching exercises should always be below the pain threshold of the individual. Some mild discomfort will occur, especially during the PNF exercises when the target muscle is contracted isometrically. However, the joint should not be stretched beyond its pain-free ROM (ACSM 2000).

▪ *How long does each stretch need to be held?*

To date there is a limited amount of research concerning the optimal time that a static stretch should be sustained to improve ROM. In the past, some experts have suggested varying lengths of static stretch, ranging from 10 to 60 sec (Beaulieu 1980). The ACSM (2000) recommends holding the stretched position only as long as it feels comfortable (usually 10 to 30 sec).

Borms, Van Roy, Santens, and Haentjens (1987) compared the effects of 10, 20, and 30 sec of static stretching on hip flexibility of women engaging in a 10-week (two sessions a week) static flexibility training program. They reported similar improvements in hip flexibility for all three groups, suggesting that a duration of 10 sec of static stretching is sufficient for improving hip flexibility.

Another study compared the effect of three static stretching durations (15, 30, and 60 sec) on the hip flexibility of men and women with "tight" hamstring muscles (Bandy and Irion 1994). The subjects participated in a six-week static flexibility training program, stretching five times a week. The authors noted that 30 and 60 sec of static stretching were more effective than stretching 15 sec for increasing hip flexibility. They observed no significant difference between stretching for 30 sec and for 60 sec, indicating that a 30-sec stretch of the hamstring muscles was as effective as the longer-duration stretch.

Roberts and Wilson (1999) compared the effects of stretching 5 or 15 sec on active and passive ROM in the lower extremity. The treatment groups participated in a static stretching program three times a week for a five-week period. The investigators controlled the total amount of time spent stretching (45 sec) by having the 5-sec group perform nine repetitions and the 15-sec group three repetitions for each exercise. The improvement in passive ROM was similar for the 5- and 15-sec groups; however, the 15-sec group showed significantly greater improvement in active ROM.

In light of these findings, it is recommended that the stretch be sustained at least 10 to 15 sec during the initial stages of the static stretching program. As flexibility improves, the muscle group may be progressively overloaded by increasing the time that the stretched position is held up to a maximum of 30 sec for each repetition.

▪ How many repetitions of each exercise should be performed?

Beginners should start with three to four repetitions of each exercise (ACSM 2000). As flexibility improves during the training program, the number of repetitions of each flexibility exercise may be gradually increased to five repetitions to progressively overload the muscle group.

▪ How often should flexibility exercises be performed?

Flexibility exercises should be performed a minimum of two to three days a week (ACSM 2000) but preferably daily (Knudson 2000). Flexibility exercises should be performed after moderate or vigorous physical activity and are often an integral part of the cool-down segments of aerobic exercise and resistance training workouts. Stretching during the warm-up phase for most physical activities is controversial. There is a lack of scientific support for the idea that stretching prior to physical activity prevents injury or increases physical performance (Pope, Herbert, Kirwan, and Graham 2000). In fact, Knudson (1999) noted that stretching may have a detrimental effect on performance and recommended stretching during warm-up only when engaging in activities that require beyond normal ROM such as dance, diving, and gymnastics.

GUIDELINES FOR DESIGNING FLEXIBILITY PROGRAMS

- **Mode:** Static or PNF stretching
- **Number of exercises:** 10 to 12
- **Frequency:** Minimum of two to three days a week, preferably daily
- **Intensity:** Slowly stretch the muscle to a position of mild discomfort
- **Time of stretch:** 10 to 30 sec for static stretching; 6-sec contraction, followed by 10 to 30 sec of assisted stretching for PNF
- **Repetitions:** Three to five for each stretch
- **Duration:** 15 to 30 min per session

Instruct clients who are engaging in stretching programs to adhere to the following guidelines (Kravitz and Heyward 1995):

CLIENT GUIDELINES FOR STRETCHING PROGRAMS

- Perform a general warm-up before stretching to increase body temperature and to warm the muscles to be stretched.
- Stretch all major muscle groups, as well as opposing muscle groups.
- Focus on the target muscles involved in the stretch, relax the target muscle, and minimize the movement of other body parts.
- Hold the stretch for 10 to 30 sec.
- Stretch to the limit (end point) of the movement, not to the point of pain.
- Keep breathing slowly and rhythmically while holding the stretch.
- Stretch the target muscle groups in different planes to improve overall ROM at the joint.

DESIGNING LOW BACK CARE EXERCISE PROGRAMS

Low back pain frequently causes activity restrictions for middle-aged and older adults, disabling 3 to 4 million people each year. Chronic low back pain is the number-one cause of disability in the working population (Carpenter and Nelson 1999). The safest and most effective way to prevent and rehabilitate low back injuries remains controversial. This section describes two approaches for low back care programs. The approach you select depends on your client's needs, health/fitness status, and training objective (e.g., reducing low back pain, lowering the risk of low back injury, or maximizing athletic performance).

Traditional Approach

Traditionally, low back care programs have been designed to correct improper alignment and support of the spinal column and pelvis. Generally, a combination of stretching and strengthening exercises is prescribed to increase (a) the ROM of the hip flexors, hamstrings, and low back extensor muscles and (b) the strength of the abdominal muscles.

Exercise professionals have focused primarily on strengthening the abdominal muscles in order to prevent low back pain and injury, giving little or no attention to the low back muscles. Recent research, however, suggests that low-back-strengthening programs are effective for relieving and preventing low back pain and injury (Carpenter and Nelson 1999). A current practice in some low back care programs is to include exercises to increase the strength and endurance of both the abdominal and low back extensor muscles.

To strengthen the low back (lumbar extensor) muscles, **pelvic stabilization** is a key requirement. If the pelvis is not stabilized during extension of the trunk, the hip extensor muscles rotate the pelvis (~110°), and the lumbar vertebrae maintain their relative position to each other (do not extend). On the other hand, when the pelvis is immobilized, the lumbar vertebrae extend (~72°) as the low back extensor muscles contract (Carpenter and Nelson 1999). Most calisthenic-type floor exercises do not isolate the low back muscles because the pelvis is free to move. Using a lumbar extension machine, with thigh and femur restraints to stabilize the pelvis, prevents hip extension and isolates the low back muscles during the movement. Exercising on a lumbar extension machine with a minimal training volume (one set of 8 to 15

repetitions of lumbar extension exercise to fatigue per week) significantly improves lumbar muscle strength and bone mineral density (Graves et al. 1994; Pollock, Garzarella, and Graves 1992) and reduces the incidence of back injuries (Mooney, Kron, Rummerfield, and Holmes 1995). Individuals with chronic low back pain who participate in this type of low-back-strengthening program can expect significant improvements in joint mobility and muscular strength and endurance, as well as relief from pain (Carpenter and Nelson 1999).

To strengthen the abdominal muscles, select exercises that maximize the activation of the abdominal muscles but minimize the compression (load) of the lumbar vertebrae (i.e., a high challenge : compression ratio). Since the psoas muscle (prime mover for hip flexion) is a major source of spinal loading, choose exercises that minimize the activation of this muscle, such as bent-knee curl-ups (feet free or anchored), dynamic cross-knee curl-ups (curl-ups with a twist), isometric side support (side bridge), and dynamic sideward curl exercises (Axler and McGill 1997; Juker, McGill, Kropf, and Steffen 1998; Knudson 1999). The bent-knee curl-up exercise emphasizes the rectus abdominis, while the isometric side support emphasizes the abdominal oblique and quadratus lumborum muscles. Because of their low challenge : compression ratios, the following abdominal exercises are not recommended: straight-leg or bent-knee sit-ups, supine straight-leg raises, and hanging bent-knee raises (Axler and McGill 1997).

Using the traditional approach, the following exercises are recommended for low back care. Some of these exercises are described and illustrated in appendix F.3, "Exercises for Low Back Care," page 344.

- Pelvic tilt (supine-lying position) to stretch the abdominal muscles
- Knee-to-chest (supine-lying position) to stretch the hamstring, buttock, and low back muscles
- Trunk flex (on hands and knees) to stretch the back, abdominal, and hamstring muscles
- Lumbar extension exercises with pelvic stabilization (on machine) to strengthen the low back extensors
- Curl-ups, dynamic cross-knee curl-ups, and isometric side-support exercises to strengthen the abdominal and quadratus lumborum muscles
- Single-leg extension (prone-lying position) to strengthen the hamstring and buttock muscles and to stretch the hip flexor muscles

A New Approach

Recent studies suggest that the major cause of low back injury during exercise or performance of activities of daily living is lumbar instability, rather than improper alignment of the spinal column and pelvis per se (McGill 2001). Research also indicates that muscle *endurance* is more protective than muscle *strength* for reducing low back injury and that greater lumbar mobility (ROM) actually increases one's risk of low back injury (McGill 1998, 2001). Thus, sufficient stability of the lumbar spine (i.e., **lumbar stabilization**) is the major emphasis in this new approach to low back care. Norris (2000) provides a detailed discussion and suggestions for applying the concept of lumbar stabilization to low back care programs.

To develop and maintain lumbar stability, experts (McGill 2001) recommend:

- "Bracing" the lumbar spine during activity by isometrically co-contracting the abdominal wall and low back muscles
- Maintaining a "neutral" spine (i.e., the natural lordotic curve in the lumbar spine while standing upright) during activity
- Avoiding end ROM positions (fully flexed or extended) of the trunk while lifting or exercising
- Performing exercises that emphasize the development of muscle endurance rather than strength

The following sequence of exercises is specifically recommended for beginners who are starting a low back care program. These exercises are illustrated in appendix F.3, "Exercises for Low Back Care," page 344.

- Cat-camel exercise to slowly and dynamically move through the full range of spinal flexion and extension, with emphasis on spinal mobility rather than pressing and holding the trunk position at the ends of the ROM (usually five to six cycles of this exercise are sufficient)
- Stretching exercises to increase mobility at the hip and knee joints
- Curl-ups with one leg flexed and hands placed underneath the lumbar spine to help in maintaining a neutral spine
- Isometric side support (side bridge) exercises for the quadratus lumborum and abdominal oblique muscles
- Single-leg extension holds while on hands and knees for the low back and hip extensor muscles
- Isometric stabilization exercises requiring simultaneous contraction of the abdominal muscles to generate an abdominal "brace" during performance of other exercises
- Dynamic "hollowing" or drawing of the navel toward the spine for the deeper abdominal wall muscles (i.e., transverse abdominis and internal obliques)

SOURCES FOR EQUIPMENT

Product	Manufacturer's Address
Flexometer Inclinometer Sit-and-reach box Universal goniometer	Country Technology Inc. P.O. Box 87 Gay Mills, WI 54631 Phone: (608) 735-4718 www.fitnessmart.com

KEY POINTS

- Static flexibility is a measure of the total ROM at the joint.
- Dynamic flexibility is a measure of the rate of torque or resistance developed during movement through the ROM.
- Flexibility is highly joint specific, and the ROM depends, in part, on the structure of the joint.
- Lack of physical activity is a major cause of inflexibility.

- A universal goniometer, flexometer, or inclinometer can be used to obtain direct measures of ROM.

- A yardstick and anthropometric tape measure can be used to obtain indirect measures of ROM.

- The principles of specificity and progressive overload must be applied to the design of flexibility exercise programs.

- Static, ballistic, and PNF stretching techniques are equally effective in increasing ROM. Ballistic stretching, however, increases the risk of injury and muscle soreness.

- A well-rounded flexibility program includes at least one exercise for each major muscle group of the body.

- A way to overload the muscle group is to progressively increase the length of time that the stretched position is held (10 to 30 sec) and the number of repetitions (three to five repetitions) performed.

- Flexibility exercises should be performed at least two to three days a week, but preferably daily.

- Lumbar instability is a major cause of low back problems.

- Exercises designed to develop and maintain lumbar stability are recommended for low back care programs.

- Exercises to develop muscle endurance may be more effective than muscle-strengthening exercises for prevention and treatment of low back injuries.

KEY TERMS

Learn the definition for each of the following key terms. Definitions of terms can be found in "Glossary of Terms," page 349.

ankylosis
ballistic stretching
biaxial joint
contract-relax agonist contract (CRAC) technique
contract-relax technique
contracture
dynamic flexibility
elastic deformation
flexibility
flexometer
goniometer
hypermobility

inclinometer
joint laxity
lumbar stabilization
pelvic stabilization
proprioceptive neuromuscular facilitation (PNF)
range of motion
static flexibility
static stretching
stress relaxation
triaxial joint
uniaxial joint
viscoelastic properties
viscous deformation

REVIEW QUESTIONS

In addition to being able to define each of the key terms, test your knowledge and understanding of the material by answering the following review questions.

1. Why are flexibility tests included in most health-related fitness test batteries?

2. Identify and explain how morphological factors affect range of joint motion.

3. How do age, gender, and physical activity (or lack thereof) affect flexibility?

4. Identify and briefly describe three direct methods for measuring static flexibility.

5. Do sit-and-reach tests yield valid measures of hamstring and low back flexibility? Explain.

6. Is the modified standard sit-and-reach test more valid than the standard sit-and-reach test for assessing hamstring and low back flexibility?

7. Describe two methods of stretching that are recommended for increasing flexibility.

8. Explain why ballistic stretching is not recommended for flexibility programs.

9. Describe the basic guidelines for designing flexibility programs. How do the specificity and overload training principles apply?

10. Describe three abdominal exercises that have high challenge-to-compression ratios.

11. What are the similarities and differences between the traditional approach and the new approach for low back care exercise programs?

12. Describe the recommended sequence of exercises for beginners starting a low back care program.

REFERENCES

Ahlback, S.O., and Lindahl, O. 1964. Sagittal mobility of the hip-joint. *Acta Orthopaedica Scandinavica* 34: 310–313.

Alter, M.J. 1996. *Science of flexibility and stretching.* Champaign, IL: Human Kinetics.

American College of Sports Medicine (ACSM). 2000. *ACSM's guidelines for exercise testing and prescription.* Philadelphia: Lippincott Williams & Wilkins.

American Medical Association. 1988. *Guides to the evaluation of permanent impairment,* 3rd ed. Chicago, IL: Author.

Anderson, R. 1980. *Stretching.* Fullerton, CA: Shelter.

Axler, C.T., and McGill, S.M. 1997. Low back loads over a variety of abdominal exercises: Searching for the safest abdominal challenge. *Medicine & Science in Sports & Exercise* 29: 804–810.

Bandy, W.D., and Irion, J.M. 1994. The effect of time on static stretch on the flexibility of the hamstring muscles. *Physical Therapy* 74: 845–851.

Beaulieu, J.E. 1980. *Stretching for all sports.* Pasadena, CA: Athletic Press.

Borms, J., Van Roy, P., Santens, J.P., and Haentjens, A. 1987. Optimal duration of static stretching exercises for improvement of coxo-femoral flexibility. *Journal of Sports Science* 5: 39–47.

Brown, D.A., and Miller, W.C. 1998. Normative data for strength and flexibility of women throughout life. *European Journal of Applied Physiology* 78: 77–82.

Canadian Society for Exercise Physiology. 1998. *The Canadian physical activity, fitness and lifestyle appraisal.* 2nd ed. Ottawa, ON: author.

Carpenter, D.M., and Nelson, B.W. 1999. Low back strengthening for the prevention and treatment of low back pain. *Medicine & Science in Sports & Exercise* 31: 18–24.

Chapman, E.A., deVries, H.A., and Swezey, R. 1972. Joint stiffness: Effects of exercise on young and old men. *Journal of Gerontology* 27: 218–221.

Cooper Institute for Aerobics Research. 1992. *The Prudential FITNESSGRAM test administration manual.* Dallas: Author.

Cotten, D.J. 1972. A comparison of selected trunk flexibility tests. *American Corrective Therapy Journal* 26: 24.

deVries, H.A. 1962. Evaluation of static stretching procedures for improvement of flexibility. *Research Quarterly* 33: 222–229.

Dickinson, R.V. 1968. The specificity of flexibility. *Research Quarterly* 39: 792–793.

Enwemeka, C.S. 1986. Radiographic verification of knee goniometry. *Scandinavian Journal of Rehabilitation Medicine* 18: 47–49.

Fitness Canada. 1986. *Canadian standardized test of fitness (CSTF) operations manual,* 3rd ed. Ottawa, ON: Fitness and Amateur Sport Canada.

Gajdosik, R.L., Vander Linden, D.W., and Williams, A.K. 1999. Influence of age on length and passive elastic stiffness characteristics of the calf muscle-tendon unit of women. *Physical Therapy* 79: 827–838.

Girouard, C.K., and Hurley, B.F. 1995. Does strength training inhibit gains in range of motion from flexibility training in older adults? *Medicine & Science in Sports & Exercise* 27: 1444–1449.

Graves, J.D., Webb, D.C., Pollock, M.L. Matkozich, J., Leggett, S.H., Carpenter, D.M., Foster, D.N., and Cirulli, J. 1994. Pelvic stabilization during resistance training: Its effect on the development of lumbar extension strength. *Archives of Physical Medicine and Rehabilitation* 75: 210–215.

Greene, W.B., and Heckman, J.D. 1994. *The clinical measurement of joint motion.* Rosemont, IL: American Academy of Orthopaedic Surgeons.

Harris, M.L. 1969. A factor analytic study of flexibility. *Research Quarterly* 40: 62–70.

Hartley-O'Brien, S.J. 1980. Six mobilization exercises for active range of hip flexion. *Research Quarterly for Exercise and Sport* 51: 625–635.

Hoeger, W.W.K. 1989. *Lifetime physical fitness and wellness.* Englewood Cliffs, NJ: Morton.

Hoeger, W.W.K., and Hopkins, D.R. 1992. A comparison of the sit-and-reach and the modified sit-and-reach in the measurement of flexibility in women. *Research Quarterly for Exercise and Sport* 63: 191–195.

Hoeger, W.W.K., Hopkins, D.R., Button, S., and Palmer, T.A. 1990. Comparing the sit and reach with the modified sit and reach in measuring flexibility in adolescents. *Pediatric Exercise Science* 2: 156–162.

Holt, L.E., Travis, T.M., and Okita, T. 1970. Comparative study of three stretching techniques. *Perceptual and Motor Skills* 31: 611–616.

Hubley-Kozey, C.L. 1991. Testing flexibility. In *Physiological testing of the high-performance athlete,* ed. J.D. MacDougall, H.A. Wenger, and H.J. Green, 309–359. Champaign, IL: Human Kinetics.

Hui, S.C., and Yuen, P.Y. 2000. Validity of the modified back-saver sit-and-reach test: A comparison with other protocols. *Medicine & Science in Sports & Exercise* 32: 1655–1659.

Hui, S.C., Yuen, P.Y., Morrow, J.R., and Jackson, A.W. 1999. Comparison of the criterion-related validity of sit-and-reach tests with and without limb length adjustment in Asian adults. *Research Quarterly for Exercise and Sport* 70: 401–406.

Hultborn, H., Illert, M., and Santini, M. 1974. Disynaptic inhibition of the interneurons mediating the reciprocal Ia inhibition of motor neurones. *Acta Physiologica Scandinavica* 91: 14A–16A.

Jackson, A.W., and Langford, N.J. 1989. The criterion-related validity of the sit-and-reach test: Replication and extension of previous findings. *Research Quarterly for Exercise and Sport* 60: 384–387.

Jackson, A.W., Morrow, J.R., Brill, P.A., Kohl, H.W., Gordon, N.F., and Blair, S.N. 1998. Relations of sit-up and sit-and-reach tests to low back pain in adults. *Journal of Orthopaedic and Sports Physical Therapy* 27: 22–26.

Johns, R.J., and Wright, V. 1962. Relative importance of various tissues in joint stiffness. *Journal of Applied Physiology* 17: 824–828.

Jones, B.H., and Knapik, J.J. 1999. Physical training and exercise-related injuries. *Sports Medicine* 27: 111–125.

Jones, C.J., Rikli, R.E., Max, J., and Noffal, G. 1998. The reliability and validity of a chair sit-and-reach test as a measure of hamstring flexibility in older adults. *Research Quarterly for Exercise and Sport* 69: 338–343.

Juker, D., McGill, S., Kropf, P., and Steffen, T. 1998. Quantitative intramuscular myoelectric activity of lumbar portions of psoas and the abdominal wall during a wide variety of tasks. *Medicine & Science in Sports & Exercise* 30: 301–310.

Kirby, R.L., Simms, F.C., Symington, V.J., and Garner, J.B. 1981. Flexibility and musculoskeletal symptomatology in female gymnasts and age-matched controls. *American Journal of Sports Medicine* 9: 160–164.

Knudson, D.V. 1999. Issues in abdominal fitness: Testing and technique. *Journal of Physical Education, Recreation and Dance* 70(3): 49–55.

Knudson, D.V., Magnusson, P., and McHugh, M. 2000. Current issues in flexibility fitness. *President's Council on Physical Fitness and Sports Research Digest* 3(10): 1–8.

Kravitz, L., and Heyward, V.H. 1995. Flexibility training. *Fitness Management* 11(2): 32–38.

Kubo, K., Kaneshisa, H., Takeshita, D., Kawakami, Y., Fukashiro, S., and Fukunaga, T. 2000. In vivo dynamics of human medial gastrocnemius muscle-tendon complex curing stretch-shortening cycle exercise. *Acta Physiologica Scandinavica* 170: 127–135.

Kubo, K., Kawakami, Y., and Fukunaga, T. 1999. Influence of elastic properties of tendon structures on jump performance in humans. *Journal of Applied Physiology* 87: 2090–2096.

Leighton, J.R. 1955. An instrument and technique for measurement of range of joint motion. *Archives of Physical Medicine and Rehabilitation* 36: 571–578.

Magnusson, S.P. 1998. Passive properties of human skeletal muscle during stretch maneuvers. A review. *Scandinavian Journal of Medicine and Science in Sports* 8(2): 65–77.

Magnusson, S.P., Simonsen, E.B., Aagaard, P., Bueson, J., Johannson, F., and Kjaer, M. 1997. Determinants of musculoskeletal flexibility: Visoelastic properties, cross-sectional area, EMG and stretch tolerance. *Scandinavian Journal of Medicine and Science in Sports* 7: 195–202.

Martin, S.B., Jackson, A.W., Morrow, J.R., and Liemohn, W. 1998. The rationale for the sit and reach test revisited. *Measurement in Physical Education and Exercise Science* 2: 85–92.

Mayer, T.G., Tencer, A.F., and Kristoferson, S. 1984. Use of noninvasive technique for quantification of spinal range-of-motion in normal subjects and chronic low back dysfunction patients. *Spine* 9: 588–595.

McCue, B.F. 1953. Flexibility of college women. *Research Quarterly* 24: 316–324.

McGill, S.M. 1998. Low back exercises: Prescription for the healthy back and when recovering from injury. In *ACSM's resource manual for guidelines for exercise testing and prescription,* 3rd ed., 116–126. Philadelphia: Lippincott Williams & Wilkins.

McGill, S.M. 2001. Low back stability: From formal description to issues for performance and rehabilitation. *Exercise and Sport Sciences Reviews* 29(1): 26–31.

McHugh, M.P. Kremenic, I.J., Fox, M.B., and Gleim, G.W. 1998. The role of mechanical and neural restraints to joint range of motion during passive stretch. *Medicine & Science in Sports & Exercise* 30: 928–932.

McHugh, M.P., Magnusson, S.P., Gleim, G.W., and Nicholas, J.A. 1992. Viscoelastic stress relaxation in human skeletal muscle. *Medicine & Science in Sports & Exercise* 24: 1375–1382.

Mcrae, I.F., and Wright, V. 1969. Measurement of back movement. *Annals of Rheumatic Diseases* 28: 584–589.

Minkler, S., and Patterson, P. 1994. The validity of the modified sit-and-reach test in college-age students. *Research Quarterly for Exercise and Sport* 65: 189–192.

Mooney, V., Kron, M., Rummerfield, P., and Holmes, B. 1995. The effect of workplace based strengthening on low back injury rates: A case study in the strip mining industry. *Journal of Occupational Rehabilitation* 5: 157–167.

Moore, M.A., and Hutton, R.S. 1980. Electromyographic investigation of muscle stretching techniques. *Medicine & Science in Sports & Exercise* 12: 322–329.

Munroe, R.A., and Romance, T.J. 1975. Use of the Leighton flexometer in the development of a short flexibility test battery. *American Corrective Therapy Journal* 29: 22.

Norkin, C.C., and White, D.J. 1995. *Measurement of joint motion: A guide to goniometry.* Philadelphia: Davis.

Norris, C. 2000. *Back stability.* Champaign, IL: Human Kinetics.

Patterson, P., Wiksten, D.L., Ray, L., Flanders, C., and Sanphy, D. 1996. The validity and reliability of the backsaver sit-and-reach test in middle school girls and boys. *Research Quarterly for Exercise and Sport* 67: 448–451.

Payne, N., Gledhill, N., Kazmarzyk, P.T., Jamnik, V., and Keir, P.J. 2000. Canadian musculoskeletal fitness norms. *Canadian Journal of Applied Physiology* 25: 430–442.

Plowman, S.A. 1992. Physical activity, physical fitness, and low-back pain. *Exercise and Sport Sciences Reviews* 20: 221–242.

Pollock, M., Garzarella, L., and Graves, J. 1992. Effects of isolated lumbar extension resistance training on BMD of the elderly. *Medicine & Science in Sports & Exercise* 24: S66 [abstract].

Pope, R.P., Herbert, R.D., Kirwan, J.D., and Graham, B.J. 2000. A randomized trial of pre-exercise stretching for prevention of lower-limb injury. *Medicine & Science in Sports & Exercise* 32: 271–277.

Rikli, R.E., and Jones, C.J. 2001. *Senior fitness test manual.* Champaign, IL: Human Kinetics.

Roberts, J.M., and Wilson, K. 1999. Effect of stretching duration on active and passive range of motion in the lower extremity. *British Journal of Sports Medicine* 33: 259–263.

Sell, K.E., Verity, T.M., Worrell, T.W., Pease, B.J., and Wigglesworth, J. 1994. Two measurement techniques for assessing subtalar joint position: A reliability study. *Journal of Orthopaedic and Sports Physical Therapy* 19: 162–167.

Van Adrichem, J.A.M., and van der Korst, J.K. 1973. Assessment of flexibility of the lumbar spine: A pilot study in children and adolescents. *Scandinavian Journal of Rheumatology* 2: 87–91.

Wallin, D., Ekblom, B., Grahn, R., and Nordenborg, T. 1985. Improvement of muscle flexibility. A comparison between two techniques. *American Journal of Sports Medicine* 13: 263–268.

Williams, R., Binkley, J., Bloch, R., Goldsmith, C.H., and Minuk, T. 1993. Reliability of the modified-modified Schober and double inclinometer methods for measuring lumbar flexion and extension. *Physical Therapy* 73: 26–37.

Worrell, T.W., Smith, T.L., and Winegardner, J. 1994. Effect of hamstring stretching on hamstring muscle performance. *Journal of Orthopaedic and Sports Physical Therapy* 20: 154–159.

Wright, V., and Johns, R.J. 1960. Physical factors concerned with the stiffness of normal and diseased joints. *Bulletin of Johns Hopkins Hospital* 106: 215–231.

YMCA of the USA. 2000. *YMCA fitness testing and assessment manual.* 4th ed. Champaign, IL: Human Kinetics.

chapter 11

Assessing and Managing Stress

KEY QUESTIONS

- What causes stress?
- How does the body respond and adapt to acute and chronic stress?
- What are the signs and symptoms of excessive stress?

- How is stress measured?
- What techniques may be used to effectively manage stress?
- What is the role of exercise in stress management?

Stress evokes a generalized physiological response of the body to physical, psychological, or environmental demands. Throughout life, everyone encounters both good and bad changes that produce stress. Everything from the death of a family member, the loss of a job, or the birth of a child, to a change in one's eating or exercise habits is a potentially stressful event. People differ, however, in what they perceive as stressful and how they cope with stress-producing situations. It is important for each person to find ways to manage stress effectively, because constant stress or overstress may lead to disease or illness (Selye 1956).

This chapter discusses the body's response to stress and the role of exercise in alleviating stress. It also deals with techniques for assessing stress and neuromuscular tension and with methods of relaxation for relieving tension.

PHYSIOLOGICAL RESPONSE TO STRESS

Stressors may be physiological or psychological. Activities such as weightlifting, jogging, and swimming, as well as changes in temperature or altitude, are examples of physiological stressors. Psychological stressors include such life-event changes as a new job, family illness, or final examinations.

The body does not differentiate between physiological and psychological stressors. Instead, the immediate response of the body to stress is generalized and prepares the body to fight or flee from potentially threatening situations. The fight-or-flight response is characterized by increases in heart rate, breathing rate, body temperature, blood flow to muscles, sweating, oxygen utilization, and muscle tension.

These changes are mediated through the activation of the sympathetic nervous system and the adrenal glands. The glucocorticoids from the adrenal cortex promote fat utilization, protein catabolism, and carbohydrate conservation. An elevated blood glucose level supplies energy to the brain and nervous tissue and may increase the body's ability to resist stress. In addition, the glucocorticoids are known to enhance the effect of the adrenal medulla hormones—norepinephrine and epinephrine. These catecholamines produce physiological changes that are similar to those produced by the neurotransmitters of the sympathetic nervous system.

Selye (1956) hypothesized three stages that describe the body's reaction to stress. In the first stage, known as the **alarm reaction stage,** the body perceives the stress, and the fight-or-flight response is activated. In the second stage, **resistance and adaptation,** the body continues to resist and adapt to the stressor. If the stress is too intense or prolonged, the body may lose its ability to resist the stressor and enter the third, or **exhaustive,** stage, which is characterized by illness or even death in some cases.

STRESS AND DISEASE

Excessive stress from any source may lead to sickness and disease. Insomnia, diarrhea, loss of appetite, muscular tension, and headaches are physical symptoms of stress. Colitis, ulcers, hypertension, stroke, and coronary artery disease are also associated with excessive stress. Some of the psychological effects of excessive stress are anxiety, depression, decreased concentration, irritability, poor memory, and anger. In the workplace, signs of excessive stress are increased absenteeism, tardiness, accidents, and turnover, as well as poor communication among employees and decreased productivity.

Researchers are investigating the links among psychological stress, behavior profiles, and disease risk. Friedman and Rosenman (1975) identified behavior profiles that represent two extremes on a behavior continuum. **Type A behavior** is characterized by an extreme need to achieve, competitiveness, impatience, overcommitment to work, explosive speech patterns, and aggressiveness. At the other extreme, the **type B behavior** profile is characterized by a relaxed and easygoing nature. The type A behavior pattern is positively associated with stress in black and white women (Adams-Campbell, Washburn, and Haile 1990), and with increased risk of coronary heart disease (CHD) risk in middle-aged men (Hendrix and Hughes 1997). Interventions aimed at healthy lifestyles favorably modify type A behavior in CHD patients (Sebregts, Falger, and Bar 2000). In addition, type A behavior counseling may also lead to reduced morbidity and mortality due to CHD (Friedman et al. 1996; Sebregts et al. 2000).

ASSESSMENT OF STRESS AND NEUROMUSCULAR TENSION

You may use data from questionnaires to assess the stress level and behavior characteristics of your clients. Computer software is available that generates a stress profile to help identify sources of stress for each individual. Also, you may use electromyography or manual tension tests to evaluate neuromuscular tension due to stress.

Stress

Questionnaires have been developed for self-assessment of stress (Orioli, Jaffe, and Scott 1987) and identification of overt characteristics associated with type A behavior patterns (Jenkins, Rosenman, and Zyzanski 1974). The StressMap Questionnaire (Orioli et al. 1987), divided into four parts, uses 21 scales to assess the following:

- Environmental pressures
- Coping responses
- Inner thoughts and feelings
- Signals of distress

This comprehensive questionnaire provides a valid and reliable (r's ranging from 0.72 to 0.93) assessment of stress.

The Jenkins Activity Survey (Jenkins et al. 1974) consists of 52 multiple-choice questions and provides a type A behavior standard score as well as three factor scores:

- Speed and impatience
- Job involvement
- Hard-driving behavior and competitiveness

Various forms of the Jenkins Activity Survey have been validated for different groups, including employed men and women, housewives, college students, and retired persons. There are also many computerized health risk appraisals you can use to evaluate the stress profiles of your clients.

You can use a four-part inventory developed by Girdano and Everly (1979) to assess the stress level and coping strategies of your clients. Tests 1 to 3 measure your client's degree of stress due to frustration and inhibition; vulnerability to overload; and compulsive, time-urgent, and aggressive behavioral traits. Test 4 identifies the strategies that your client uses to cope with common sources of stress.

Neuromuscular Tension

Neuromuscular tension is associated with acute and chronic stress. The degree of tension in skeletal muscles is increased as part of the fight-or-flight response to stress. Chronic or prolonged stress also may increase neuromuscular tension levels.

Electromyography (EMG) is the most valid method for measuring muscle activity at rest. There is a direct relationship between the frequency and amplitude of EMG signals and the degree of tension in the resting muscle. Electromyographic equipment is relatively expensive, and the technique is time consuming. Thus, for large groups, you should use alternative field techniques to evaluate muscular tension.

One such technique is the Rathbone **manual tension test** (Rathbone and Hunt 1965). This test assesses the muscular tension during passive movement of the wrist, elbow, shoulder, neck, hip, and knee joints (see appendix F.4, "Rathbone Manual Tension Test," p. 346). The validity of this test was established using EMG as the criterion for 11 muscle groups ($r = 0.97$). The test evaluates four manifestations of muscular tension:

1. **Assistance**—Client aids the tester in moving the body segment.

2. **Resistance**—Client resists the movement of the body segment.

3. **Posturing**—Client maintains the new position after the limb is released by the tester.

4. **Perseveration**—Client continues to move or repeats the movement of the body segment after it is released by the tester.

For each movement, you assign a numerical value that corresponds to the degree of tension observed in the limb:

0 = none
1 = slight
2 = moderate
3 = marked tension

In addition to manual symptoms, you can use visual signs to detect the presence of neuromuscular tension. Visual symptoms include frowning, twitching, fluttering eyelids, rapid breathing, tightness of the mouth, and repeated swallowing.

EXERCISE AND STRESS

Exercise is a physiological stressor that evokes an acute **stress response**, such as increased heart rate, blood pressure, breathing rate, blood flow to muscles, oxygen consumption, and metabolic rate. Intense and prolonged exercise (usually > 30 min) increases the plasma levels of cortisol (Hartley et al. 1972; Shephard and Sidney 1975; Tharp 1975), epinephrine, and norepinephrine

(Hartley et al. 1972; VonEuler 1974). It appears that a minimum exercise intensity of 60% $\dot{V}O_2$max is needed to produce these hormonal responses (Davies and Few 1973; Hartley 1975; VonEuler 1974).

The response patterns of corticosteroids and norepinephrine to exercise are partly dependent on the fitness status of the individual and may be modified by physical conditioning (Hartley et al. 1972; Hartley 1975; White, Ismail, and Bottoms 1976). The lower plasma corticosteroid and norepinephrine levels at a given submaximal workload in endurance-trained individuals suggests that they are better able to tolerate the physiological stress produced by exercise than are sedentary individuals.

Exercise also plays an important role in the management of psychological stress (Brehm 2000). Mental and emotional stress may lead to states of anxiety and depression. Vigorous physical activity reduces state anxiety in both highly anxious and normally anxious men and women (Morgan 1973; Wertz, Koltyn, and Morgan 1997); this effect may persist for up to several hours (Petruzzello, Landers, Hatfield, Kubitz, and Salazar 1991). Raglin and Wilson (1996) reported significant reductions in state anxiety following 20 min of cycle ergometer exercise performed at 40%, 60%, and 70% $\dot{V}O_2$max. The reduction in state anxiety is dependent on the duration of the aerobic exercise (i.e., at least 21 min) (Petruzzello et al. 1991). Focht and Koltyn (1999) recently reported that an acute bout of resistance exercise performed at 50% one-repetition maximum is associated with significant postexercise reductions in state anxiety of experienced and novice weight lifters 180 min after the cessation of activity.

Regular participation in an aerobic exercise program also appears to reduce symptoms of moderate depression (Martinsen and Morgan 1997) and to enhance psychological fitness. Highly trained, world-class athletes tend to be less anxious, depressed, and confused than the average person (Morgan 1979). Participation in exercise programs may improve mood states by reducing state anxiety and enhancing one's sense of vigor (Jin 1992). Many people who participate in a regular program of exercise report that they feel better after exercising (Hoffmann 1997). Thus, exercise appears to be an effective technique for reducing stress, coping with stress, and regulating mood behaviors (Anthony 1991; Severtsen and Bruya 1986; Thayer, Newman, and McClain 1994). In fact, a recent study (Babyak et al. 2000) of adults diagnosed with major depressive disorder indicated that individuals who participated in 30 min of aerobic exercise (i.e., brisk walking, stationary cycling, or jogging), three times a week for four months, showed improvements in symptoms of depression that equaled those of individuals taking either a prescription drug (i.e., Zoloft) or a combination of the drug and exercise. Moreover, individuals in the exercise-only group were far less likely to see their depression return after 10 months compared to people taking the drug or the combination therapy.

The underlying psychophysiological mechanisms, however, are not fully understood. Some factors that may explain, in part, the effectiveness of exercise for reducing psychological stress and altering mood states are the following:

- Exercise is a diversion that enables the person to relax due to a change in environment or routine.

- Exercise serves as an outlet to dissipate emotions such as anger, fear, and frustration.

- Exercise enhances one's self-esteem and increases confidence in one's ability to deal with stress-producing situations (Sonstroem 1997).

- Exercise produces biochemical changes that alter psychological states. For example, a low level of norepinephrine is associated with depression. During exercise, plasma levels of norepinephrine increase, which may help to alleviate symptoms of depression (Dishman 1997). Exercise may also increase the levels of beta-endorphins in the blood. These opioid substances have a narcotic effect that induces feelings of pleasure and wellness, referred to as "endorphin calm" or "jogger's high" (Hoffman 1997; Wildmann, Kruger, Schmole, Niemann, and Matthaei 1986).

RELAXATION TECHNIQUES

A number of relaxation techniques can relieve muscular tension and stress. The goal of these techniques is to elicit a relaxation response that is characterized by decreases in EMG activity, heart rate, blood pressure, breathing rate, and oxygen consumption. You can use physical, mental, or a combination of approaches to achieve the relaxation response.

Physical Approach

Aerobic exercise and the progressive relaxation technique (Jacobson 1978) are two methods that produce relaxation through the physical mode. Regular aerobic exercise is effective for reducing psychological stress and increasing the body's resistance to many types of stressors. For tense individuals, low-intensity (30% to 60% maximum heart rate) rhythmic exercise, such as jogging, cycling, and walking, performed 5 to 30 min per day, lowers muscular tension levels at rest (deVries 1975). Participation in an aerobic exercise program enables one to reduce stress and tension while enjoying the cardiorespiratory, body composition, and weight control benefits of the exercise. Because of these multiple benefits, aerobic exercise is a highly recommended relaxation technique.

In the **progressive relaxation technique,** the client learns to identify muscular tension in the major muscle groups and to relax these muscles consciously. According to Jacobson (1978), progressive relaxation refers to the individual's ability to

- relax major muscle groups one after the other,

- relax each muscle group further and further, and

- progress toward a habit of effortless relaxation.

The relaxation response is developed by deliberately contracting, and then relaxing ("letting it go"), each muscle group, starting with the muscles of the feet and ending with the facial muscles. Daily practice of this technique is recommended to achieve effortless relaxation. For detailed information about the progressive relaxation technique, see Jacobson (1978).

Mental Approach

Meditation, imagery, biofeedback, and autogenic relaxation training use a mind-over-matter approach to relaxation (Curtis, Detert, Schindler, and Zirkel 1985). Meditation produces a hypometabolic state in which oxygen consumption is reduced by 10% to 20%, and heart rate is decreased 3 bpm on the average (Benson 1975). There is also an increase in the alpha brain wave activity, which is indicative of a relaxed state. With this technique, relaxation is achieved through the continued repetition of a word or phrase.

The Benson technique (Benson 1975) also uses meditation to promote relaxation. Bahrke and Morgan (1978) noted that the Benson relaxation technique and aerobic exercise were equally effective in reducing state anxiety. The basic elements of this technique are

- a quiet environment,
- a comfortable position,
- repetition of a word or phrase, and
- a passive, let-it-happen attitude.

Imagery is a form of autosuggestion or self-hypnosis that uses visual images to produce a relaxed state. The person visualizes floating or sinking images and obtains temporary relief from tension, worry, and anxiety. A number of excellent sources deal with visualization to induce relaxation (Bry 1979; Curtis, Detert, Schindler, and Zirkel 1985).

In **biofeedback,** the individual uses visual and auditory signals to control unconscious bodily functions, such as heart rate, blood pressure, body temperature, and muscular tension. This technique can effectively reduce neuromuscular tension and promote relaxation. Detailed descriptions of the use of various methods of biofeedback training for relaxation are provided elsewhere (Basmajian 1983; Brown 1981; Curtis et al. 1985; Danskin and Crow 1981).

Autogenic relaxation training consists of a series of six mental exercises that the person practices several times daily to elicit the relaxation response (Benson 1975). Lying in a quiet room with the eyes closed, the client focuses on the following:

- a sensation of heaviness in the limbs,
- a sensation of warmth in the limbs,
- breathing,

- regulation of heart rate,
- feelings of coolness in the forehead, and
- a passive, let-it-happen attitude.

Combination Approach

Some experts recommend using a combination of aerobic exercise and meditation to reduce stress. Severtsen and Bruya (1986) noted that the combination of daily meditation and aerobic exercise increased ability to cope with stress. Likewise, Thayer, Newman, and McClain (1994) recommended a combination of relaxation, stress management, and cognitive and exercise techniques to self-regulate bad moods, to increase energy levels and vigor, and to reduce tension.

Hatha yoga is a combination of physical and mental exercise that is sometimes used to achieve a state of total relaxation. Stretching exercises, poses, and breathing exercises are performed to relieve muscular tension. Mental relaxation is produced through concentration and autosuggestion techniques (Barney and Frauenglass 1980).

Tai chi has been promoted as an activity that has a positive impact on mental and physical health. Brown, Wang, and Ward (1995) found that women participating in a tai chi exercise program for 16 weeks have reduced tension, depression, anger, confusion, and mood disturbance, as well as an improved general mood. Jin (1992) reported that the stress-reduction effect of tai chi was similar to that produced by brisk walking.

KEY POINTS

- Stress is a state that evokes a generalized physiological response of the body to physical, psychological, or environmental demands.

- The immediate, generalized response of the body to physiological and psychological stressors is known as the fight-or-flight response.

- The physiological changes associated with the fight-or-flight response are mediated through the sympathetic nervous system and adrenal glands.

- The three stages of stress are alarm reaction, resistance, and exhaustion.

- Excessive stress may lead to illness, disease, or death.

- Type A behavior is associated with high levels of stress and an increased risk of coronary artery disease.

- The Jenkins Activity Survey may be used to assess type A behavior patterns.

- Neuromuscular tension is associated with acute and chronic stress.

- Electromyography is a valid method of assessing tension levels in skeletal muscles.

- The Rathbone manual tension test evaluates muscular tension during passive movements of body segments.

- Exercise is a physiological stressor that evokes an acute stress response.

- The hormonal response to exercise stress depends on the fitness status of the individual and may be modified by physical training.

- Exercise produces biochemical changes that may alter psychological states of anxiety and depression.

- Relaxation may be induced through physical and mental exercise.
- Aerobic exercise, progressive relaxation, meditation, imagery, biofeedback, autogenic relaxation training, yoga, and tai chi are effective relaxation techniques.

KEY TERMS

Learn the definition for each of the following key terms. Definitions of terms can be found in "Glossary of Terms," page 349.

alarm reaction stage
assistance
autogenic relaxation
biofeedback
electromyography (EMG)
exhaustive stage
imagery
manual tension test

perseveration
posturing
progressive relaxation technique
resistance
resistance and adaptation stage
stress response
type A behavior
type B behavior

REVIEW QUESTIONS

In addition to being able to define each of the key terms, test your knowledge and understanding of the material by answering the following review questions.

1. What is the difference between physiological and psychological stressors? Give examples of each.

2. Describe Selye's theory of stress.

3. Describe some of the physiological and psychological symptoms and signs of stress.

4. What is the relationship between behavior profiles (type A or type B behavior) and disease risk?

5. Identify and briefly describe two paper-and-pencil tests that you can use to assess your client's stress level.

6. Describe two methods that you can use to assess your client's neuromuscular tension.

7. Describe the underlying mechanisms that may explain why exercise and physical activity are often effective in reducing psychological stress and altering mood states.

8. Physical, mental, and combination approaches are often used to induce a relaxation response. Describe some of these techniques and compare their effectiveness as relaxation techniques.

REFERENCES

Adams-Campbell, L.L., Washburn, R.A., and Haile, G.T. 1990. Physical activity, stress, and type A behavior in blacks. *Journal of the National Medical Association* 82: 701–705.

Anthony, J. 1991. Psychologic aspects of exercise. *Clinics in Sports Medicine* 10: 171–180.

Babyak, M., Blumenthal, J.A., Herman, S., Khatri, P., Doraiswamy, M., Moore, K., Craighead, E., Baldewicz, T., and Krishnan, K.R. 2000. Exercise treatment for major depression: Maintenance of therapeutic benefit at 10 months. *Psychosomatic Medicine* 62: 633–638.

Bahrke, M.S., and Morgan, W.P. 1978. Influence of acute physical activity and non-cultic meditation on state anxiety. *Cognitive Therapy and Research* 2: 323.

Barney, K., and Frauenglass, D. 1980. Introductory yoga. In *Fitness and movement,* ed. W.L. DeGroot, 137–167. Winston-Salem, NC: Hunter.

Basmajian, J., ed. 1983. *Biofeedback: Principles and practice for clinicians.* Baltimore: Williams & Wilkins.

Benson, H. 1975. *The relaxation response.* New York: Morrow.

Brehm, B.A. 2000. Maximizing the psychological benefits of physical activity. *ACSM's Health & Fitness Journal* 4(6): 7–11, 26.

Brown, B. 1981. *Stress and the art of biofeedback.* New York: Bantam Books.

Brown, D.R., Wang, Y., and Ward, A. 1995. Chronic psychological effects of exercise and exercise plus cognitive strategies. *Medicine & Science in Sports & Exercise* 27: 765–775.

Bry, A. 1979. *Visualization—directing the movies of your mind.* New York: Harper & Row.

Curtis, J.D., Detert, R.A., Schindler, J., and Zirkel, K. 1985. *Teaching stress management and relaxation skills: An instructor's guide.* LaCrosse, WI: Coulee Press.

Danskin, D., and Crow, M. 1981. *Biofeedback: An introduction and guide.* Palo Alto, CA: Mayfield.

Davies, C.T.M., and Few, J.D. 1973. Effects of exercise on adrenocortical function. *Journal of Applied Physiology* 35: 887–891.

deVries, H.A. 1975. Physical education, adult fitness programs: Does physical activity promote relaxation? *Journal of Physical Education and Recreation* 46: 53–54.

Dishman, R.K. 1997. The norepinephrine hypothesis. In *Physical activity and mental health,* ed. W.P. Morgan, 199–212. Washington, D.C.: Taylor & Francis.

Focht, B.C., and Koltyn, K.F. 1999. Influence of resistance exercise of different intensities on state anxiety and blood pressure. *Medicine & Science in Sports & Exercise* 31: 456–463.

Friedman, M., Breall, W.S., Goodwin, M.L., Sparagon, B.J., Ghandour, G., and Fleischmann, N. 1996. Effect of type A behavioral counseling on frequency of episodes of silent myocardial ischemia in coronary patients. *American Heart Journal* 132: 933–937.

Friedman, M., and Rosenman, R.H. 1975. *Type A behavior and your heart.* New York: Knopf.

Girdano, D.A., and Everly, G.S. 1979. *Controlling stress and tension: A holistic approach.* Englewood Cliffs, NJ: Prentice-Hall.

Hartley, L.H. 1975. Growth hormone and catecholamine response to exercise in relation to physical training. *Medicine and Science in Sports* 7: 34–36.

Hartley, L.H., Mason, J.W., Mougey, E.H., Wherry, F.E., Pennington, L.L., and Ricketts, P.T. 1972. Multiple hormonal responses to prolonged exercise in relation to physical training. *Journal of Applied Physiology* 33: 607–610.

Hendrix, W.H., and Hughes, R.L. 1997. Relationship of trait, Type A behavior, and physical fitness variables to cardiovascular reactivity and coronary heart disease potential. *American Journal of Health Promotion* 11: 264–271.

Hoffmann, P. 1997. The endorphin hypothesis. In *Physical activity and mental health,* ed. W.P. Morgan, 163–177. Washington, D.C.: Taylor & Francis.

Jacobson, E. 1978. *You must relax.* New York: McGraw-Hill.

Jenkins, C.D., Rosenman, R.H., and Zyzanski, S.J. 1974. Prediction of clinical coronary heart disease by a test for the coronary-prone behavior pattern. *New England Journal of Medicine* 290: 1271–1275.

Jin, P. 1992. Efficacy of Tai Chi, brisk walking, meditation, and reading in reducing mental and emotional stress. *Journal of Psychosomatic Research* 36: 361–370.

Martinsen, E.W., and Morgan, W.P. 1997. Antidepressant effects of physical activity. In *Physical activity and mental health,* ed. W.P. Morgan, 93–106. Washington, D.C.: Taylor & Francis.

Morgan, W.P. 1973. Influence of acute physical activity on state anxiety. *NCPEAM Proceedings* 76: 113.

Morgan, W.P. 1979. Prediction of performance in athletics. In *Coach, athlete, and the sports psychologist,* ed. P. Klavora and J.V. Daniel, 173–186. Champaign, IL: Human Kinetics.

Orioli, E.M., Jaffe, D.T., and Scott, C.D. 1987. *StressMap.* New York: Newmarket.

Petruzzello, S.J., Landers, D.M., Hatfield, B.D., Kubitz, K.A., and Salazar, W. 1991. A meta-analysis on the anxiety reducing effects of acute and chronic exercise: Outcomes and mechanisms. *Sports Medicine* 11: 143–182.

Raglin, J.S., and Wilson, M. 1996. State anxiety following 20 min of leg ergometry at differing intensities. *International Journal of Sports Medicine* 17: 467–471.

Rathbone, J., and Hunt, V. 1965. *Corrective physical education.* Philadelphia: Saunders.

Sebregts, E.H., Falger, P.R., and Bar, F.W. 2000. Risk factor modification through nonpharmacological interventions in patients with coronary heart disease. *Journal of Psychosomatic Research* 48: 425–441.

Selye, H. 1956. *The stress of life.* New York: McGraw-Hill.

Severtsen, B., and Bruya, M.A. 1986. Effects of meditation and aerobic exercise on EEG patterns. *Journal of Neuroscience Nursing* 18: 206–210.

Shephard, R.J., and Sidney, K.H. 1975. Effects of physical exercise on plasma growth hormone and cortisol levels in human subjects. *Exercise and Sport Sciences Reviews* 3: 1–30.

Sonstroem, R.J. 1997. Physical activity and self-esteem. In *Physical activity and mental health,* ed. W.P. Morgan, 127–143. Washington, D.C.: Taylor & Francis.

Tharp, G.D. 1975. The role of glucocorticoids in exercise. *Medicine and Science in Sports* 7: 6–11.

Thayer, R.E., Newman, J.R., and McClain, T.M. 1994. Self-regulation of mood: Strategies for changing a bad mood, raising energy, and reducing tension. *Journal of Personality and Social Psychology* 67: 910–925.

VonEuler, U.S. 1974. Sympatho-adrenal activity in physical exercise. *Medicine and Science in Sports* 6: 165–173.

Wertz, A.L., Koltyn, K.F., and Morgan, W.P. 1997. Influence of acute physical activity and relaxation on state anxiety and blood lactate. *International Journal of Sports Medicine* 18: 470–476.

White, J.A., Ismail, A.H., and Bottoms, G.D. 1976. Effect of physical fitness on the adrenocortical response to exercise stress. *Medicine and Science in Sports* 8: 113–118.

Wildmann, J., Kruger, A., Schmole, M., Niemann, J., and Matthaei, H. 1986. Increase of circulating beta-endorphin-like immunoreactivity correlates with the change in feeling of pleasantness after running. *Life Sciences* 38: 997–1003.

Health and Fitness Appraisal

This appendix includes questionnaires and forms that you can duplicate and use for the pretest health screening of your clients. The PAR-Q (Appendix A.1) is used to identify individuals who need medical clearance from their physicians before taking any physical fitness tests or starting an exercise program. The Medical History Questionnaire (Appendix A.2) is used to obtain a personal and family health history for your client. As part of the pretest health screening, ask your clients if they have any of the conditions or symptoms listed in the Checklist for Signs and Symptoms of Disease (Appendix A.3). The PARmed-X (Appendix A.4) may be used by physicians to assess and convey medi-

cal clearance for physical activity participation of your clients.

You can obtain a lifestyle profile for your clients by using either the Lifestyle Evaluation form or the FANTASTIC Lifestyle Checklist provided in Appendix A.5. Be sure that each participant signs the Informed Consent (Appendix A.6) before conducting any physical fitness tests or allowing your client to engage in an exercise program.

You can use the Sample ECG Tracings (Appendix A.7) to practice measuring heart rates. Appendix A.8 provides the answers to the questions posed in the sample case study presented in chapter 5 (see p. 104). Appendix A.9 includes web sites for selected professional organizations and institutes.

PAR - Q & YOU

(A Questionnaire for People Aged 15 to 69)

Regular physical activity is fun and healthy, and increasingly more people are starting to become more active every day. Being more active is very safe for most people. However, some people should check with their doctor before they start becoming much more physically active.

If you are planning to become much more physically active than you are now, start by answering the seven questions in the box below. If you are between the ages of 15 and 69, the PAR-Q will tell you if you should check with your doctor before you start. If you are over 69 years of age, and you are not used to being very active, check with your doctor.

Common sense is your best guide when you answer these questions. Please read the questions carefully and answer each one honestly: check YES or NO.

YES	NO		
☐	☐	1.	Has your doctor ever said that you have a heart condition <u>and</u> that you should only do physical activity recommended by a doctor?
☐	☐	2.	Do you feel pain in your chest when you do physical activity?
☐	☐	3.	In the past month, have you had chest pain when you were not doing physical activity?
☐	☐	4.	Do you lose your balance because of dizziness or do you ever lose consciousness?
☐	☐	5.	Do you have a bone or joint problem that could be made worse by a change in your physical activity?
☐	☐	6.	Is your doctor currently prescribing drugs (for example, water pills) for your blood pressure or heart condition?
☐	☐	7.	Do you know of <u>any other reason</u> why you should not do physical activity?

If
you
answered

YES to one or more questions

Talk with your doctor by phone or in person BEFORE you start becoming much more physically active or BEFORE you have a fitness appraisal. Tell your doctor about the PAR-Q and which questions you answered YES.

- You may be able to do any activity you want — as long as you start slowly and build up gradually. Or, you may need to restrict your activities to those which are safe for you. Talk with your doctor about the kinds of activities you wish to participate in and follow his/her advice.
- Find out which community programs are safe and helpful for you.

NO to all questions

If you answered NO honestly to <u>all</u> PAR-Q questions, you can be reasonably sure that you can:

- start becoming much more physically active — begin slowly and build up gradually. This is the safest and easiest way to go.
- take part in a fitness appraisal — this is an excellent way to determine your basic fitness so that you can plan the best way for you to live actively. It is also highly recommended that you have your blood pressure evaluated. If your reading is over 144/94, talk with your doctor before you start becoming much more physically active.

DELAY BECOMING MUCH MORE ACTIVE:

- if you are not feeling well because of a temporary illness such as a cold or a fever — wait until you feel better; or
- if you are or may be pregnant — talk to your doctor before you start becoming more active.

Please note: If your health changes so that you then answer YES to any of the above questions, tell your fitness or health professional. Ask whether you should change your physical activity plan.

<u>Informed Use of the PAR-Q</u>: The Canadian Society for Exercise Physiology, Health Canada, and their agents assume no liability for persons who undertake physical activity, and if in doubt after completing this questionnaire, consult your doctor prior to physical activity.

You are encouraged to copy the PAR-Q but only if you use the entire form

NOTE: If the PAR-Q is being given to a person before he or she participates in a physical activity program or a fitness appraisal, this section may be used for legal or administrative purposes.

I have read, understood and completed this questionnaire. Any questions I had were answered to my full satisfaction.

NAME _____

SIGNATURE _____ DATE _____

SIGNATURE OF PARENT _____ WITNESS _____
or GUARDIAN (for participants under the age of majority)

continued on other side...

© *Canadian Society for Exercise Physiology*
Société canadienne de physiologie de l'exercice

Supported by: Health   Santé
Canada   Canada

From Vivian H. Heyward, 2002, *Advanced Fitness Assessment and Exercise Prescription*, 4th ed. (Champaign, IL: Human Kinetics). Reprinted from the 1994 revised version of the Physical Activity Readiness Questionnaire (PAR-Q and You). Par-Q and You is a copyrighted pre-exercise screen owned by the Canadian Society for Exercise Physiology.

APPENDIX A.1

...continued from other side

PAR - Q & YOU

We know that being physically active provides benefits for all of us. Not being physically active is recognized by the Heart and Stroke Foundation of Canada as one of the four modifiable primary risk factors for coronary heart disease (along with high blood pressure, high blood cholesterol, and smoking). People are physically active for many reasons — play, work, competition, health, creativity, enjoying the outdoors, being with friends. There are also as many ways of being active as there are reasons. What we choose to do depends on our own abilities and desires. No matter what the reason or type of activity, physical activity can improve our well-being and quality of life. Well-being can also be enhanced by integrating physical activity with enjoyable healthy eating and positive self and body image. Together, all three equal VITALITY. So take a fresh approach to living. Check out the VITALITY tips below!

Active Living:

- accumulate 30 minutes or more of moderate physical activity most days of the week
- take the stairs instead of an elevator
- get off the bus early and walk home
- join friends in a sport activity
- take the dog for a walk with the family
- follow a fitness program

Healthy Eating:

- follow Canada's Food Guide to Healthy Eating
- enjoy a variety of foods
- emphasize cereals, breads, other grain products, vegetables and fruit
- choose lower-fat dairy products, leaner meats and foods prepared with little or no fat
- achieve and maintain a healthy body weight by enjoying regular physical activity and healthy eating
- limit salt, alcohol and caffeine
- don't give up foods you enjoy — aim for moderation and variety

Positive Self and Body Image:

- accept who you are and how you look
- remember, a healthy weight range is one that is realistic for your own body make-up (body fat levels should neither be too high nor too low)
- try a new challenge
- compliment yourself
- reflect positively on your abilities
- laugh a lot

Enjoy eating well, being active and feeling good about yourself. That's VITALITY®

FITNESS AND HEALTH PROFESSIONALS MAY BE INTERESTED IN THE INFORMATION BELOW.

The following companion forms are available for doctors' use by contacting the Canadian Society for Exercise Physiology (address below):

The **Physical Activity Readiness Medical Examination (PARmed-X)** - to be used by doctors with people who answer YES to one or more questions on the PAR-Q.

The **Physical Activity Readiness Medical Examination for Pregnancy (PARmed-X for PREGNANCY)** - to be used by doctors with pregnant patients who wish to become more active.

References:
Arraix, G.A., Wigle, D.T., Mao, Y. (1992). Risk Assessment of Physical Activity and Physical Fitness in the Canada Health Survey Follow-Up Study. **J. Clin. Epidemiol.** 45:4 419-428.
Mottola, M., Wolfe, L.A. (1994). Active Living and Pregnancy, In: A. Quinney, L. Gauvin, T. Wall (eds.), **Toward Active Living: Proceedings of the International Conference on Physical Activity, Fitness and Health**. Champaign, IL: Human Kinetics.
PAR-Q Validation Report, British Columbia Ministry of Health, 1978.
Thomas, S., Reading, J., Shephard, R.J. (1992). Revision of the Physical Activity Readiness Questionnaire (PAR-Q). **Can. J. Spt. Sci.** 17:4 338-345.

To order multiple printed copies of the PAR-Q, please contact the

Canadian Society for Exercise Physiology
185 Somerset St. West, Suite 202
Ottawa, Ontario CANADA K2P 0J2
Tel. (613) 234-3755 FAX: (613) 234-3565

The original PAR-Q was developed by the British Columbia Ministry of Health. It has been revised by an Expert Advisory Committee assembled by the Canadian Society for Exercise Physiology and Fitness Canada (1994).

Disponible en français sous le titre «Questionnaire sur l'aptitude à l'activité physique - Q-AAP (revisé 1994)».

Supported by: Health   Santé
Canada   Canada

From Vivian H. Heyward, 2002, *Advanced Fitness Assessment and Exercise Prescription*, 4th ed. (Champaign, IL: Human Kinetics). Reprinted from the 1994 revised version of the Physical Activity Readiness Questionnaire (PAR-Q and You). Par-Q and You is a copyrighted pre-exercise screen owned by the Canadian Society for Exercise Physiology.

Medical History Questionnaire

Demographic Information

Last name	First name	Middle initial

Date of birth	Sex	Home phone

Address	City, State	Zip code

Work phone	Family physician

Section A

1. When was the last time you had a physical examination?

2. If you are allergic to any medications, foods, or other substances, please name them.

3. If you have been told that you have any chronic or serious illnesses, please list them.

4. Give the following information pertaining to the last 3 times you have been hospitalized. *Note*: Women, do not list normal pregnancies.

	Hospitalization 1	Hospitalization 2	Hospitalization 3
Reason for hospitalization	_____	_____	_____
Month and year of hospitalization	_____	_____	_____
Hospital	_____	_____	_____
City and state	_____	_____	_____

Section B

During the past 12 months

1. Has a physician prescribed any form of medication for you?	Yes	No
2. Has your weight fluctuated more than a few pounds?	Yes	No
3. Did you attempt to bring about this weight change through diet or exercise?	Yes	No
4. Have you experienced any faintness, light-headedness, or blackouts?	Yes	No
5. Have you occasionally had trouble sleeping?	Yes	No
6. Have you experienced any blurred vision?	Yes	No
7. Have you had any severe headaches?	Yes	No
8. Have you experienced chronic morning cough?	Yes	No
9. Have you experienced any temporary change in your speech pattern, such as slurring or loss of speech?	Yes	No
10. Have you felt unusually nervous or anxious for no apparent reason?	Yes	No
11. Have you experienced unusual heartbeats such as skipped beats or palpitations?	Yes	No
12. Have you experienced periods in which your heart felt as though it were racing for no apparent reason?	Yes	No

From Vivian H. Heyward, 2002, *Advanced Fitness Assessment and Exercise Prescription,* 4th ed. (Champaign, IL: Human Kinetics).

APPENDIX A.2

At present

1. Do you experience shortness or loss of breath while walking with others your own age?   Yes   No

2. Do you experience sudden tingling, numbness, or loss of feeling in your arms, hands, legs, feet, or face?   Yes   No

3. Have you ever noticed that your hands or feet sometimes feel cooler than other parts of your body?   Yes   No

4. Do you experience swelling of your feet and ankles?   Yes   No

5. Do you get pains or cramps in your legs?   Yes   No

6. Do you experience any pain or discomfort in your chest?   Yes   No

7. Do you experience any pressure or heaviness in your chest?   Yes   No

8. Have you ever been told that your blood pressure was abnormal?   Yes   No

9. Have you ever been told that your serum cholesterol or triglyceride level was high?   Yes   No

10. Do you have diabetes?   Yes   No

    If yes, how is it controlled?

    ❐ Dietary means   ❐ Insulin injection

    ❐ Oral medication   ❐ Uncontrolled

11. How often would you characterize your stress level as being high?   Yes   No

    ❐ Occasionally   ❐ Frequently   ❐ Constantly

12. Have you ever been told that you have any of the following illnesses?   Yes   No

    ❐ Myocardial infarction   ❐ Arteriosclerosis   ❐ Heart disease

    ❐ Coronary thrombosis   ❐ Rheumatic heart   ❐ Heart attack

    ❐ Coronary occlusion   ❐ Heart failure   ❐ Heart murmer

    ❐ Heart block   ❐ Aneurysm   ❐ Angina

Section C

Has any member of your immediate family been treated for or suspected to have had any of these conditions? Please identify their relationship to you (father, mother, sister, brother, etc.).

A. Diabetes

B. Heart disease

C. Stroke

D. High blood pressure

From Vivian H. Heyward, 2002, *Advanced Fitness Assessment and Exercise Prescription,* 4th ed. (Champaign, IL: Human Kinetics).

Checklist for Signs and Symptoms of Disease

Instructions: Ask your clients if they have any of the following conditions. If so, refer them to their physicians to obtain a signed medical clearance prior to any exercise testing or participation. See "Glossary of Terms" (p. 349) for definitions of terms.

Client's name _____ Date _____

Condition	Yes	No	Comments
Cardiovascular			
Hypertension			
Hypercholesterolemia			
Heart murmurs			
Myocardial infarction			
Fainting/dizziness			
Claudication			
Chest pain			
Palpitations			
Ischemia			
Tachycardia			
Ankle edema			
Stroke			
Pulmonary			
Asthma			
Bronchitis			
Emphysema			
Nocturnal dyspnea			
Coughing up blood			
Exercise-induced asthma			
Breathlessness during or after mild exertion			
Metabolic			
Diabetes			
Obesity			
Glucose intolerance			
McArdle's syndrome			

From Vivian H. Heyward, 2002, *Advanced Fitness Assessment and Exercise Prescription,* 4th ed. (Champaign, IL: Human Kinetics).

Condition	Yes	No	Comments
Metabolic *(continued)*			
Hypoglycemia			
Thyroid disease			
Cirrhosis			
Musculoskeletal			
Osteoporosis			
Osteoarthritis			
Low back pain			
Prosthesis			
Muscular atrophy			
Swollen joints			
Orthopedic pain			
Artificial joints			

From Vivian H. Heyward, 2002, *Advanced Fitness Assessment and Exercise Prescription,* 4th ed. (Champaign, IL: Human Kinetics).

PARmed-X PHYSICAL ACTIVITY READINESS MEDICAL EXAMINATION

The PARmed-X is a physical activity-specific checklist to be used by a physician with patients who have had positive responses to the Physical Activity Readiness Questionnaire (PAR-Q). In addition, the Conveyance/Referral Form in the PARmed-X can be used to convey clearance for physical activity participation, or to make a referral to a medically-supervised exercise program.

Regular physical activity is fun and healthy, and increasingly more people are starting to become more active every day. Being more active is very safe for most people. The PAR-Q by itself provides adequate screening for the majority of people. However, some individuals may require a medical evaluation and specific advice (exercise prescription) due to one or more positive responses to the PAR-Q.

Following the participant's evaluation by a physician, a physical activity plan should be devised in consultation with a physical activity professional (CSEP-Professional Fitness and Lifestyle Consultant). To assist in this, the following instructions are provided:

PAGE 1: • Sections A, B, C, and D should be completed by the participant BEFORE the examination by the physician. The bottom section is to be completed by the examining physician.

PAGES 2 & 3: • A checklist of medical conditions requiring special consideration and management.

PAGE 4: • Physical Activity & Lifestyle Advice for people who do not require specific instructions or prescribed exercise.

• Physical Activity Readiness Conveyance/Referral Form - an optional tear-off tab for the physician to convey clearance for physical activity participation, or to make a referral to a medically-supervised exercise program.

This section to be completed by the participant

A PERSONAL INFORMATION:

NAME _____

ADDRESS _____

_____

TELEPHONE _____

BIRTHDATE _____ GENDER _____

MEDICAL No. _____

B PAR-Q: Please indicate the PAR-Q questions to which you answered YES

- ❏ Q 1 Heart condition
- ❏ Q 2 Chest pain during activity
- ❏ Q 3 Chest pain at rest
- ❏ Q 4 Loss of balance, dizziness
- ❏ Q 5 Bone or joint problem
- ❏ Q 6 Blood pressure or heart drugs
- ❏ Q 7 Other reason:

_____

C RISK FACTORS FOR CARDIOVASCULAR DISEASE:
Check all that apply

- ❏ Less than 30 minutes of moderate physical activity most days of the week.
- ❏ Currently smoker (tobacco smoking 1 or more times per week).
- ❏ High blood pressure reported by physician after repeated measurements.
- ❏ High cholesterol level reported by physician.
- ❏ Excessive accumulation of fat around waist.
- ❏ Family history of heart disease.

Please note: *Many of these risk factors are modifiable. Please refer to page 4 and discuss with your physician.*

D PHYSICAL ACTIVITY INTENTIONS:

What physical activity do you intend to do?

_____

_____

_____

This section to be completed by the examining physician

Physical Exam:

Ht	Wt	BP i)	/
		BP ii)	/

Conditions limiting physical activity:

- ❏ Cardiovascular
- ❏ Musculoskeletal
- ❏ Respiratory
- ❏ Abdominal
- ❏ Other

Tests required:

- ❏ Resting ECG
- ❏ Blood
- ❏ Exercise Stress Test
- ❏ Urinalysis
- ❏ X-Ray
- ❏ Other

Physical Activity Readiness Conveyance/Referral:

Based upon a current review of health status, I recommend:

- ❏ No physical activity
- ❏ Progressive physical activity
  - ❏ with avoidance of: _____
  - ❏ with inclusion of: _____
  - ❏ with Physical Therapy: _____
- ❏ Unrestricted physical activity — start slowly and build up gradually
- ❏ Only a medically-supervised exercise program until further medical clearance

Further Information:
- ❏ Attached
- ❏ To be forwarded
- ❏ Available on request

CSEP SCPE
© *Canadian Society for Exercise Physiology*
Société Canadienne de Physiologie de l'Exercice

Supported by: Health Santé
Canada Canada

From Vivian H. Heyward, 2002, *Advanced Fitness Assessment and Exercise Prescription*, 4th ed. (Champaign, IL: Human Kinetics). Source: Physical Activity Readiness Medical Examination (PARmed-X), ©1995. Reprinted with permission from the Canadian Society for Exercise Physiology.

PARmed-X
PHYSICAL ACTIVITY READINESS
MEDICAL EXAMINATION

Following is a checklist of medical conditions for which a degree of precaution and/or special advice should be considered for those who answered "YES" to one or more questions on the PAR-Q, and people over the age of 69. Conditions are grouped by system. Three categories of precautions are provided. Comments under Advice are general, since details and alternatives require clinical judgement in each individual instance.

	Absolute Contraindications	Relative Contraindications	Special Prescriptive Conditions	
	Permanent restriction or temporary restriction until condition is treated, stable, and/or past acute phase.	Highly variable. Value of exercise testing and/or program may exceed risk. Activity may be restricted. Desirable to maximize control of condition. Direct or indirect medical supervision of exercise program may be desirable.	Individualized prescriptive advice generally appropriate: • limitations imposed; and/or • special exercises prescribed. May require medical monitoring and/or initial supervision in exercise program.	**ADVICE**
Cardiovascular	❏ aortic aneurysm (dissecting) ❏ aortic stenosis (severe) ❏ congestive heart failure ❏ crescendo angina ❏ myocardial infarction (acute) ❏ myocarditis (active or recent) ❏ pulmonary or systemic embolism—acute ❏ thrombophlebitis ❏ ventricular tachycardia and other dangerous dysrhythmias (e.g., multi-focal ventricular activity)	❏ aortic stenosis (moderate) ❏ subaortic stenosis (severe) ❏ marked cardiac enlargement ❏ supraventricular dysrhythmias (uncontrolled or high rate) ❏ ventricular ectopic activity (repetitive or frequent) ❏ ventricular aneurysm ❏ hypertension—untreated or uncontrolled severe (systemic or pulmonary) ❏ hypertrophic cardiomyopathy ❏ compensated congestive heart failure	❏ aortic (or pulmonary) stenosis—mild angina pectoris and other manifestations of coronary insufficiency (e.g., post-acute infarct) ❏ cyanotic heart disease ❏ shunts (intermittent or fixed) ❏ conduction disturbances • complete AV block • left BBB • Wolff-Parkinson-White syndrome ❏ dysrhythmias—controlled ❏ fixed rate pacemakers	• clinical exercise test may be warranted in selected cases, for specific determination of functional capacity and limitations and precautions (if any). • slow progression of exercise to levels based on test performance and individual tolerance. • consider individual need for initial conditioning program under medical supervision (indirect or direct).
			❏ intermittent claudication	progressive exercise to tolerance
			❏ hypertension: systolic 160-180; diastolic 105+	progressive exercise; care with medications (serum electrolytes; post-exercise syncope; etc.)
Infections	❏ acute infectious disease (regardless of etiology)	❏ subacute/chronic/recurrent infectious diseases (e.g., malaria, others)	❏ chronic infections ❏ HIV	variable as to condition
Metabolic		❏ uncontrolled metabolic disorders (diabetes mellitus, thyrotoxicosis, myxedema)	❏ renal, hepatic & other metabolic insufficiency	variable as to status
			❏ obesity ❏ single kidney	dietary moderation, and initial light exercises with slow progression (walking, swimming, cycling)
Pregnancy		❏ complicated pregnancy (e.g., toxemia, hemorrhage, incompetent cervix, etc.)	❏ advanced pregnancy (late 3rd trimester)	refer to the "PARmed-X for PREGNANCY"

References:

Arraix, G.A., Wigle, D.T., Mao, Y. (1992). Risk Assessment of Physical Activity and Physical Fitness in the Canada Health Survey Follow-Up Study. **J. Clin. Epidemiol.** 45:4 419-428.

Mottola, M., Wolfe, L.A. (1994). Active Living and Pregnancy, In: A. Quinney, L. Gauvin, T. Wall (eds.), **Toward Active Living: Proceedings of the International Conference on Physical Activity, Fitness and Health.** Champaign, IL: Human Kinetics.

PAR-Q Validation Report, British Columbia Ministry of Health, 1978.

Thomas, S., Reading, J., Shephard, R.J. (1992). Revision of the Physical Activity Readiness Questionnaire (PAR-Q). **Can. J. Spt. Sci.** 17:4 338-345.

The PAR-Q and PARmed-X were developed by the British Columbia Ministry of Health. They have been revised by an Expert Advisory Committee assembled by the Canadian Society for Exercise Physiology and the Fitness Program, Health Canada (1995).

You are encouraged to copy the PARmed-X, but only if you use the entire form

Disponible en français sous le titre

«Évaluation médicale de l'aptitude à l'activité physique (X-AAP)».

Physical Activity Readiness
Medical Examination
(revised 1995)

	Special Prescriptive Conditions	**ADVICE**
Lung	❑ chronic pulmonary disorders	special relaxation and breathing exercises
	❑ obstructive lung disease	breath control during endurance exercises to tolerance; avoid polluted air
	❑ asthma	
	❑ exercise-induced bronchospasm	avoid hyperventilation during exercise; avoid extremely cold conditions; warm up adequately; utilize appropriate medication.
Musculoskeletal	❑ low back conditions (pathological, functional)	avoid or minimize exercise that precipitates or exasperates e.g., forced extreme flexion, extension, and violent twisting; correct posture, proper back exercises
	❑ arthritis---acute (infective, rheumatoid; gout)	treatment, plus judicious blend of rest, splinting and gentle movement
	❑ arthritis---subacute	progressive increase of active exercise therapy
	❑ arthritis---chronic (osteoarthritis and above conditions)	maintenance of mobility and strength; non-weightbearing exercises to minimize joint trauma (e.g., cycling, aquatic activity, etc.)
	❑ orthopaedic	highly variable and individualized
	❑ hernia	minimize straining and isometrics; stregthen abdominal muscles
	❑ osteoporosis or low bone density	avoid exercise with high risk for fracture such as push-ups, curl-ups, vertical jump and trunk forward flexion.
CNS	❑ convulsive disorder not completely controlled by medication	minimize or avoid exercise in hazardous environments and/or exercising alone (e.g., swimming, mountainclimbing, etc.)
	❑ recent concussion	thorough examination if history of two concussions; review for discontinuation of contact sport if three concussions, depending on duration of unconsciousness, retrograde amnesia, persistent headaches, and other objective evidence of cerebral damage
Blood	❑ anemia—severe (< 10 Gm/dl)	control preferred; exercise as tolerated
	❑ electrolyte disturbances	
Medications	❑ antianginal ❑ antiarrhythmic ❑ antihypertensive ❑ anticonvulsant ❑ beta-blockers ❑ digitalis preparations ❑ diuretics ❑ ganglionic blockers ❑ others	NOTE: consider underlying condition. Potential for: exertional syncope, electrolyte imbalance, bradycardia, dysrhythmias, impaired coordination and reaction time, heat intolerance. May alter resting and exercise ECG's and exercise test performance.
Other	❑ post-exercise syncope	moderate program
	❑ heat intolerance	prolong cool-down with light activities; avoid exercise in extreme heat
	❑ temporary minor illness	postpone until recovered
	❑ cancer	if potential metastases, test by cycle ergometry, consider non-weight bearing exercises; exercise at lower end of prescriptive range (40-65% of heart rate reserve), depending on condition and recent treatment (radiation, chemotherapy); monitor hemoglobin and lymphocyte counts; add dynamic lifting exercise to strengthen muscles, using machines rather than weights.

*Refer to special publications for elaboration as required

The following companion forms are available by contacting the Canadian Society for Exercise Physiology (address below):

The **Physical Activity Readiness Questionnaire (PAR-Q)** - a questionnaire for people aged 15-69 to complete before becoming much more physically active.

The **Physical Activity Readiness Medical Examination for Pregnancy (PARmed-X for PREGNANCY)** - to be used by physicians with pregnant patients who wish to become more physically active.

To order multiple printed copies of the PARmed-X and/or any of the companion forms (for a nominal charge), please contact the:

Canadian Society for Exercise Physiology
185 Somerset St. West., Suite 202
Ottawa, Ontario CANADA K2P OJ2
Tel. (613) 234-3755   FAX: (613) 234-3565

Note to physical activity professionals...

It is a prudent practice to retain the completed Physical Activity Readiness Conveyance/Referral Form in the participant's file.

© Canadian Society for Exercise Physiology
Société Canadienne de Physiologie de l'Exercice

Supported by: Health   Santé
Canada   Canada

From Vivian H. Heyward, 2002, *Advanced Fitness Assessment and Exercise Prescription*, 4th ed. (Champaign, IL: Human Kinetics). Source: Physical Activity Readiness Medical Examination (PARmed-X), ©1995. Reprinted with permission from the Canadian Society for Exercise Physiology.

       APPENDIX A.4

Physical Activity & Lifestyle Advice

We know that being physically active provides benefits for all of us. Physical inactivity is recognized by the Heart and Stroke Foundation of Canada as one of the four modifiable primary risk factors for coronary heart disease (along with high blood pressure, high blood cholesterol, and smoking). Physical activity has also been shown to reduce the incidence of hypertension, colon cancer, maturity onset diabetes mellitus, and osteoporosis. It can also reduce stress and anxiety, relieve depression, and improve self-esteem.

People are physically active for many reasons — play, work, competition, health, creativity, enjoying the outdoors, being with friends. There are also as many ways of being active as there are reasons. What we choose to do depends on our own abilities and desires. No matter what the reason or type of activity, physical activity can improve our well-being and quality of life. Well-being can also be enhanced by integrating physical activity with enjoyable healthy eating and positive self and body image. Together, all three equal VITALITY. So take a fresh approach to living. Check out the VITALITY tips below!

Active Living:

➤ make meaningful and satisfying physical activities a valued and integral part of daily living
➤ accumulate 30 minutes or more of moderate physical activity most days of the week
➤ choose from an endless range of opportunities to be active according to your own abilities and desires:
  ♦ take the stairs instead of an elevator
  ♦ get off the bus early and walk home
  ♦ join friends in a sport activity
  ♦ take the dog for a walk with the family
  ♦ follow a fitness program

Healthy Eating:

➤ follow Canada's Food Guide to Healthy Eating
➤ enjoy a variety of foods
➤ emphasize cereals, breads, other grain products, vegetables and fruit
➤ choose lower-fat dairy products, leaner meats and foods prepared with little or no fat
➤ achieve and maintain a healthy body weight by enjoying regular physical activity and healthy eating
➤ limit salt, alcohol and caffeine
➤ don't give up foods you enjoy — aim for moderation and variety

Positive Self and Body Image:

➤ accept who you are and how you look
➤ remember, a healthy weight range is one that is realistic for your own body make-up (body fat levels should neither be too high nor too low)
➤ try a new challenge
➤ compliment yourself
➤ reflect positively on your abilities
➤ laugh a lot

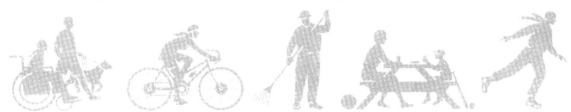

Enjoy eating well, being active and feeling good about yourself. That's VITALITY®

✂ · ·

Physical Activity Readiness Conveyance/Referral Form

Based upon a current review of the health status of _____, I recommend:

❏ No physical activity

❏ Only a medically-supervised exercise program until further medical clearance

❏ Progressive physical activity

  ❏ with avoidance of: _____

  ❏ with inclusion of: _____

  ❏ with Physical Therapy: _____

❏ Unrestricted physical activity — start slowly and build up gradually

Further Information:
❏ Attached
❏ To be forwarded
❏ Available on request

_____ M.D.

_____ 19 _____
(date)

Physician/clinic stamp:

From Vivian H. Heyward, 2002, *Advanced Fitness Assessment and Exercise Prescription*, 4th ed. (Champaign, IL: Human Kinetics). Source: Physical Activity Readiness Medical Examination (PARmed-X), © 1995. Reprinted with permission from the Canadian Society for Exercise Physiology.

Lifestyle Evaluation

Smoking habits

1. Have you ever smoked cigarettes, cigars, or a pipe?   Yes   No
2. Do you smoke presently?   Yes   No

        Cigarettes _____ a day

        Cigars _____ a day

        Pipefuls _____ a day

3. At what age did you start smoking? _____ years
4. If you have quit smoking, when did you quit? _____

Drinking habits

1. During the past month, how many days did you drink alcoholic beverages? _____
2. During the past month, how many times did you have 5 or more drinks per occasion? _____
3. On the average, how many glasses of beer, wine, or highballs do you consume a week?

        Beer _____ glasses or cans

        Wine _____ glasses

        Highballs _____ glasses

        Other _____ glasses

Exercise habits

1. Do you exercise vigorously on a regular basis?   Yes   No
2. What activities do you engage in on a regular basis?

3. If you walk, run, or jog, what is the average number of miles you cover each workout? _____ miles
4. How many minutes on the average is each of your exercise workouts? _____ minutes
5. How many workouts a week do you participate in on the average? _____ workouts
6. Is your occupation?

        _____ Inactive (e.g., desk job)

        _____ Light work (e.g., housework, light carpentry)

        _____ Heavy work (e.g., heavy carpentry, lifting)

7. Check those activities that you would prefer in a regular exercise program for yourself:

_____ Walking, running, or jogging	_____ Handball, racquetball, or squash
_____ Stationary running	_____ Basketball
_____ Jumping rope	_____ Swimming
_____ Bicycling	_____ Tennis
_____ Stationary cycling	_____ Aerobic dance
_____ Step aerobics	_____ Stair climbing
	_____ Other (specify)

From Vivian H. Heyward, 2002, *Advanced Fitness Assessment and Exercise Prescription,* 4th ed. (Champaign, IL: Human Kinetics).

Dietary habits

1. What is your current weight? ____ lb ____ kg height? ____ in. ____ cm
2. What would you like to weigh? ____ lb ____ kg
3. What is the most you ever weighed as an adult? ____ lb ____ kg
4. What is the least you ever weighed as an adult? ____ lb ____ kg
5. What weight loss methods have you tried? _____

_____

6. Which do you eat regularly?

    ❏ Breakfast   ❏ Midafternoon snack

    ❏ Midmorning snack   ❏ Dinner

    ❏ Lunch   ❏ After-dinner snack

7. How often do you eat out each week? _____ times
8. What size portions do you normally have?

    ❏ Small ❏ Moderate ❏ Large ❏ Extra large ❏ Uncertain

9. How often do you eat more than one serving?

    ❏ Always ❏ Usually ❏ Sometimes ❏ Never

10. How long does it usually take you to eat a meal? _____ minutes
11. Do you eat while doing other activities (e.g., watching TV, reading, working)? _____
12. When you snack, how many times a week do you eat the following?

    Cookies, cake, pie ____   Candy ____   Diet soda ____

    Soft drinks ____   Doughnuts ____   Fruit ____

    Milk or milk beverage ____   Potato chips, pretzels, etc. ____

    Peanuts or other nuts ____   Ice cream ____

    Cheese and crackers ____   Other _____

13. How often do you eat dessert? _____ times a day _____ times a week
14. What dessert do you eat most often? _____
15. How often do you eat fried foods? _____ times a week
16. Do you salt your food at the table? ❏ Yes ❏ No

    ❏ Before tasting it   ❏ After tasting it

From Vivian H. Heyward, 2002, *Advanced Fitness Assessment and Exercise Prescription,* 4th ed. (Champaign, IL: Human Kinetics).

Fantastic Lifestyle Checklist

INSTRUCTIONS: Unless otherwise specified, place an 'X' beside the box which best describes your behaviour or situation in the past month. Explanations of questions and scoring are provided on the next page.

FAMILY FRIENDS	I have someone to talk to about things that are important to me	almost never	seldom	some of the time	fairly often	almost always	
	I give and receive affection	almost never	seldom	some of the time	fairly often	almost always	
ACTIVITY	I am vigorously active for at least 30 minutes per day e.g., running, cycling, etc.	less than once/week	1-2 times/week	3 times/week	4 times/week	5 or more times/week	
	I am moderately active (gardening, climbing stairs, walking, housework)	less than once/week	1-2 times/week	3 times/week	4 times/week	5 or more times/week	
NUTRITION	I eat a balanced diet (see explanation)	almost never	seldom	some of the time	fairly often	almost always	
	I often eat excess 1) sugar, or 2) salt, or 3) animal fats, or 4) junk foods.	four of these	three of these	two of these	one of these	none of these	
	I am within____kg of my healthy weight	not within 8 kg	8 kg (20 lbs)	6 kg (15 lbs)	4 kg (10 lbs)	2 kg (5 lbs)	
TOBACCO TOXICS	I smoke tobacco	more than 10 times/week	1 - 10 times/week	none in the past 6 months	none in the past year	none in the past 5 years	
	I use drugs such as marijuana, cocaine	sometimes				never	
	I overuse prescribed or 'over the counter' drugs	almost daily	fairly often	only occasionally	almost never	never	
	I drink caffeine-containing coffee, tea, or cola	more than 10/day	7-10/day	3-6/day	1-2/day	never	
ALCOHOL	My average alcohol intake per week is____ (see explanation)	more than 20 drinks	13-20 drinks	11-12 drinks	8-10 drinks	0-7 drinks	
	I drink more than four drinks on an occasion	almost daily	fairly often	only occasionally	almost never	never	
	I drive after drinking	sometimes				never	
SLEEP SEATBELTS STRESS SAFE SEX	I sleep well and feel rested	almost never	seldom	some of the time	fairly often	almost always	
	I use seatbelts	never	seldom	some of the time	most of the time	always	
	I am able to cope with the stresses in my life	almost never	seldom	some of the time	fairly often	almost always	
	I relax and enjoy leisure time	almost never	seldom	some of the time	fairly often	almost always	
	I practice safe sex (see explanation)	almost never	seldom	some of the time	fairly often	always	
TYPE of behaviour	I seem to be in a hurry	almost always	fairly often	some of the time	seldom	almost never	
	I feel angry or hostile	almost always	fairly often	some of the time	seldom	almost never	
INSIGHT	I am a postive or optimistic thinker	almost never	seldom	some of the time	fairly often	almost always	
	I feel tense or uptight	almost always	fairly often	some of the time	seldom	almost never	
	I feel sad or depressed	almost always	fairly often	some of the time	seldom	almost never	
CAREER	I am satisfied with my job or role	almost never	seldom	some of the time	fairly often	almost always	

STEP 1   Total the X's in each column → [ ] [ ] [ ] [ ] [ ]

STEP 2   Multiply the totals by the numbers indicated (write your answer in the box below) →   0   x 1   x 2   x 3   x 4

STEP 3   Add your scores across the bottom for your grand total →   [ ] + [ ] + [ ] + [ ] = [ ]

Grand total
(see explantion)

From Vivian H. Heyward, 2002, *Advanced Fitness Assessment and Exercise Prescription*, 4th ed. (Champaign, IL: Human Kinetics). Adapted, by permission, from D. Wilson, 1998, *Fantastic lifestyle assessment*, as it appears in CSEP's *The Canadian physical activity, fitness, and lifestyle appraisal* 2nd ed.

A BALANCED DIET:

According to Canada's Food Guide to Healthy Eating (for people four years and over):

Different People Need Different Amounts of Food

The amount of food you need every day from the 4 food groups and other foods depends on your age, body size, activity level, whether you are male or female and if your are pregnant or breast feeding. That's why the Food Guide gives a lower and higher number of servings for each food group. For example, young children can choose the lower number of servings, while male teenagers can select the higher number. Most other people can choose servings somewhere in between.

Grain Products	Vegetables & Fruit	Milk Products	Meat & Alternatives	Other Foods
Choose whole grain and enriched products more often.	Choose dark green and orange vegetables more often.	Choose lower fat milk products more often.	Choose leaner meats, poultry and fish, as well as dried peas, beans and lentils more often.	Taste and enjoyment can also come from other foods and beverages that are not part of the 4 food groups. Some of these are higher in fat or calories, so use these foods in moderation.

recommended number of servings per day:

5-12	**5-10**	Children 4-9 years: 2-3 Youth 10-16 years: 3-4 Adults: 2-4 Pregnant and breast-feeding women: 3-4	**2-3**	

ALCOHOL INTAKE:

1 drink equals:

		Canadian	Metric	U.S.
1 bottle of beer	5% alcohol	12 oz.	340.8 ml	10 oz.
1 glass wine	12% alcohol	5 oz.	142 ml	4.5 oz
1 shot spirits	40% alcohol	1.5 oz	42.6 ml	1.25 oz.

SAFE SEX:

Refers to the use of methods of preventing infection or conception.

WHAT DOES THE SCORE MEAN?

85-100	70-84	55-69	35-54	0-34
EXCELLENT	VERY GOOD	GOOD	FAIR	NEEDS IMPROVEMENT

NOTE: A low total score does not mean that you have failed. There is always the chance to change your lifestyle — starting now. Look at the areas where you scored a 0 or 1 and decide which areas you want to work on first.

TIPS:

1   Don't try to change all the areas at once. This will be too overwhelming for you.

2   Writing down your proposed changes and your overall goal will help you to succeed.

3   Make changes in small steps towards the overall goal.

4   Enlist the help of a friend to make similar changes and/or to support you in your attempts.

5   Congratulate yourself for achieving each step. Give yourself appropriate rewards.

6   Ask your physical activity professional (CSEP-Professional Fitness and Lifestyle Consultant), family physician, nurse or health department for more information on any of these areas.

From Vivian H. Heyward, 2002, *Advanced Fitness Assessment and Exercise Prescription*, 4th ed. (Champaign, IL: Human Kinetics). Adapted, by permission, from D. Wilson, 1998, *Fantastic lifestyle assessment*, as it appears in CSEP's *The Canadian physical activity, fitness, and lifestyle appraisal* 2nd ed.

Informed Consent

In order to assess cardiovascular function, body composition, and other physical fitness components, the undersigned hereby voluntarily consents to engage in one or more of the following tests (check the appropriate boxes):

- ❐ Graded exercise stress test
- ❐ Body composition tests
- ❐ Muscle fitness tests
- ❐ Flexibility tests

Explanation of the tests

The graded exercise test is performed on a bicycle ergometer or motor-driven treadmill. The workload is increased every few minutes until exhaustion or until other symptoms dictate that we terminate the test. You may stop the test at any time because of fatigue or discomfort.

The underwater weighing procedure involves being completely submerged in a tank or tub after fully exhaling the air from your lungs. You will be submerged for 3 to 5 seconds while we measure your underwater weight. This test provides an accurate assessment of your body composition.

For muscle fitness testing, you lift weights for a number of repetitions using barbells or exercise machines. These tests assess the strength and endurance of the major muscle groups in the body.

For evaluation of flexibility, you perform a number of tests. During these tests, we measure the range of motion in your joints.

Risks and discomforts

During the graded exercise test, certain changes may occur. These changes include abnormal blood pressure responses, fainting, irregularities in heartbeat, and heart attack. Every effort is made to minimize these occurrences. Emergency equipment and trained personnel are available to deal with these situations if they occur.

You may experience some discomfort during the underwater weighing, especially after you expire all the air from your lungs. However, this discomfort is momentary, lasting only 3 to 5 seconds. If this test causes you too much discomfort, an alternative procedure (e.g., skinfold or bioelectrical impedance test) can be used to estimate your body composition.

There is a slight possibility of pulling a muscle or spraining a ligament during the muscle fitness and flexibility testing. In addition, you may experience muscle soreness 24 or 48 hours after testing. These risks can be minimized by performing warm-up exercises prior to taking the tests. If muscle soreness occurs, appropriate stretching exercises to relieve this soreness will be demonstrated.

Expected benefits from testing

These tests allow us to assess your physical working capacity and to appraise your physical fitness status. The results are used to prescribe a safe, sound exercise program for you. Records are kept strictly confidential unless you consent to release this information.

Inquiries

Questions about the procedures used in the physical fitness tests are encouraged. If you have any questions or need additional information, please ask us to explain further.

From Vivian H. Heyward, 2002, *Advanced Fitness Assessment and Exercise Prescription,* 4th ed. (Champaign, IL: Human Kinetics).

APPENDIX A.6

Freedom of Consent

Your permission to perform these physical fitness tests is strictly voluntary. You are free to stop the tests at any point, if you so desire.

I have read this form carefully and I fully understand the test procedures that I will perform and the risks and discomforts. Knowing these risks and having had the opportunity to ask questions that have been answered to my satisfaction, I consent to participate in these tests.

Date	Signature of patient

Date	Signature of witness

Date	Signature of supervisor

From Vivian H. Heyward, 2002, *Advanced Fitness Assessment and Exercise Prescription,* 4th ed. (Champaign, IL: Human Kinetics).

Sample ECG Tracings

Directions: Use these ECG tracings to practice techniques described in chapter 2 for measuring heart rate from ECG recordings.

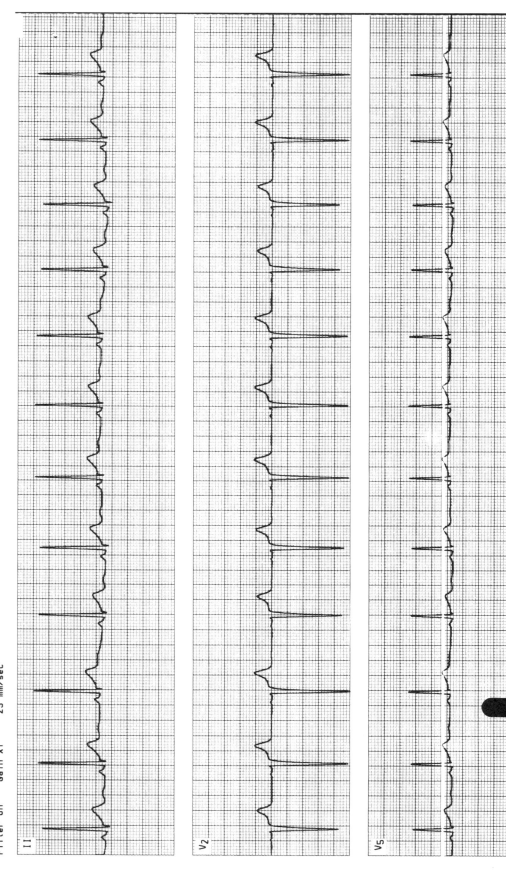

```
3 Lead                    Date  1/27/1995   9:48A
ST Lead   V5    Resting
               Level +0.7  Slope  +4   HR   65
Speed          MPH  Grade  0.0%
Filter on      Gain x1     25 mm/sec
```

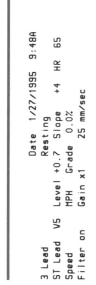

From Vivian H. Heyward, 2002, *Advanced Fitness Assessment and Exercise Prescription*, 4th ed. (Champaign, IL: Human Kinetics).

Date 11/06/1996 11:44A

12 Lead Sml
ST Lead V5   Level -0.1 Slope +4 HR 106
Speed   MPH   Grade 0.0%
                   Gain x1   25 mm/sec

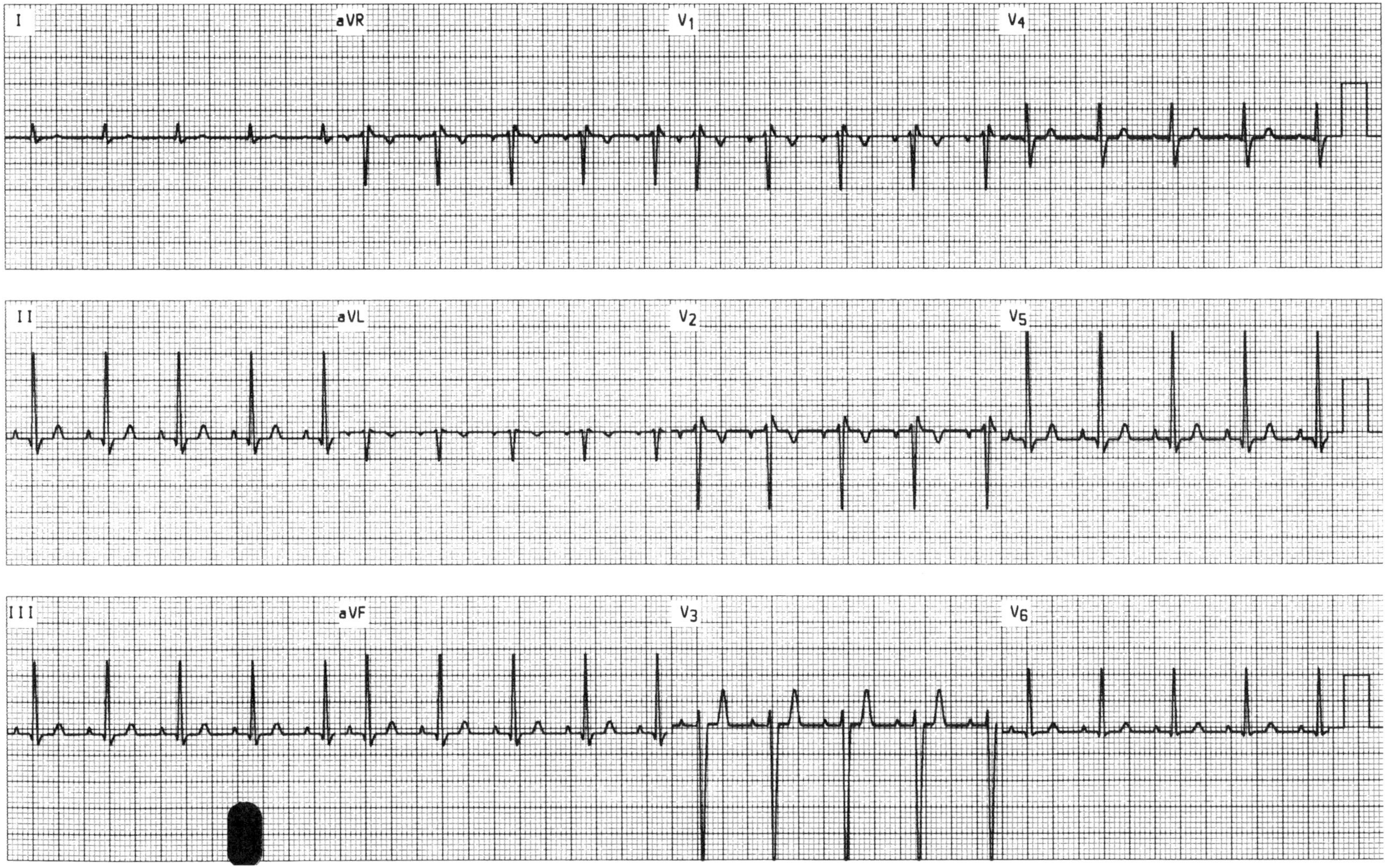

Resting

I   aVR   V1   V4

II   aVL   V2   V5

III   aVF   V3   V6

From Vivian H. Heyward, 2002, *Advanced Fitness Assessment and Exercise Prescription*, 4th ed. (Champaign, IL: Human Kinetics).

12 Lead Sml
ST Lead V5   Level +0.0   Slope   +8   HR 122
Speed   MPH   Grade 0.0%
              Gain x1   25 mm/sec

Date 11/06/1996 11:47A
Resting

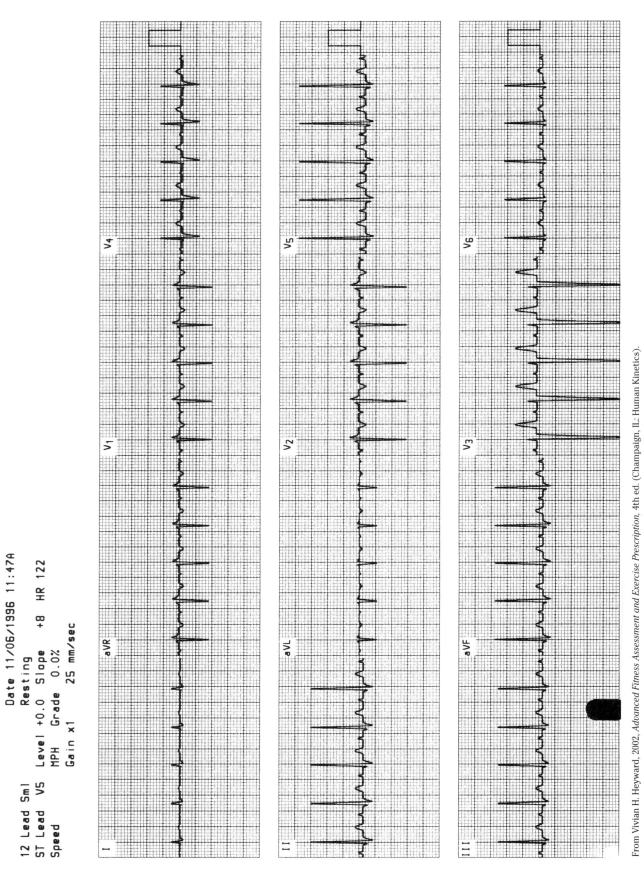

From Vivian H. Heyward, 2002, *Advanced Fitness Assessment and Exercise Prescription*, 4th ed. (Champaign, IL: Human Kinetics).

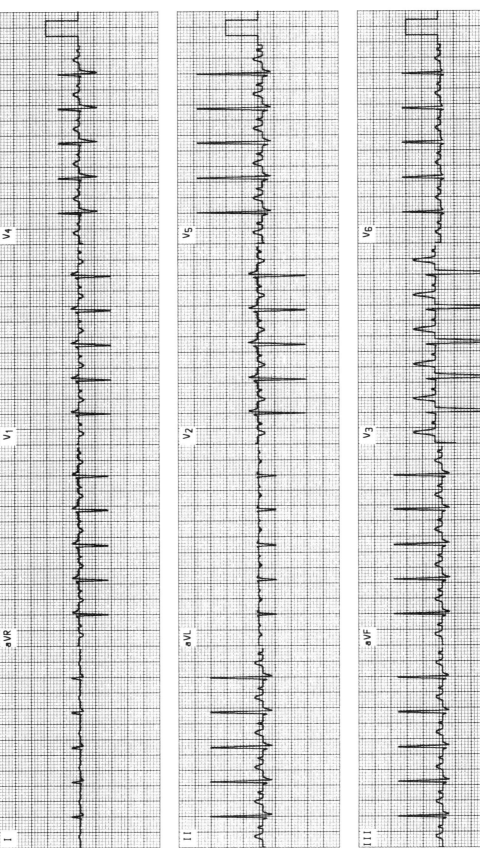

Date 11/06/1996 11:48A

Resting

12 Lead Sml
ST Lead   VS   Level -0.1 Slope   +2   HR 134
Speed   MPH   Grade   0.0%
                 Gain x1   25 mm/sec

I   aVR   V1   V4

II   aVL   V2   V5

III   aVF   V3   V6

From Vivian H. Heyward, 2002, *Advanced Fitness Assessment and Exercise Prescription*, 4th ed. (Champaign, IL: Human Kinetics).

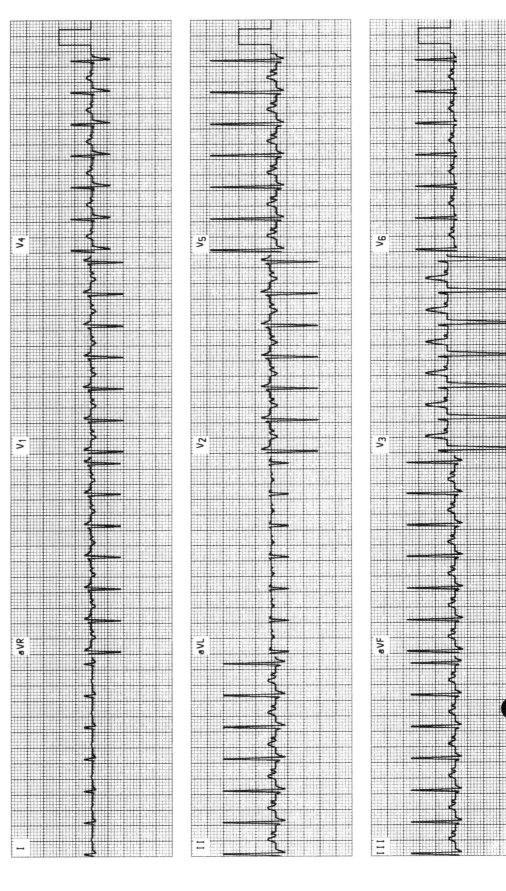

12 Lead Sml
ST Lead V5
Speed

Date 11/06/1996 11:49A
Resting
Level −0.1 Slope +2 HR 147
MPH Grade 0.0%
Gain x1 25 mm/sec

I

aVR

V1

V4

II

aVL

V2

V5

III

aVF

V3

V6

From Vivian H. Heyward, 2002, *Advanced Fitness Assessment and Exercise Prescription*, 4th ed. (Champaign, IL: Human Kinetics).

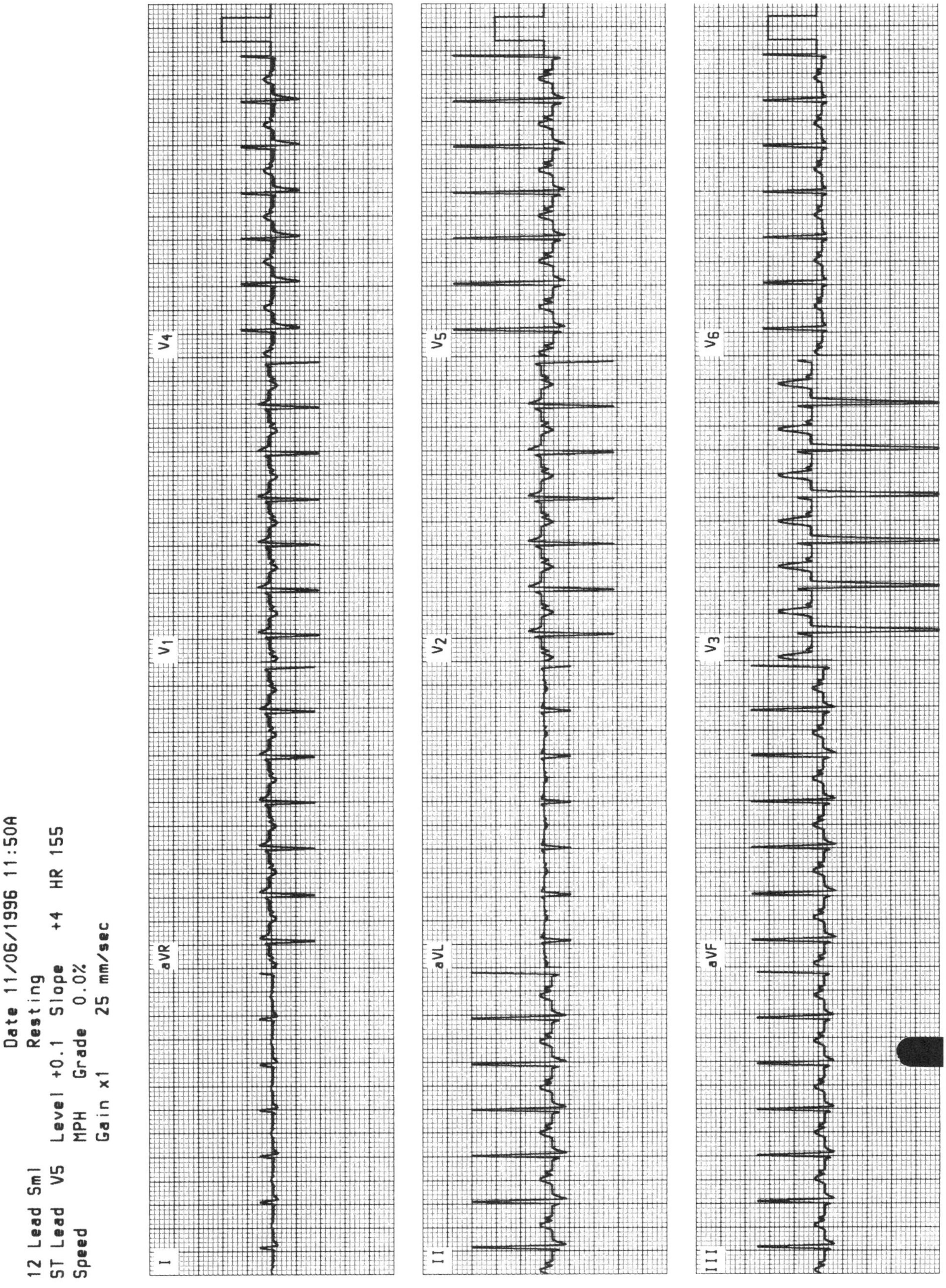

Date 11/06/1996 11:50A

12 Lead Sml
ST Lead V5   Level +0.1 Slope   +4   HR 155
              MPH   Grade 0.0%
Speed   Gain x1   25 mm/sec

Resting

I

II

III

aVR

aVL

aVF

V1

V2

V3

V4

V5

V6

From Vivian H. Heyward, 2002, *Advanced Fitness Assessment and Exercise Prescription*, 4th ed. (Champaign, IL: Human Kinetics).

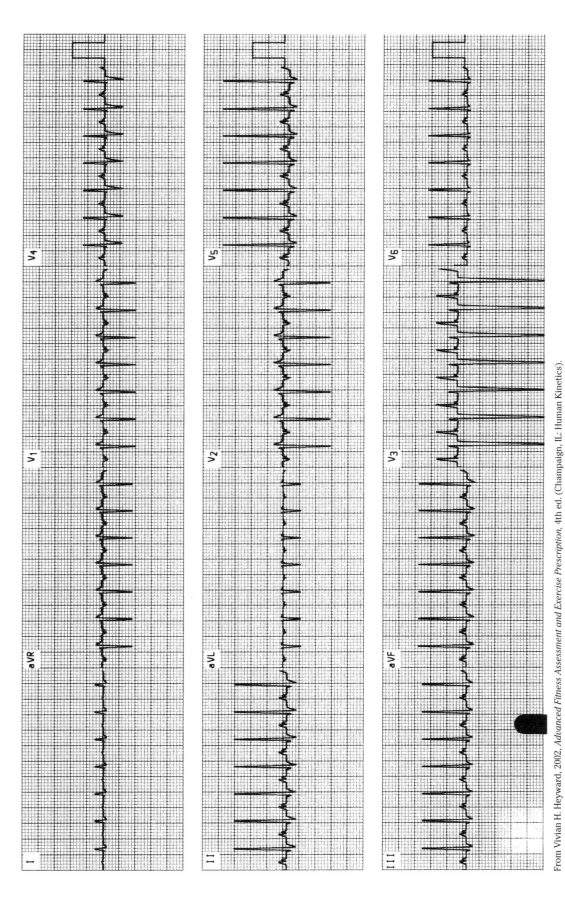

From Vivian H. Heyward, 2002, *Advanced Fitness Assessment and Exercise Prescription*, 4th ed. (Champaign, IL: Human Kinetics).

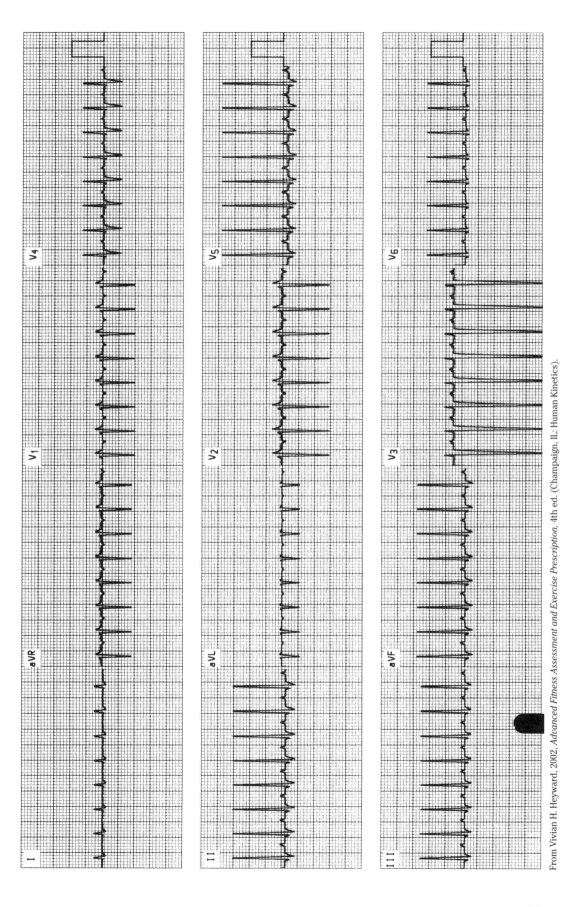

Date 11/06/1996 11:54A

12 Lead Sml   Resting
ST Lead V5   Level -0.1 Slope   +4   HR 190
Speed   MPH   Grade 0.0%
               Gain x1   25 mm/sec

I

aVR

V1

V4

II

aVL

V2

V5

III

aVF

V3

V6

From Vivian H. Heyward, 2002, *Advanced Fitness Assessment and Exercise Prescription*, 4th ed. (Champaign, IL: Human Kinetics).

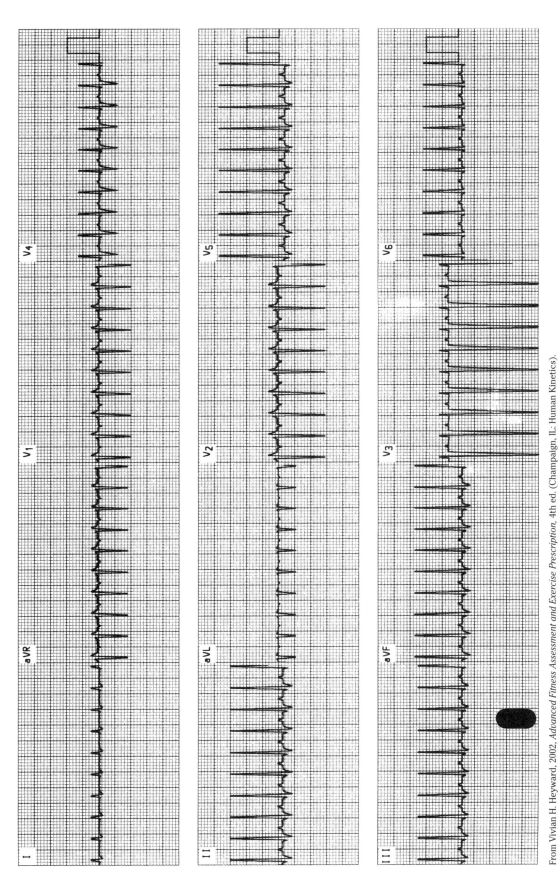

12 Lead Sml

Date 11/06/1996 11:57A

Resting

ST Lead V5   Level +0.0 Slope   +2 HR 217

Speed   MPH   Grade 0.0%

Gain x1   25 mm/sec

From Vivian H. Heyward, 2002, *Advanced Fitness Assessment and Exercise Prescription*, 4th ed. (Champaign, IL: Human Kinetics).

Analysis of Sample Case Study in Chapter 5

1. CHD Risk Profile

This client has risk factors for CHD. Her total cholesterol (TC; 220 mg · dl^{-1}) is borderline high (200 to 230 mg · dl^{-1}), and her blood pressure (140/82 mm Hg) is categorized as Stage I hypertension (140 to 159 mm Hg). Also, her HDL-C (37 mg · dl^{-1}) and TC/HDL ratio (5.9) place her at higher risk (<40 mg · dl^{-1} and >5.0, respectively). She quit smoking cigarettes (one pack a day) three years ago, which is a step in the right direction. Following the National Cholesterol Education Program's recommendation, you should encourage this client to have her LDL-C assessed to determine if she needs a cholesterol treatment program. Engaging in an aerobic exercise program should lower her systolic blood pressure. Her triglycerides and blood glucose levels are normal. She should be encouraged to dine out less frequently and to eat three well-balanced meals a day. When dining out, she should select foods that are low in saturated fat, cholesterol, and sodium. This may help to lower her blood cholesterol and blood pressure.

The client is also at greater risk because of

- the high stress associated with her job (police officer) and lifestyle (divorced parent raising two children),
- family history of cardiovascular disease, and
- physical inactivity (she does not exercise regularly outside of work-related physical activity).

2. Special Considerations

The client has not exercised aerobically for the past six years, and she has gained 15 lb during that time. It is likely that she will experience some discomfort when she starts her aerobic exercise program. Thus, it is important to initially prescribe low-intensity exercise to minimize her physical discomfort.

You also need to consider her busy schedule to find a convenient time for her to exercise. She reports feeling dizzy after eating. The likely reason is that she is eating only one meal a day, and the insulin surge after eating is lowering her blood glucose level. It is important to convince this client to start eating at least three meals a day to avoid this problem.

3. HR, BP, and RPE Responses to Graded Exercise Test

The client's HR response to the graded exercise test was normal. The exercise HR increased during each stage of the exercise test. The maximal heart rate (190 bpm) was very close to her age-predicted maximal HR (220 − 28 = 192 bpm). The client's BP response to the graded exercise test was normal. The diastolic BP remained fairly constant (78 to 82 mm Hg), and the systolic BP increased with each stage of the exercise test. The RPEs were normal. The ratings increased linearly with exercise intensity.

4. Functional Aerobic Capacity

The graded exercise test was voluntarily terminated by the client due to fatigue. This was most likely a maximal-effort exercise test as indicated by the RPE (18) and the exercise heart rate (190 bpm) during the last stage of the graded exercise test. The treadmill speed and grade during the last stage of the protocol was 2.5 mph and 12%, respectively. This corresponds to a functional aerobic capacity of 7.0 METs or 24.5 ml · kg^{-1}. According to the norms, this client's cardiorespiratory fitness level is *poor* for her age.

5. & 6. Training HRs

The graph of the client's HR and RPE responses to the graded exercise test is presented in figure A.8 (see p. 287).

From Vivian H. Heyward, 2002, *Advanced Fitness Assessment and Exercise Prescription,* 4th ed. (Champaign, IL: Human Kinetics).

Given the client's poor cardiorespiratory fitness level and her lack of regular aerobic exercise, the initial minimal training intensity will be 50% $\dot{V}O_2R$ (4.0 METs), gradually increasing to a maximum intensity of 75% $\dot{V}O_2R$ (5.5 METs). The corresponding training HRs, extrapolated from figure A.8, are 152 bpm (50% $\dot{V}O_2R$ or 4.0 METs) and 174 bpm (75% $\dot{V}O_2R$ or 5.5 METs). The HRs and RPEs corresponding to the relative exercise intensities in the following chart were extrapolated from the graph.

%$\dot{V}O_2R$	METs	HR (bpm)	RPE
50%	4.0	152	12
60%	4.6	165	14
70%	5.2	170	15
75%	5.5	174	16

7. Speed Calculations (ACSM Formula for Walking on Level Course)

To calculate walking speed corresponding to 60% of client's $\dot{V}O_2R$ [.60 × (7 − 1) + 1] = 4.6 METs):

a. Convert METs into ml · kg^{-1} · min^{-1}.

$$4.6 \text{ METs} \times 3.5 \text{ ml} \cdot \text{kg}^{-1} \cdot \text{min}^{-1} = 16.1 \text{ ml} \cdot \text{kg}^{-1} \cdot \text{min}^{-1}$$

b. Substitute into ACSM walking equation and solve for speed (m·min^{-1}).

$$\dot{V}O_2 = [\text{speed} \times 0.1] + [1.8 \times \text{speed} \times \text{grade}] + \text{resting } \dot{V}O_2$$

$$16.1 \text{ ml} \cdot \text{kg}^{-1} \cdot \text{min}^{-1} = [\text{speed} \times 0.1] + [1.8 \times \text{speed} \times 0\% \text{ grade}] + 3.5 \text{ ml} \cdot \text{kg}^{-1} \cdot \text{min}^{-1}$$

$$12.6 \text{ ml} \cdot \text{kg}^{-1} \cdot \text{min}^{-1} = \text{m} \cdot \text{min}^{-1} \times 0.1$$

$$126 \text{ m} \cdot \text{min}^{-1} = \text{speed}$$

c. Convert speed (m · min^{-1}) into miles per hour (26.8 m · min^{-1} = 1 mph).

$$126 \text{ m} \cdot \text{min}^{-1}/26.8 \text{ m} \cdot \text{min}^{-1} = 4.7 \text{ mph}$$

d. Convert miles per hour into minutes per mile walking pace.

$$60 \text{ min} \cdot \text{hr}^{-1}/4.7 \text{ mph} = 12.8 \text{ min} \cdot \text{mile}^{-1}, \text{ or } 12:48 \text{ (12 min, 48 sec per mile)}$$

Follow these same steps to calculate the walking speed corresponding to 70% $\dot{V}O_2R$ and 75% $\dot{V}O_2R$.

(Answers: 70% $\dot{V}O_2R$ = 5.5 mph; 75% $\dot{V}O_2R$ = 5.9 mph.)

8. Lifestyle Modifications

- Eat three well-balanced meals a day.
- Avoid fried foods high in saturated fats, cholesterol, and sodium.
- Dine out less frequently and select restaurants offering healthy food choices (e.g., salad bar, grilled skinless chicken, or fish).
- Exercise aerobically at least three days a week.
- Try using relaxation techniques (e.g., stretching, progressive relaxation, mental imagery) to relax in the evening instead of drinking wine.

From Vivian H. Heyward, 2002, *Advanced Fitness Assessment and Exercise Prescription,* 4th ed. (Champaign, IL: Human Kinetics).

APPENDIX A.8

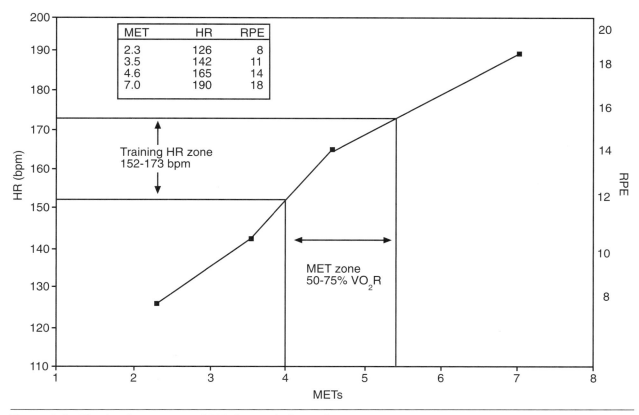

Figure A.8 Plotting heart rate vs METs for graded exercise test.

From Vivian H. Heyward, 2002, *Advanced Fitness Assessment and Exercise Prescription,* 4th ed. (Champaign, IL: Human Kinetics).

Web Sites for Selected Professional Organizations and Institutes[a]

Name	Web site address
Aerobics and Fitness Association of America (AFAA)	www.afaa.com
American Association for Health, Physical Education, Recreation and Dance (AAHPERD)	www.aapherd.org
American Association of Cardiovascular and Pulmonary Rehabilitation (AACPR)	www.aacvpr.org
American College of Sports Medicine (ACSM)	www.acsm.org
American Council on Exercise (ACE)	www.acefitness.org
American Fitness Professionals and Associates (AFPA)	www.afpafitness.org
American Society of Exercise Physiologists (ASEP)	www.css.edu/asep
Australian Association for Exercise and Sport Sciences (AAESS)	www.aaess.com.au
Canadian Academy of Sports Medicine (CASM)	www.casm-acms.org
Canadian Society for Exercise Physiology (CSEP)	www.csep.ca
Cooper Institute for Aerobics Research	www.cooperinst.org
Gatorade Sport Science Institute (GSSI)	www.gssiweb.com
IDEA Health and Fitness Association	www.ideafit.com
International Federation of Sports Medicine (FIMS)	www.fims.org
International Fitness Professionals Association (IFPA)	www.ifpa-fitness.com
International Society for Aging and Physical Activity (ISAPA)	www.isapa.org
National Athletic Trainers Association (NATA)	www.nata.org
National Strength and Conditioning Association (NSCA)	www.nsca-lift.org
North American Society for Pediatric Exercise Medicine (NASPEM)	www.naspem.org
Sports Medicine Australia	www.sma.org.au
Sports Medicine New Zealand	www.sportsmedicine.co.nz

[a]Organizations and institutes dealing with exercise physiology, sports medicine, and/or physical fitness.

From Vivian H. Heyward, 2002, *Advanced Fitness Assessment and Exercise Prescription,* 4th ed. (Champaign, IL: Human Kinetics).

APPENDIX A.9

Cardiorespiratory Assessments

Appendix B.1 includes a Summary of GXT and Cardiorespiratory Field Test Protocols that are presented in more detail in chapter 4. This appendix summarizes popular maximal and submaximal protocols for treadmill, bicycle ergometer, bench stepping, stairclimbing, rowing ergometer, and distance run/walk tests, as well as methods that you can use to obtain an estimate of your client's $\dot{V}O_2$max for each protocol.

Appendix B.2, the Rockport Fitness Charts, provides age-gender norms for the Rockport Walking Test. These charts may be used to classify your client's aerobic capacity.

Appendix B.3 presents a variety of step test protocols. Testing and scoring procedures are included for each protocol. For some protocols, prediction equations are available to estimate your client's $\dot{V}O_2$max.

Summary of Graded Exercise Test and Cardiorespiratory Field Test Protocols

Test mode/Protocol	Population	Type	Method to estimate $\dot{V}O_2$max	Description (page)
Treadmill				
Balke	Active/sedentary men and women	Max or submax	Prediction equation Multistage equation/graphing	58
Modified Balke	Children	Max or submax	ACSM equations (walk/run) Multistage equations/graphing	79
Bruce	Active/sedentary men and women	Max or submax	Prediction equation Multistage equation/graphing	58
	Elderly	Max or submax	Prediction equation Multistage equation/graphing	
	Cardiac patients	Max or submax	Prediction equation Multistage equation/graphing	
Modified Bruce	High-risk and elderly	Max or submax	ACSM walking equation Multistage equation/graphing	60
Ebbeling (single-stage walking)	Healthy adults (20-59 years)	Submax	Prediction equation	68
George (single-stage jogging)	Healthy adults (18-28 years)	Submax	Prediction equation	68
Latin and Elias (single-stage walking or jogging)	Healthy adults (19-40 years)	Submax	Prediction equation	68
Naughton	Male cardiac patients	Max or submax	Prediction equation Multistage equation/graphing	61
Bicycle ergometer				
Åstrand	Healthy adults	Max	ACSM leg ergometry equation	64
ACSM	Healthy adults	Submax	Multistage equation/graphing	69
Åstrand-Ryhming	Healthy adults	Submax	Nomogram	71
Fox	Healthy adults	Max or submax	ACSM leg ergometry equation Prediction equation	65
YMCA	Healthy adults	Submax	Multistage equation/graphing	69
McMaster	Children	Max or submax	ACSM leg ergometry equation Multistage equation/graphing	79
Bench stepping				
Åstrand-Ryhming	Healthy adults	Submax	Nomogram	73
Nagle	Healthy adults	Max	ACSM stepping equation	66
Queens College	Healthy adults (college age)	Submax	Prediction equation	73

From Vivian H. Heyward, 2002, *Advanced Fitness Assessment and Exercise Prescription,* 4th ed. (Champaign, IL: Human Kinetics).

Test mode/Protocol	Population	Type	Method to estimate $\dot{V}O_2max$	Description (page)
Stair climbing				
Howley	Healthy adults	Submax	Multistage equation/graphing	74
Rowing ergometer				
Hagerman	Noncompetitive and unskilled rowers	Submax	Nomogram	74
Lakomy	Noncompetitive and skilled rowers	Submax	Nomogram	75
Distance run/walk				
1.0-mile run/walk	Children (8-17 years)	Submax	Prediction equation	78
1.0-mile steady-state jog	Healthy adults (college age)	Submax	Prediction equation	77
1.5-mile run/walk	Healthy adults	Submax	Prediction equation	77
1.0-mile walk	Healthy adults	Submax	Prediction equation	77
12-min run	Healthy adults	Submax	Prediction equation	77
15-min run	Healthy adults	Submax	Prediction equation	73

From Vivian H. Heyward, 2002, *Advanced Fitness Assessment and Exercise Prescription,* 4th ed. (Champaign, IL: Human Kinetics).

Rockport Fitness Charts

Age-Gender Norms for the Rockport Walking Test

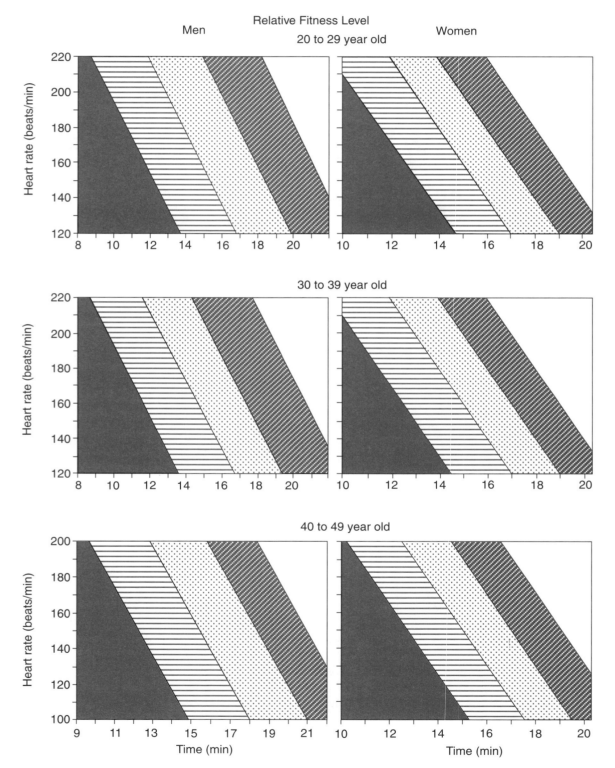

Relative Fitness Level

From Vivian H. Heyward, 2002, *Advanced Fitness Assessment and Exercise Prescription,* 4th ed. (Champaign, IL: Human Kinetics). Reprinted with the permission of The Rockport Company, Inc.

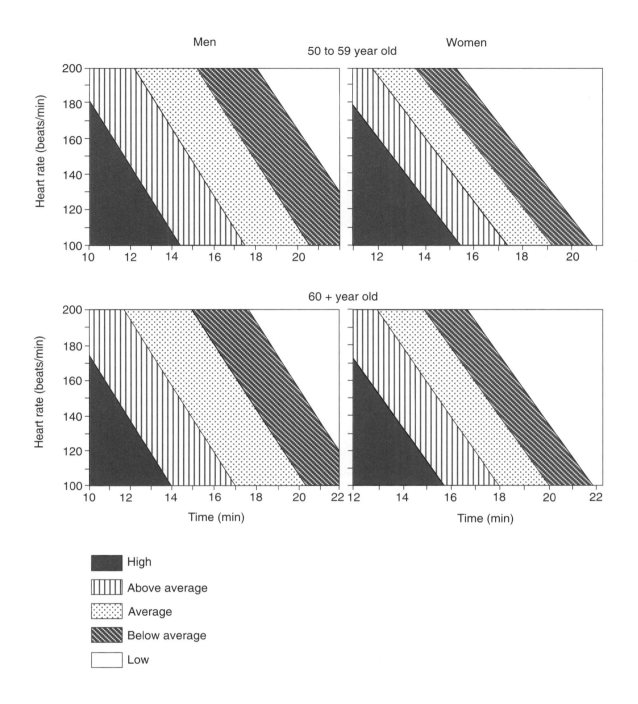

From Vivian H. Heyward, 2002, *Advanced Fitness Assessment and Exercise Prescription,* 4th ed. (Champaign, IL: Human Kinetics). Reprinted with the permission of The Rockport Company, Inc.

Step Test Protocols

Harvard Step Test (Brouha 1943)

Age and sex: Young men
Stepping rate: 30 steps · min^{-1}
Bench height: 20 in.
Duration of exercise: 5 min

Scoring procedures: Sit down immediately after exercise. The pulse rate is counted in 1/2-min counts, from 1 to 1 1/2, 2 to 2 1/2, and 3 to 3 1/2 min after exercise. The three 1/2-min pulse counts are summed and used in the following equation to determine physical efficiency index (PEI):

$$PEI = \frac{\text{duration of exercise (sec)} \times 100}{2 \times \text{sum of recovery HRs}}$$

You can evaluate the performance of college-age males using the following PEI classifications: <55 = poor, 55-64 = low average, 65-79 = average, 80-89 = good, and ≥90 = excellent.

Three-Minute Step Test (Hodgkins and Skubic 1963)

Age and sex: High school- and college-age women
Stepping rate: 24 steps · min^{-1}
Bench height: 18 in.
Duration of exercise: 3 min

Scoring procedures: Sit down immediately after exercise. The pulse rate is counted for 30 sec after 1 min of rest (1 to 1 1/2 min after exercise). Use the recovery pulse count in the following equation:

$$CV \text{ efficiency} = \frac{\text{duration of exercise (sec)} \times 100}{\text{recovery pulse} \times 5.6}$$

You can evaluate the performance of college-age women using the following classifications for cardiovascular (CV) efficiency: 0-27 = very poor, 28-38 = poor, 39-48 = fair, 49-59 = good, 60-70 = very good, and 71-100 = excellent.

OSU Step Test (Kurucz, Fox, and Mathews 1969)

Age and sex: Men 19-56 years
Stepping rate: 24 to 30 steps · min^{-1}
Bench height: Split-level bench 15 and 20 in. high with an adjustable hand bar
Duration of exercise: 18 innings, 50 sec each
  Phase I: 6 innings, 24 steps · min^{-1}, 15-in. bench
  Phase II: 6 innings, 30 steps · min^{-1}, 15-in. bench
  Phase III: 6 innings, 30 steps · min^{-1}, 20-in. bench
  (Each inning consists of 30 sec of stepping and 20 sec of rest.)

Scoring procedures: Exactly 5 sec into each rest period, take a 10-sec pulse count. Terminate the test when the heart rate reaches 150 bpm (25 counts × 6). The score is the inning during which the heart rate reaches 150 bpm.

Eastern Michigan University Step Test (Witten 1973)

Age and sex: College-age women
Stepping rate: 24 to 30 steps · min^{-1}
Bench height: Tri-level bench 14 to 20 in.

From Vivian H. Heyward, 2002, *Advanced Fitness Assessment and Exercise Prescription,* 4th ed. (Champaign, IL: Human Kinetics).

Duration of exercise: 20 innings, 50 sec each

  Phase I: 5 innings, 24 steps · min^{-1}, 14-in. bench

  Phase II: 5 innings, 30 steps · min^{-1}, 14-in. bench

  Phase III: 5 innings, 30 steps · min^{-1}, 17-in. bench

  Phase IV: 5 innings, 30 steps · min^{-1}, 20-in. bench

  (Each inning consists of 30 sec of stepping and 20 sec of rest.)

Scoring procedures: Exactly 5 sec into each rest period, take a 10-sec pulse count. Terminate the test when the heart rate reaches 168 bpm (28 counts $\times$ 6). The score is the inning during which the heart rate reaches 168 bpm.

Cotten Revision of OSU Step Test (Cotten 1971)

Age and sex: High school- and college-age men

Stepping rate: 24 to 36 steps · min^{-1}

Bench height: 17 in.

Duration of exercise: 18 innings, 50 sec each

  Phase I: 6 innings, 24 steps · min^{-1}, 17-in. bench

  Phase II: 6 innings, 30 steps · min^{-1}, 17-in. bench

  Phase III: 6 innings, 36 steps · min^{-1}, 17-in. bench

  (Each inning consists of 30 sec of stepping and 20 sec of rest.)

Scoring procedures: As with the OSU Step Test, the score is the inning during which the heart rate reaches 150 bpm (25 counts in 10 sec). $\dot{V}O_2$max in ml · kg^{-1} · min^{-1} can be estimated using the following equation:

$$\dot{V}O_2\text{max} = (1.69978 \times \text{step test score}) - (0.06252 \times \text{body weight in lb}) + 47.12525$$

Queens College Step Test (McArdle et al. 1972)

Age and sex: College-age women and men

Stepping rate: 22 steps · min^{-1} for women; 24 steps · min^{-1} for men

Bench height: 16 1/4 in.

Duration of exercise: 3 min

Scoring procedures: Remain standing after exercise. Beginning 5 sec after the cessation of exercise, take a 15-sec pulse count. Multiply the 15-sec count by 4 to express the score in beats per minute (bpm). $\dot{V}O_2$max in ml · kg^{-1} · min^{-1} can be estimated using the following equations:

  Women: $\dot{V}O_2$max = 65.81 − (0.1847 $\times$ HR)

  Men: $\dot{V}O_2$max = 111.33 − (0.42 $\times$ HR)

References

Brouha, L. 1943. The step test: A simple method of measuring physical fitness for muscular work in young men. *Research Quarterly* 14: 31–36.

Cotten, D.J. 1971. A modified step test for group cardiovascular testing. *Research Quarterly* 42: 91–95.

Hodgkins, J. and Skubic, V. 1963. Cardiovascular efficiency test scores for college women in the United States. *Research Quarterly* 34: 454–461.

Kurucz, R., Fox, E.L., and Mathews, D.K. 1969. Construction of a submaximal cardiovascular step test. *Research Quarterly* 40: 115–122.

McArdle, W.D., Katch, F.I., Pechar, G.S., Jacobson, L., and Ruck, S. 1972. Reliability and interrelationships between maximal oxygen intake, physical working capacity and step-test scores in college women. *Medicine and Science in Sports* 4: 182–186.

Witten, C. 1973. Construction of a submaximal cardiovascular step test for college females. *Research Quarterly* 44: 46–50.

From Vivian H. Heyward, 2002, *Advanced Fitness Assessment and Exercise Prescription,* 4th ed. (Champaign, IL: Human Kinetics).

Muscular Fitness Exercises and Norms

Appendix C.1 includes norms for isokinetic (Omnitron) muscular fitness tests. Average strength, endurance, and power values are presented for young adults, older adults, and weight-trained individuals.

Appendix C.2 describes and illustrates some sample basic static (isometric) exercises for a variety of muscle groups.

Appendix C.3 provides an extensive list of dynamic resistance training exercises. Exercises for the upper and lower extremities are organized by body region (e.g., chest, upper arm, thigh, etc.). For each exercise, equipment, body positions, joint actions, prime movers, and exercise variations are presented.

Average Strength, Endurance, and Power Values for Isokinetic (Omni-Tron) Tests

Strength[a]	Young adult[b]	Older adult[c]	Weight trained[d]
Females			
Chest press	88.1	76.7	131.8
Lateral row	82.6	77.4	111.4
Shoulder press	32.9	30.4	60.1
Lateral pull-down	70.8	66.3	101.2
Knee extension	67.7	59.3	82.7
Knee flexion	51.5	43.3	64.3
Males			
Chest press	173.8	154.9	218.6
Lateral row	153.5	143.2	178.6
Shoulder press	69.2	62.4	102.6
Lateral pull-down	134.8	115.3	176.0
Knee extension	110.9	95.5	127.2
Knee flexion	75.9	67.3	89.9

Note: Data courtesy of Hydra-Fitnesss, Belton, TX: 1988.
[a]Values of strength measured in foot-pounds at dial setting 10.
[b]Average age for females = 15.1 ± 2.6 years; for males = 15.8 ± 2.7 years.
[c]Average age for females = 38.2 ± 9.7 years; for males = 37.6 ± 9.6 years.
[d]Average age for females = 21.2 ± 2.0 years; for males = 20.6 ± 2.1 years.

Endurance[a]	Young adult[b]	Older adult[c]	Weight trained[d]
Females			
Chest press	64.3	53.4	125.7
Lateral row	102.4	85.7	143.7
Shoulder press	28.1	25.1	56.3
Lateral pull-down	109.1	91.5	216.3
Knee extension	88.7	86.6	111.6
Knee flexion	114.3	89.2	148.2
Males			
Chest press	211.8	167.3	321.1
Lateral row	266.9	221.2	312.5
Shoulder press	112.4	94.2	170.9
Lateral pull-down	352.2	296.3	501.5
Knee extension	72.9	80.8	98.9
Knee flexion	83.5	84.2	130.9

[a]Values of endurance measured in foot-pounds at dial setting 3.
[b]Average age for females = 15.1 ± 2.6 years; for males = 15.8 ± 2.7 years.
[c]Average age for females = 38.2 ± 9.7 years; for males = 37.6 ± 9.6 years.
[d]Average age for females = 21.2 ± 2.0 years; for males = 20.6 ± 2.1 years.

From Vivian H. Heyward, 2002, *Advanced Fitness Assessment and Exercise Prescription,* 4th ed. (Champaign, IL: Human Kinetics).

APPENDIX C.1

Power[a]	Young adult[b]	Older adult[c]	Weight trained[d]
Females			
Chest press	86.3	73.7	163.0
Lateral row	121.3	113.6	156.3
Shoulder press	39.5	32.9	81.9
Lateral pull-down	165.4	128.4	254.1
Knee extension	101.9	73.4	122.5
Knee flexion	103.5	74.6	142.1
Males			
Chest press	264.9	228.4	392.3
Lateral row	302.4	268.4	345.0
Shoulder press	130.7	122.0	224.5
Lateral pull-down	430.9	354.7	550.9
Knee extension	198.4	159.4	233.5
Knee flexion	182.0	155.5	259.5

[a]Values of power measured in foot-pounds at dial setting 6.
[b]Average age for females = 15.1 ± 2.6 years; for males = 15.8 ± 2.7 years.
[c]Average age for females = 38.2 ± 9.7 years; for males = 37.6 ± 9.6 years.
[d]Average age for females = 21.2 ± 2.0 years; for males = 20.6 ± 2.1 years.

From Vivian H. Heyward, 2002, *Advanced Fitness Assessment and Exercise Prescription,* 4th ed. (Champaign, IL: Human Kinetics).

Basic Static (Isometric) Exercises

Exercise 1: Chest Push

Muscle groups: Shoulder and elbow flexors

Equipment: None

Description:

1. Lock hands together.
2. Keep forearms parallel to ground and hands close to chest.
3. Push hands together.

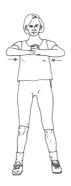

Exercise 2: Shoulder Pull

Muscle groups: Shoulder and elbow flexors

Equipment: None

Description:

1. Using same position as in chest push, attempt to pull hands apart

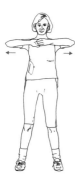

Exercise 3: Triceps Extension

Muscle groups: Elbow extensors

Equipment: Towel or rope

Description:

1. Placing left hand over shoulder and right hand at small of back, grasp rope or towel behind back.
2. Attempt to pull towel upward with left hand.
3. Change position of hands.

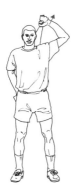

Exercise 4: Arm Curls

Muscle groups: Elbow flexors

Equipment: Towel or rope

Description:

1. Stand with knees flexed about 45°.
2. Place rope or towel behind thighs and grasp each end with hands shoulder-width apart.
3. Attempt to flex elbows.

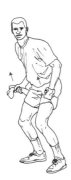

From Vivian H. Heyward, 2002, *Advanced Fitness Assessment and Exercise Prescription,* 4th ed. (Champaign, IL: Human Kinetics).

Exercise 5: Ball Squeeze

Muscle groups: Wrist and finger flexors

Equipment: Tennis ball

Description:

1. Hold tennis ball firmly in hand and squeeze maximally.

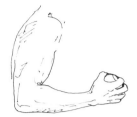

Exercise 6: Leg and Thigh Extensions

Muscle groups: Hip and knee extensors

Equipment: Rope

Description:

1. Stand on rope with knees flexed.
2. Grasp rope firmly with hands at sides, elbows fully extended.
3. Keeping trunk erect, attempt to extend legs by lifting upward.

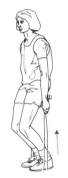

Exercise 7: Leg Press

Muscle groups: Hip and knee extensors

Equipment: Doorway

Description:

1. Sit in doorway facing side of door frame.
2. Grasp door frame behind head.
3. Attempt to extend legs by pushing feet against door frame.

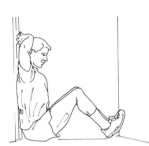

Exercise 8: Leg Curl

Muscle groups: Knee flexors

Equipment: Dresser

Description:

1. Pull out lower dresser drawer slightly.
2. Lying prone, with knees flexed, hook heels under bottom of drawer.
3. Attempt to pull heels toward head.

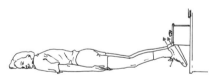

Exercise 9: Knee Squeeze or Pull

Muscle groups: Hip adductors or abductors

Equipment: Chair

Description:

1. Sitting on chair with forearms crossed and hands on inside of knees, attempt to squeeze knees together (adductors).
2. Same position but place hands on outside of knees; attempt to pull knees apart (abductors).

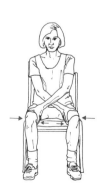

From Vivian H. Heyward, 2002, *Advanced Fitness Assessment and Exercise Prescription,* 4th ed. (Champaign, IL: Human Kinetics).

Exercise 10: Pelvic Tilt

Muscle groups: Abdominals

Equipment: None

Description:

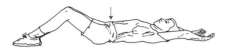

1. Supine with knees flexed and arms overhead.
2. Tighten abdominal muscles while pressing lower back into floor.

Exercise 11: Gluteal Squeeze

Muscle groups: Hip extensors and abductors

Equipment: None

Description:

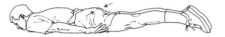

1. Lie prone with legs together and fully extended.
2. Tighten and squeeze the buttocks together.

From Vivian H. Heyward, 2002, *Advanced Fitness Assessment and Exercise Prescription,* 4th ed. (Champaign, IL: Human Kinetics).

APPENDIX C.2

Dynamic Resistance Training Exercises

Exercise	Type[a]	Variations	Equipment[b]	Body position	Joint actions	Prime movers
Upper extremity						
Chest						
Bench press	M-J	Flat	B, D, M	Supine lying on flat bench	Shoulder horizontal adduction, elbow extension	Pectoralis major (midsternal), triceps brachii
		Incline	B, D, M	Sitting on incline bench	Shoulder flexion, elbow extension	Pectoralis major (clavicular), triceps brachii
		Decline	B, D	Supine lying on decline bench	Shoulder flexion, elbow extension	Pectoralis major (lower sternal), triceps brachii
Push-up	M-J	Hands wider than shoulders	None	Prone; BW supported by hands and feet	Shoulder horizontal adduction, elbow extension	Pectoralis major (midsternal), triceps brachii
		Hands narrower than shoulders	None	Same as above	Shoulder flexion, elbow extension	Pectoralis major (clavicular), ant deltoid, triceps brachii
Bar dip	M-J	Neutral grip	Parallel bars	Vertically supported by bars	Shoulder flexion, elbow extension	Pectoralis major (clavicular), ant deltoid, triceps brachii
		Pronated grip		Same as above	Shoulder adduction, elbow extension	Pectoralis major (midsternal), triceps brachii
Fly	S	Flat	D	Supine lying on flat bench	Shoulder adduction	Pectoralis major (midsternal)
Pullover (bent arm)	S	Flat	B, D	Supine lying on flat bench	Shoulder extension	Pectoralis major (lower sternal), post deltoid, latissimus dorsi

(continued)

From Vivian H. Heyward, 2002, *Advanced Fitness Assessment and Exercise Prescription*, 4th ed. (Champaign, IL: Human Kinetics).

Dynamic Resistance Training Exercises *(continued)*

Exercise	Type[a]	Variations	Equipment[b]	Body position	Joint actions	Prime movers
Upper extremity *(cont.)*						
Shoulders						
Overhead press	M-J	Military	B, D, M	Sitting or standing	Shoulder flexion, elbow extension	Pectoralis major (clavicular), ant deltoid, triceps brachii
		Behind the head	B	Sitting	Shoulder abduction, elbow extension	Ant/mid deltoid, supraspinatus
Upright row	M-J		B, D	Standing	Shoulder abduction, scapula upward rotation, elbow flexion	Mid deltoid, supraspinatus, trapezius (upper), brachialis
Front arm raise	S		B, C, D	Standing	Shoulder flexion	Pectoralis major (clavicular), ant deltoid
Lateral arm raise	S		C, D, M	Sitting or standing	Shoulder abduction	Mid deltoid, supraspinatus, pectoralis major (clavicular)
Reverse fly	S		C, D	Standing	Shoulder horizontal extension	Post deltoid, infraspinatus, teres minor
Upper arm						
Arm curl	S	Supinated grip	B, D, M	Standing or sitting on incline bench or preacher bench	Elbow flexion	Biceps brachii, brachialis
	S	Neutral grip	Same as above		Elbow flexion	Brachioradialis, brachialis, biceps brachii
	S	Pronated grip	Same as above		Elbow flexion	Brachialis
Triceps press-down	M-J		M	Seated	Shoulder flexion, elbow extension	Ant deltoid, pectoralis major (clavicular), triceps brachii

From Vivian H. Heyward, 2002, *Advanced Fitness Assessment and Exercise Prescription*, 4th ed. (Champaign, IL: Human Kinetics).

Exercise	Type[a]	Variations	Equipment[b]	Body position	Joint actions	Prime movers
Upper extremity (cont.)						
Upper arm (cont.)						
Triceps extension	S		B	Supine lying on flat bench	Elbow extension	Triceps brachii
Triceps push-down	S	V-bar or strength bar	C	Standing	Elbow extension	Triceps brachii
French press	S		D	Standing or sitting	Elbow extension	Triceps brachii (medial head)
Overhead press	S		C, R	Standing with trunk flexed 45°	Elbow extension	Triceps brachii
Triceps kickback	S		D	Standing with one knee/hand on flat bench and trunk horizontal to floor	Elbow extension	Triceps brachii (long head)
Forearm						
Radioulnar rotation	S		D	Forearm/elbow supported on bench; hand free	Supination and pronation	Supinator, pronator teres, biceps brachii, brachioradialis
Wrist curl	S		D	Same as above	Wrist flexion	FCU, FCR
Reverse wrist curl	S		D	Same as above	Wrist extension	ECU, ECR (longus, brevis)
Radioulnar flexion	S		D	Standing with arm at side	Radial flexion, ulna flexion	FCR, ECR, FCU, ECU
Upper-mid back						
Lat pull-down	M-J	Pronated, wide grip	M	Sitting	Shoulder adduction, scapula adduction	Latissimus dorsi (upper), teres major, pectoralis major (upper), trapezius, rhomboids
	M-J	Narrow, neutral grip	M	Sitting	Shoulder extension, elbow flexion	Latissimus dorsi (lower), pectoralis major (lower sternal), biceps brachii

(continued)

From Vivian H. Heyward, 2002, *Advanced Fitness Assessment and Exercise Prescription*, 4th ed. (Champaign, IL: Human Kinetics).

Dynamic Resistance Training Exercises (*continued*)

Exercise	Type[a]	Variations	Equipment[b]	Body position	Joint actions	Prime movers
Upper mid-back (cont.)						
Seated row	M-J	Neutral grip	M	Sitting	Shoulder extension, elbow flexion	Latissimus dorsi (lower), biceps brachii
	M-J	Pronated grip	M	Sitting with elbows horizontal to floor	Shoulder horizontal extension, elbow flexion	Post deltoid, latissimus dorsi (upper), infraspinatus, brachialis
Bent-over row	M-J	Neutral grip	D	Standing with trunk flexed 90°	Shoulder extension, elbow flexion	Latissimus dorsi, biceps brachii
	M-J	Pronated grip	D	Standing with trunk flexed 90° and elbows out	Shoulder horizontal extension, elbow flexion	Post deltoid, infraspinatus, latissimus dorsi, brachialis
Pull-up	M-J	Pronated grip	Pull-up bar	Vertically hanging from bar	Shoulder adduction, elbow flexion	Latissimus dorsi (upper), pectoralis major (sternal), brachialis
Chin-up	M-J	Supinated or neutral grip	Pull-up bar	Vertically hanging from bar	Shoulder extension, elbow flexion	Latissimus dorsi (lower), pectoralis major (sternal), biceps brachii
Shoulder shrug	S	Regular	B, D, M	Standing	Shoulder girdle (scapula and clavicle) elevation	Trapezius (upper), levator scapulae, rhomboids
	S	Elevation with shoulder roll		Standing	Shoulder girdle elevation, scapula adduction	Trapezius (mid), rhomboids
Lower back						
Trunk extension	M-J		M	Sitting with pelvis/thighs stabilized	Spinal extension	Erector spinae
Back raise	M-J		Glut-ham developer	Prone with pelvis supported; trunk flexed	Spinal extension	Erector spinae
Side bends	M-J		D	Standing	Spinal lateral flexion	Quadratus lumborum

From Vivian H. Heyward, 2002, *Advanced Fitness Assessment and Exercise Prescription*, 4th ed. (Champaign, IL: Human Kinetics).

Exercise	Type[a]	Variations	Equipment[b]	Body position	Joint actions	Prime movers
Lower back (cont.)						
Isometric side support (side bridge)	M-J		None	Side-lying with BW supported by forearm and feet	None	Quadratus lumborum, abdominal obliques
Single-leg extension	M-J		None	Hands and knees	Spinal extension, hip extension	Erector spinae, gluteus maximus, hamstrings (upper)
Abdomen						
Curl-up	M-J	Bent knee	None	Supine lying with knees bent	Spinal flexion	Rectus abdominis
	M-J	With twist	None	Same as above	Spinal flexion	Abdominal obliques
Abdominal crunch	M-J		M	Sitting	Spinal flexion	Rectus abdominis
Reverse sit-up	M-J		None	Supine lying on floor on bench	Spinal flexion	Rectus abdominis (lower)
Lower extremity						
Hip						
Half squat	M-J		B, M	Standing	Hip extension, knee extension	Gluteus maximus, hamstrings (upper), quadriceps femoris
Leg press	M-J		M	Sitting	Hip extension, knee extension	Gluteus maximus, hamstrings (upper), quadriceps femoris
Lunge	M-J		B, D	Standing	Hip extension, knee extension	Gluteus maximus hamstrings (upper), quadriceps femoris
Glut-ham raise	M-J		Glut-ham developer	Prone with thighs supported and trunk flexed	Hip extension and knee flexion	Gluteus maximus, hamstrings

(continued)

Dynamic Resistance Training Exercises (continued)

Exercise	Type[a]	Variations	Equipment[b]	Body position	Joint actions	Prime movers
Lower extremity (cont.)						
Hip (cont.)						
Hip flexion	S		C, M	Standing	Hip flexion	Iliopsoas, rectus femoris (upper)
Hip extension	S		C, M	Standing	Hip extension	Gluteus maximus, hamstrings (upper)
Hip adduction	S		M	Sitting or supine lying	Hip adduction	Adductor longus, brevis, and magnus; gracilis
Hip abduction	S		M	Sitting or supine lying	Hip abduction	Gluteus medius
Side leg raise	S		None	Lying on side	Hip abduction	Gluteus medius, hamstrings (upper)
Good morning exercise	S		B, D	Standing	Hip extension	Gluteus maximus, hamstrings (upper)
Thigh						
Leg extension	S		M	Seated	Knee extension	Quadriceps femoris
Leg curl	S	Straight	M	Prone lying, seated, , or standing	Knee flexion	Hamstrings (lower)
	S	Knee externally rotated	M	Same as above	Knee flexion	Biceps femoris
	S	Knees internally rotated	M	Same as above	Knee flexion	Semitendinosus, semimembranosus
Lower leg						
Heal raise	S	Standing	D, M	Standing	Ankle plantar flexion	Gastrocnemius
	S	Seated	M	Sitting	Ankle plantar flexion	Soleus
Toe raise	S		Strength bar	Sitting	Ankle dorsiflexion	Tibialis anterior, peroneus tertius, extensor digitorum longus

Note: FCU = flexor carpi ulnaris; ECU = extensor carpi ulnaris; FCR = flexor carpi radialis; ECR = extensor carpi radialis.
[a]Type of exercise: M-J = multijoint exercise; S = single-joint exercise; [b]Equipment codes: B = barbell; C = cables; D = dumbbells; M = exercise machine; R = rope.

From Vivian H. Heyward, 2002, *Advanced Fitness Assessment and Exercise Prescription*, 4th ed. (Champaign, IL: Human Kinetics).

Body Composition Assessments

Appendix D.1 provides density constants for water temperatures. Use this table to determine water density when you are hydrostatically weighing your clients.

Appendix D.2 presents prediction equations for estimating residual lung volume. Use these equations only when it is not possible to directly measure your client's residual lung volume.

Appendix D.3 describes and illustrates the stan-

dardized sites for skinfold measurements, and Appendix D.4 describes the skinfold sites and measurement procedures for Jackson's generalized skinfold prediction equations for men and women.

Standardized sites for circumference (Appendix D.5) and bony breadth (Appendix D.6) measurements are also provided. Follow these procedures to identify and measure various sites.

Density of Water at Different Temperatures

Temperature (°C)	Density (g·cc⁻¹)
21	0.9980
22	0.9978
23	0.9975
24	0.9973
25	0.9971
26	0.9968
27	0.9965
28	0.9963
29	0.9960
30	0.9957
31	0.9954
32	0.9951
33	0.9947
34	0.9944
35	0.9941
36	0.9937
37	0.9934
38	0.9930
39	0.9926
40	0.9922

Reprinted, with permission, from R.C. Weast (ed.), *CRC Handbook of Chemistry and Physics*, 69th ed. Copyright CRC Press, Boca Raton, Florida: © 1989, F-10.

From Vivian H. Heyward, 2002, *Advanced Fitness Assessment and Exercise Prescription,* 4th ed. (Champaign, IL: Human Kinetics).

APPENDIX D.1

Prediction Equations for Residual Volume (RV)

Population	Smoking history[a]	N	Equation[b]
Men			
Boren, Kory, and Syner (1966)	Mixed	422	$RV = 0.0115(age) + 0.019(ht) - 2.24$ $r = 0.57$, *SEE* = 0.53 L
Women			
O'Brien and Drizd (1983)	Nonsmokers	926	$RV = 0.03(age) + 0.0387(ht) - 0.73(BSA) - 4.78$ $r = 0.66$, *SEE* = 0.49 L
Black, Offord, and Hyatt (1974)	Mixed	110	$RV = 0.021(age) + 0.023(ht) - 2.978$ $r = 0.70$, *SEE* = 0.46 L

[a]Mixed indicates that sample included both smokers and nonsmokers.

[b]For each equation, age (in years); ht = height (in cm); BSA = body surface area (in m^2).

References

Black, L.F., Offord, K., and Hyatt, R.E. 1974. Variability in the maximum expiratory flow volume curve in asymptomatic smokers and nonsmokers. *American Review of Respiratory Diseases* 110: 282–292.

Boren, H.G., Kory, R.C., and Syner, J.C. 1966. The Veteran's Administration-Army cooperative study of pulmonary function: II. The lung volume and its subdivisions in normal men. *American Journal of Medicine* 41: 96–114.

O'Brien, R.J., and Drizd, T.A. 1983. Roentgenographic determination of total lung capacity: Normal values from a national population survey. *American Review of Respiratory Diseases* 128: 949–952.

From Vivian H. Heyward, 2002, *Advanced Fitness Assessment and Exercise Prescription,* 4th ed. (Champaign, IL: Human Kinetics).

Standardized Sites
for Skinfold Measurements

Site	Direction of fold	Anatomical reference	Measurement
Chest	Diagonal	Axilla and nipple	Fold is taken between axilla and nipple as high as possible on anterior axillary fold, with measurement taken 1 cm below fingers.
Subscapular	Diagonal	Inferior angle of scapula	Fold is along natural cleavage line of skin just inferior to inferior angle of scapula, with caliper applied 1 cm below fingers.
Midaxillary	Horizontal	Xiphisternal junction (point where costal cartilage of ribs 5-6 articulates with sternum, slightly above inferior tip of xiphoid process)	Fold is taken on midaxillary line at level of xiphisternal junction.
Suprailiac	Oblique	Iliac crest	Fold is grasped posteriorly to midaxillary line and superiorly to iliac crest along natural cleavage of skin with caliper applied 1 cm below fingers.
Abdominal	Horizontal	Umbilicus	Fold is taken 3 cm lateral and 1 cm inferior to center of the umbilicus.
Triceps	Vertical (midline)	Acromial process of scapula and olecranon process of ulna	Using a tape measure, distance between lateral projection of acromial process and inferior margin of olecranon process is measured on lateral aspect of arm with elbow flexed 90°. Midpoint is marked on lateral side of arm. Fold is lifted 1 cm above marked line on posterior aspect of arm. Caliper is applied at marked level.
Biceps	Vertical (midline)	Biceps brachii	Fold is lifted over belly of the biceps brachii at the level marked for the triceps and on line with anterior border of the acromial process and the antecubital fossa. Caliper is applied 1 cm below fingers.
Thigh	Vertical (midline)	Inguinal crease and patella	Fold is lifted on anterior aspect of thigh midway between inguinal crease and proximal border of patella. Body weight is shifted to left foot and caliper is applied 1 cm below fingers.
Calf	Vertical (medial aspect)	Maximal calf circumference	Fold is lifted at level of maximal calf circumference on medial aspect of calf with knee and hip flexed to 90°.

Adapted from Harrison et al., (1988, pp. 55–70).

From Vivian H. Heyward, 2002, *Advanced Fitness Assessment and Exercise Prescription,* 4th ed. (Champaign, IL: Human Kinetics).

APPENDIX D.3

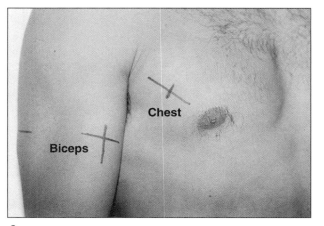 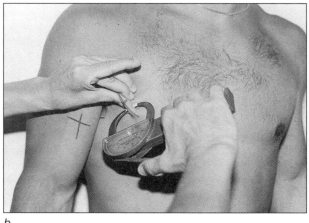

a   b

Figure D.3.1   *(a)* Site and *(b)* measurement of the chest skinfold. Photos courtesy of Linda K. Gilkey.

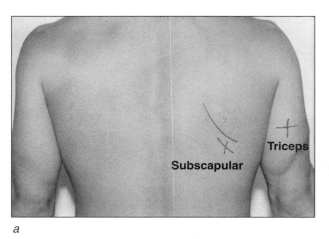 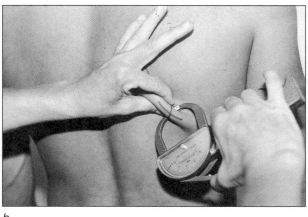

a   b

Figure D.3.2   *(a)* Site and *(b)* measurement of the subscapular skinfold. Photos courtesy of Linda K. Gilkey.

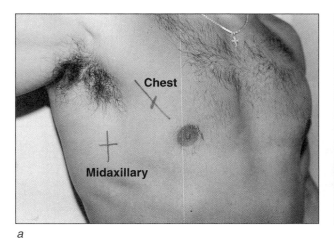 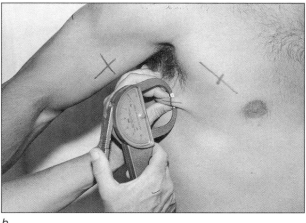

a   b

Figure D.3.3   *(a)* Site and *(b)* measurement of the midaxillary skinfold. Photos courtesy of Linda K. Gilkey.

From Vivian H. Heyward, 2002, *Advanced Fitness Assessment and Exercise Prescription,* 4th ed. (Champaign, IL: Human Kinetics).

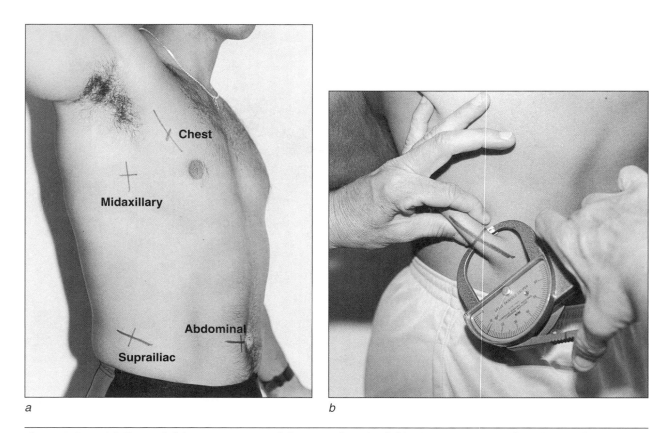

Figure D.3.4 *(a)* Site and *(b)* measurement of the suprailiac skinfold. Photos courtesy of Linda K. Gilkey.

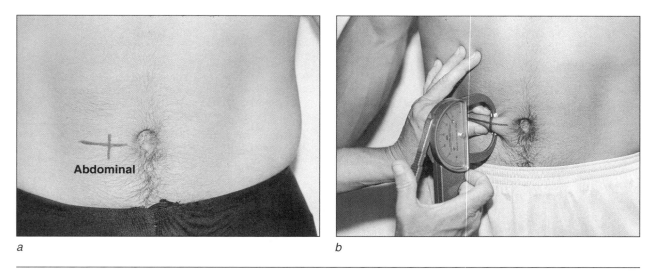

Figure D.3.5 *(a)* Site and *(b)* measurement of the abdominal skinfold. Photos courtesy of Linda K. Gilkey.

From Vivian H. Heyward, 2002, *Advanced Fitness Assessment and Exercise Prescription,* 4th ed. (Champaign, IL: Human Kinetics).

APPENDIX D.3

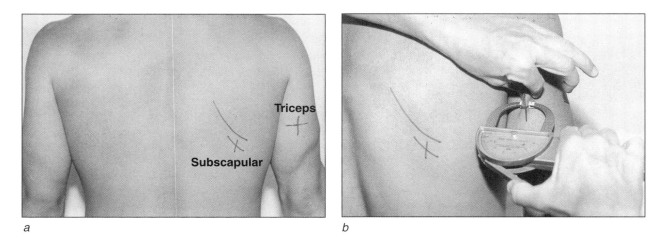

Figure D.3.6 *(a)* Site and *(b)* measurement of the triceps skinfold. Photos courtesy of Linda K. Gilkey.

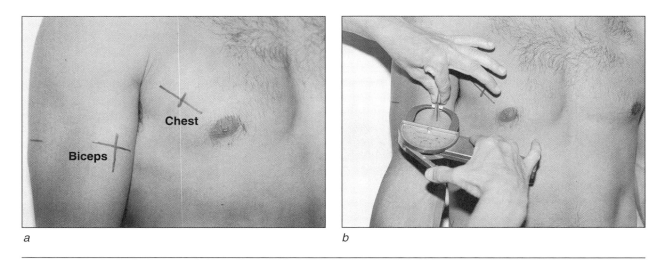

Figure D.3.7 *(a)* Site and *(b)* measurement of the biceps skinfold. Photos courtesy of Linda K. Gilkey.

From Vivian H. Heyward, 2002, *Advanced Fitness Assessment and Exercise Prescription,* 4th ed. (Champaign, IL: Human Kinetics).

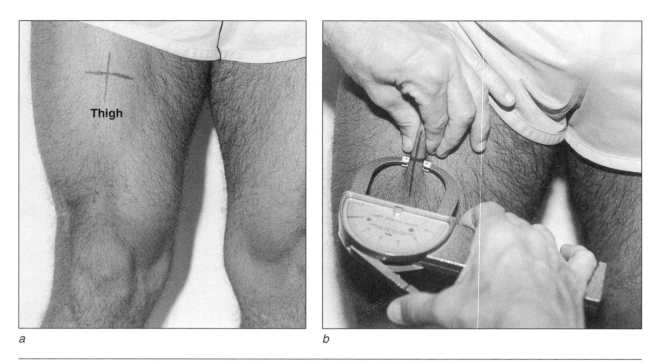

Figure D.3.8 *(a)* Site and *(b)* measurement of the thigh skinfold. Photos courtesy of Linda K. Gilkey.

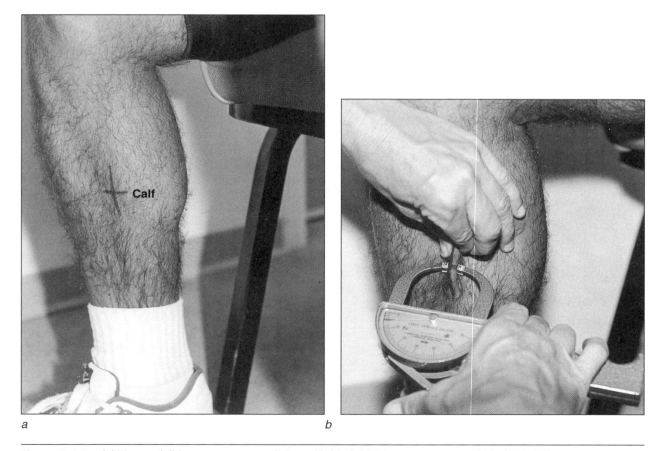

Figure D.3.9 *(a)* Site and *(b)* measurement of the calf skinfold. Photos courtesy of Linda K. Gilkey.

From Vivian H. Heyward, 2002, *Advanced Fitness Assessment and Exercise Prescription,* 4th ed. (Champaign, IL: Human Kinetics).

APPENDIX D.3

Skinfold Sites for Jackson's Generalized Skinfold Equations

Site	Direction of fold	Anatomical reference	Measurement
Chest	Diagonal	Axilla and nipple	Fold is taken 1/2 the distance between the anterior axillary line and nipple for men and 1/3 of this distance for women.
Subscapular	Oblique	Vertebral border and inferior angle of scapula	Fold is taken on diagonal line coming from the vertebral border, 1-2 cm below the inferior angle.
Midaxillary	Vertical	Xiphoid process of sternum	Fold is taken at level of xiphoid process along the midaxillary line.
Suprailiac	Diagonal	Iliac crest	Fold is taken diagonally above the iliac crest along the anterior axillary line.
Abdominal	Vertical	Umbilicus	Fold is taken vertically 2 cm lateral to the umbilicus.

Adapted from Jackson and Pollock (1978) and Jackson, Pollock, and Ward (1980).

From Vivian H. Heyward, 2002, *Advanced Fitness Assessment and Exercise Prescription,* 4th ed. (Champaign, IL: Human Kinetics).

Standardized Sites
for Circumference Measurements

Site	Anatomical reference	Position	Measurement
Neck	Laryngeal prominence ("Adam's apple")	Perpendicular to long axis of neck	Apply tape with minimal pressure just inferior to the Adam's apple.
Shoulder	Deltoid muscles and acromion processes of scapula	Horizontal	Apply tape snugly over maximum bulges of the deltoid muscles, inferior to acromion processes. Record measurement at end of normal expiration.
Chest	Fourth costosternal joints	Horizontal	Apply tape snugly around the torso at level of fourth costosternal joints. Record at end of normal expiration.
Waist	Narrowest part of torso, level of the "natural" waist between ribs and iliac crest	Horizontal	Apply tape snugly around the waist at level of narrowest part of torso. An assistant is needed to position tape behind the client. Take measurement at end of normal expiration.
Abdominal	Maximum anterior protuberance of abdomen, usually at umbilicus	Horizontal	Apply tape snugly around the abdomen at level of greatest anterior protuberance. An assistant is needed to position tape behind the client. Take measurement at end of normal expiration.
Hip (buttocks)	Maximum posterior extension of buttocks	Horizontal	Apply tape snugly around the buttocks. An assistant is needed to position tape on opposite side of body.
Thigh (proximal)	Gluteal fold	Horizontal	Apply tape snugly around thigh, just distal to the gluteal fold.
Thigh (mid)	Inguinal crease and proximal border of patella	Horizontal	With client's knee flexed 90° (right foot on bench), apply tape at level midway between inguinal crease and proximal border of patella.
Thigh (distal)	Femoral epicondyles	Horizontal	Apply tape just proximal to the femoral epicondyles.
Knee	Patella	Horizontal	Apply tape around the knee at midpatellar level with knee relaxed in slight flexion.
Calf	Maximum girth of calf muscle	Perpendicular to long axis of leg	With client sitting on end of table and legs hanging freely, apply tape horizontally around the maximum girth of calf.
Ankle	Malleoli of tibia and fibula	Perpendicular to long axis of leg	Apply tape snugly around minimum circumference of leg, just proximal to the malleoli.
Arm (biceps)	Acromion process of scapula and olecranon process of ulna	Perpendicular to long axis of arm	With client's arms hanging freely at sides and palms facing thighs, apply tape snugly around the arm at level midway between the acromion process of scapula and olecranon process of ulna (as marked for triceps and biceps skinfolds).
Forearm	Maximum girth of forearm	Perpendicular to long axis of forearm	With client's arms hanging down and away from trunk and forearm supinated, apply tape snugly around the maximum girth of the proximal part of the forearm.
Wrist	Styloid processes of radius and ulna	Perpendicular to long axis of forearm	With client's elbow flexed and forearm supinated, apply tape snugly around wrist, just distal to the styloid processes of the radius and ulna.

Adapted from Callaway et al. (1988, pp. 41–53).

From Vivian H. Heyward, 2002, *Advanced Fitness Assessment and Exercise Prescription,* 4th ed. (Champaign, IL: Human Kinetics).

APPENDIX D.5

Standardized Sites for Bony Breadth Measurements

Site	Anatomical reference	Position	Measurement
Biacromial (shoulder)	Lateral borders of acromion processes of scapula	Horizontal	With client standing, arms hanging vertically and shoulders relaxed, downward and slightly forward, apply blades of anthropometer to lateral borders of acromion processes. Measurement is taken from the rear.
Chest	Sixth rib on midaxillary line or fourth costosternal joints anteriorly	Horizontal	With client standing, arms slightly abducted, apply the large spreading caliper tips lightly on the sixth ribs on the midaxillary line. Take measurement at end of normal expiration.
Bi-iliac (bicristal)	Iliac crests	45° downward angle	With client standing, arms folded across the chest, apply anthropometer blades firmly at a 45° downward angle, at maximum breadth of iliac crest. Measurement is taken from rear.
Bitrochanteric	Greater trochanter of femur	Horizontal	With client standing, arms folded across the chest, apply anthropometer blade with considerable pressure to compress soft tissues. Measure maximum distance between the trochanters from the rear.
Knee	Femoral epicondyles	Diagonal or horizontal	With client sitting and knee flexed to 90°, apply caliper blades firmly on lateral and medial femoral epicondyles.
Ankle (bimalleolar)	Malleoli of tibia and fibula	Oblique	With client standing and weight evenly distributed, place the caliper blades on the most lateral part of lateral malleolus and most medial part of medial malleolus. Measurement is taken on an oblique plane from the rear.
Elbow	Epicondyles of humerus	Oblique	With client's elbow flexed 90°, arm raised to the horizontal, and forearm supinated, apply the caliper blades firmly to the medial and lateral humeral epicondyles at an angle that bisects the right angle at the elbow.
Wrist	Styloid process of radius and ulna, anatomical "snuff box"	Oblique	With client's elbow flexed 90°, upper arm vertical and close to torso, and forearm pronated, apply caliper tips firmly at an oblique angle to the styloid processes of the radius (at proximal part of anatomical snuff box) and ulna.

Adapted from Wilmore et al. (1988, pp. 28–38).

From Vivian H. Heyward, 2002, *Advanced Fitness Assessment and Exercise Prescription,* 4th ed. (Champaign, IL: Human Kinetics).

Energy Intake and Expenditure

You can use the Food Record and RDA Profile (Appendix E.1) to obtain information about your client's energy intake and daily energy needs. Appendix E.2 shows a sample computerized analysis of food intake that summarizes your client's recommended daily nutrients, compares the daily intake to caloric needs, and provides a detailed nutrient analysis for each food item ingested.

Your clients may use the Physical Activity Log (Appendix E.3) to record the type and duration of physical activities they engage in on a daily basis. This provides an estimate of the client's daily caloric expenditure due to activity. Appendix E.4 presents MET estimates of gross expenditure for conditioning exercises, sports, and recreational activities. You can use these estimates to calculate your client's energy expenditure (kcal/min) for a variety of activities.

Food Record and RDA Profile

Food code	Amount	Description

Food code: This is generally for office use. If you have the food code list, however, use this space to more precisely describe your food item.

Amount: You can use common measures (cup, slice, etc.) or weight for your foods.

Food description: Be specific. For example, bread choices include soft and firm textures; vegetables may be raw or cooked fresh, frozen, or canned; meats should be lean only or lean with some fat; fruit juices are fresh, frozen, or canned; and cheese might be cream or skim, soft, hard, or cottage.

From Vivian H. Heyward, 2002, *Advanced Fitness Assessment and Exercise Prescription,* 4th ed. (Champaign. IL: Human Kinetics).

APPENDIX E.1

RDA Profile Information

Name: _____

Age: _____   Height: _____

Sex: Male _____   Weight: _____

 Female _____   Activity level: _____

 Pregnant _____   (enter number from choices below)

 Nursing _____

Most people engage in a variety of activities in a 24-hr period, and each activity can use a different amount of energy. Thus, any table of activity levels must depend on averages. Choose the level that represents your *normal daily average*.

1. Sedentary

   Inactive, sometimes under someone else's care. Energy level is for basal metabolism plus about 15% for minimal activities.

2. Lightly active

   Most professionals (lawyers, doctors, accountants, architects, etc.), office workers, shop workers, teachers, homemakers with mechanical appliances, unemployed persons.

3. Moderately active

   Most persons in light industry, building workers (excluding heavy laborers), many farm workers, active students, department store workers, soldiers not in active service, people engaged in commercial fishing, homemakers without mechanical household appliances.

4. Very active

   Full-time athletes, dancers, unskilled laborers, some agricultural workers (especially in peasant farming), forestry workers, army recruits, soldiers in active service, mine workers, steel workers.

5. Exceptionally active

   Lumberjacks, blacksmiths, women construction workers, rickshaw pullers.

Courtesy of ESHA Research, 606 Juntura Way SE, Salem, OR 97302; phone: (503) 585-6242.

From Vivian H. Heyward, 2002, *Advanced Fitness Assessment and Exercise Prescription,* 4th ed. (Champaign, IL: Human Kinetics).

Sample Computerized Analysis of Food Intake

Jane Doe   Personal Profile Report

Gender:	Female
Activity Level:	Lightly Active
Height:	5 ft 3 in
Weight:	132 lbs
Age:	25 yrs
BMI:	23.38

Recommended Daily Nutrients

Basic Components				Vitamin D mcg	5.00	mcg
Calories	2044		*	Vit E-Alpha Equiv.	8.00	mg
Protein	47.9	g		Folate	180.00	mcg
Carbohydrates	296	g	**	Vitamin K	6.00	mcg
Dietary Fiber	20	g	#	Pantothenic	7.00	mg **
Fat - Total	68	g	**	**Minerals**		
Saturated Fat	20	g	**	Calcium	800.00	mg
Mono Fat	25	g	**	Chromium	125.00	mcg **
Poly Fat	23	g	**	Copper	2.50	mg **
Cholesterol	300	mg		Fluoride	2.75	mg **
Vitamins				Iodine	150	mcg
Vitamin A IU	4000	IU		Iron	15	mg
Vitamin A RE	800	RE		Magnesium	280	mg
Thiamin-B1	1.02	mg		Manganese	3.50	mg **
Riboflavin-B2	1.23	mg		Molybdenum	163	mcg **
Niacin	13.49	NE		Phosphorus	800	mg
Vitamin-B6	1.60	mg		Potassium	3750	mg
Vitamin-B12	2.00	mcg		Selenium	55	mcg
Biotin	65.00	mcg **		Sodium	2400	mg
Vitamin C	60.00	mg		Zinc	12	mg

 * Suggested values within recommended ranges
** Dietary goals   # Fiber = 1 gram/100 kcal

The Food Processor® Nutrition Analysis program from ESHA Research, Salem, Oregon.

From Vivian H. Heyward, 2002, *Advanced Fitness Assessment and Exercise Prescription,* 4th ed. (Champaign, IL: Human Kinetics).

APPENDIX E.2

Ratios and Percents

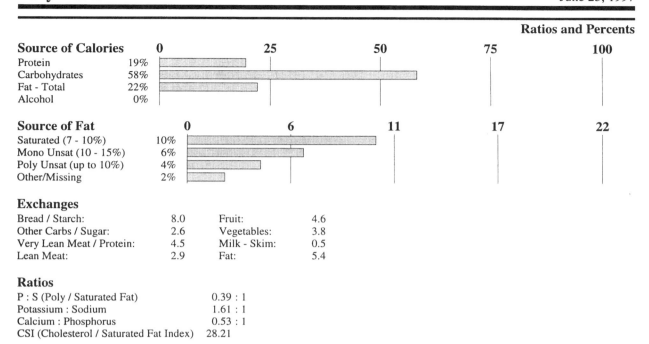

Source of Calories

		0	25	50	75	100
Protein	19%					
Carbohydrates	58%					
Fat - Total	22%					
Alcohol	0%					

Source of Fat

		0	6	11	17	22
Saturated (7 - 10%)	10%					
Mono Unsat (10 - 15%)	6%					
Poly Unsat (up to 10%)	4%					
Other/Missing	2%					

Exchanges

Bread / Starch:	8.0	Fruit:	4.6
Other Carbs / Sugar:	2.6	Vegetables:	3.8
Very Lean Meat / Protein:	4.5	Milk - Skim:	0.5
Lean Meat:	2.9	Fat:	5.4

Ratios

P : S (Poly / Saturated Fat)	0.39 : 1
Potassium : Sodium	1.61 : 1
Calcium : Phosphorus	0.53 : 1
CSI (Cholesterol / Saturated Fat Index)	28.21

Daily Intake

June 23, 1997

% comparison to: Jane Doe

Bar Graph

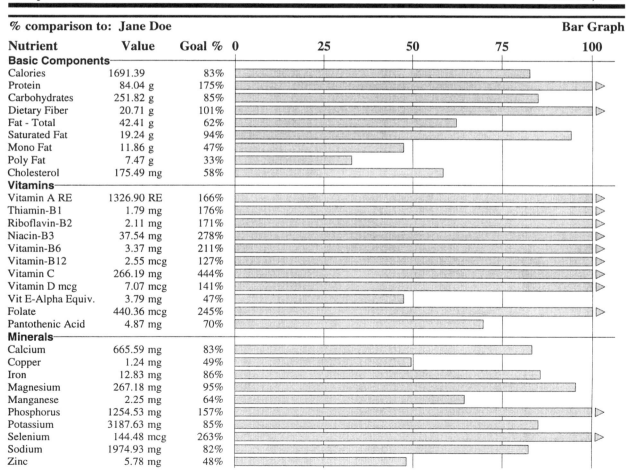

Nutrient	Value	Goal %	0	25	50	75	100
Basic Components							
Calories	1691.39	83%					
Protein	84.04 g	175%					
Carbohydrates	251.82 g	85%					
Dietary Fiber	20.71 g	101%					
Fat - Total	42.41 g	62%					
Saturated Fat	19.24 g	94%					
Mono Fat	11.86 g	47%					
Poly Fat	7.47 g	33%					
Cholesterol	175.49 mg	58%					
Vitamins							
Vitamin A RE	1326.90 RE	166%					
Thiamin-B1	1.79 mg	176%					
Riboflavin-B2	2.11 mg	171%					
Niacin-B3	37.54 mg	278%					
Vitamin-B6	3.37 mg	211%					
Vitamin-B12	2.55 mcg	127%					
Vitamin C	266.19 mg	444%					
Vitamin D mcg	7.07 mcg	141%					
Vit E-Alpha Equiv.	3.79 mg	47%					
Folate	440.36 mcg	245%					
Pantothenic Acid	4.87 mg	70%					
Minerals							
Calcium	665.59 mg	83%					
Copper	1.24 mg	49%					
Iron	12.83 mg	86%					
Magnesium	267.18 mg	95%					
Manganese	2.25 mg	64%					
Phosphorus	1254.53 mg	157%					
Potassium	3187.63 mg	85%					
Selenium	144.48 mcg	263%					
Sodium	1974.93 mg	82%					
Zinc	5.78 mg	48%					

From Vivian H. Heyward, 2002, *Advanced Fitness Assessment and Exercise Prescription,* 4th ed. (Champaign, IL: Human Kinetics).

Spreadsheet

Amount	Food Item	Weight (g)	Cals	Prot (g)	Carb (g)	Fiber (g)	Fat-T (g)
1/2 cup	Orange Juice prepared from frozen	124.50	56.03	0.85	13.45	0.25	0.07
2 oz-wt	Kelloggs Corn Flakes Cereal	56.70	220.56	4.59	48.82	1.47	0.17
1 each	Banana--Medium size	118.00	108.56	1.22	27.61	2.83	0.57
1/2 cup	Skim Milk-Vitamin A Added	122.50	42.75	4.18	5.94	0	0.22
1 piece	Whole Wheat Bread-Toasted	25.00	69.25	2.73	12.93	1.85	1.20
2 tsp	Jelly	12.67	34.33	0.05	8.97	0.13	0.01
1 each	White Pita Pocket Bread 6 1/2"diameter	60.00	165.00	5.46	33.42	1.32	0.72
1/2 cup	Tuna Salad	102.50	191.67	16.40	9.65	0	9.49
1/4 cup	Alfalfa Sprouts-Raw	8.25	2.39	0.33	0.31	0.21	0.06
2 piece	Fresh Tomato Wedge(1/4 of Medium Tomato)	62.00	13.02	0.53	2.88	0.68	0.20
8 oz-wt	Diet soda pop - average assorted	226.80	0	0	0	0	0
1 each	Medium Apple w/Peel	138.00	81.42	0.26	21.11	3.73	0.50
4 oz-wt	Chicken light meat - roasted	113.40	173.50	30.73	0	0	4.62
1 each	Baked Potato w/skin - medium	122.00	132.98	2.82	30.74	2.93	0.12
1 oz-wt	Cheddar Cheese-Shredded	28.35	114.25	7.06	0.36	0	9.38
4 oz-wt	Broccoli Pieces-Steamed	113.40	31.75	3.39	5.95	3.40	0.40
1/2 cup	Rich Vanilla Ice Cream	74.00	178.34	2.59	16.58	0	11.99
1/2 cup	Fresh Strawberries-Slices-Cup	83.00	24.90	0.51	5.83	1.91	0.31
2 tbs	Frozen Dessert Topping-Semi Solid	9.38	29.81	0.12	2.17	0	2.37
1 cup	Brewed Coffee	237.00	4.74	0.24	0.95	0	0.01
1 tsp	White Granulated Sugar	4.17	16.13	0	4.16	0	0
	Totals	1841.61	1691.39	84.04	251.82	20.71	42.41

Amount	Food Item	Fat-S (g)	Fat-M (g)	Fat-P (g)	Chol (mg)	A-RE (RE)	B1 (mg)
1/2 cup	Orange Juice prepared from frozen	0.01	0.01	0.01	0	9.96	0.10
2 oz-wt	Kelloggs Corn Flakes Cereal	0.02	0.09	0.03	0	750.71	0.74
1 each	Banana--Medium size	0.22	0.05	0.11	0	9.44	0.05
1/2 cup	Skim Milk-Vitamin A Added	0.14	0.06	0.01	2.21	74.73	0.04
1 piece	Whole Wheat Bread-Toasted	0.26	0.47	0.28	0	0	0.08
2 tsp	Jelly	0.00	0.00	0.01	0	0.25	0.00
1 each	White Pita Pocket Bread 6 1/2"diameter	0.10	0.06	0.32	0	0	0.36
1/2 cup	Tuna Salad	1.58	2.96	4.22	13.32	27.67	0.03
1/4 cup	Alfalfa Sprouts-Raw	0.01	0.00	0.03	0	1.32	0.01
2 piece	Fresh Tomato Wedge(1/4 of Medium Tomato)	0.03	0.03	0.08	0	38.44	0.04
8 oz-wt	Diet soda pop - average assorted	0	0	0	0	0	0
1 each	Medium Apple w/Peel	0.08	0.02	0.14	0	6.90	0.02
4 oz-wt	Chicken light meat - roasted	1.24	1.75	1.05	85.05	9.07	0.07
1 each	Baked Potato w/skin - medium	0.03	0.00	0.05	0	0	0.13
1 oz-wt	Cheddar Cheese-Shredded	6.01	2.66	0.27	29.77	85.90	0.01
4 oz-wt	Broccoli Pieces-Steamed	0.06	0.03	0.19	0	165.79	0.07
1/2 cup	Rich Vanilla Ice Cream	7.39	3.45	0.45	45.14	136.16	0.03
1/2 cup	Fresh Strawberries-Slices-Cup	0.02	0.04	0.15	0	2.49	0.02
2 tbs	Frozen Dessert Topping-Semi Solid	2.05	0.15	0.05	0	8.06	0
1 cup	Brewed Coffee	0.00	0	0.00	0	0	0
1 tsp	White Granulated Sugar	0	0	0	0	0	0
	Totals	19.24	11.86	7.47	175.49	1326.90	1.79

The Food Processor® Nutrition Analysis program from ESHA Research, Salem, Oregon.

From Vivian H. Heyward, 2002, *Advanced Fitness Assessment and Exercise Prescription,* 4th ed. (Champaign, IL: Human Kinetics).

Spreadsheet

Amount	Food Item	B2 (mg)	B3 (mg)	B6 (mg)	B12 (mcg)	Vit C (mg)	D-mcg (mcg)
1/2 cup	Orange Juice prepared from frozen	0.02	0.25	0.05	0	48.43	0
2 oz-wt	Kelloggs Corn Flakes Cereal	0.86	9.98	1.02	0	30.05	1.98
1 each	Banana--Medium size	0.12	0.64	0.68	0	10.74	0
1/2 cup	Skim Milk-Vitamin A Added	0.17	0.11	0.05	0.46	1.20	1.23
1 piece	Whole Wheat Bread-Toasted	0.05	0.97	0.05	0.00	0	0.05
2 tsp	Jelly	0.00	0.00	0.00	0	0.11	0
1 each	White Pita Pocket Bread 6 1/2"diameter	0.20	2.78	0.02	0	0	0
1/2 cup	Tuna Salad	0.07	6.87	0.08	1.23	2.25	3.31
1/4 cup	Alfalfa Sprouts-Raw	0.01	0.04	0.00	0	0.68	0
2 piece	Fresh Tomato Wedge(1/4 of Medium Tomato)	0.03	0.39	0.05	0	11.84	0
8 oz-wt	Diet soda pop - average assorted	0	0	0	0	0	0
1 each	Medium Apple w/Peel	0.02	0.11	0.07	0	7.87	0
4 oz-wt	Chicken light meat - roasted	0.11	11.91	0.61	0.35	0	0.34
1 each	Baked Potato w/skin - medium	0.04	2.01	0.42	0	15.74	0
1 oz-wt	Cheddar Cheese-Shredded	0.11	0.02	0.02	0.23	0	0.09
4 oz-wt	Broccoli Pieces-Steamed	0.13	0.69	0.16	0	89.70	0
1/2 cup	Rich Vanilla Ice Cream	0.12	0.06	0.03	0.27	0.52	0.07
1/2 cup	Fresh Strawberries-Slices-Cup	0.05	0.19	0.05	0	47.06	0
2 tbs	Frozen Dessert Topping-Semi Solid	0	0	0	0	0	0
1 cup	Brewed Coffee	0	0.53	0	0	0	0
1 tsp	White Granulated Sugar	0.00	0	0	0	0	0
	Totals	2.11	37.54	3.37	2.55	266.19	7.07

Amount	Food Item	E-aTE (mg)	Fola (mcg)	Panto (mg)	Calc (mg)	Copp (mg)	Iron (mg)
1/2 cup	Orange Juice prepared from frozen	0.24	54.53	0.20	11.21	0.05	0.12
2 oz-wt	Kelloggs Corn Flakes Cereal	0.14	200.15	0.10	1.70	0.04	3.58
1 each	Banana--Medium size	0.32	22.54	0.31	7.08	0.12	0.37
1/2 cup	Skim Milk-Vitamin A Added	0.05	6.37	0.40	150.68	0.01	0.05
1 piece	Whole Wheat Bread-Toasted	0.23	9.75	0.10	20.25	0.08	0.93
2 tsp	Jelly	0	0.13	0.02	1.01	0.00	0.03
1 each	White Pita Pocket Bread 6 1/2"diameter	0.02	14.40	0.24	51.60	0.10	1.57
1/2 cup	Tuna Salad	0.97	7.48	0.27	17.42	0.15	1.02
1/4 cup	Alfalfa Sprouts-Raw	0.00	2.97	0.05	2.64	0.01	0.08
2 piece	Fresh Tomato Wedge(1/4 of Medium Tomato)	0.24	9.30	0.15	3.10	0.05	0.28
8 oz-wt	Diet soda pop - average assorted	0	0	0	0	0	0
1 each	Medium Apple w/Peel	0.44	3.86	0.08	9.66	0.06	0.25
4 oz-wt	Chicken light meat - roasted	0.30	3.40	1.03	14.74	0.05	1.22
1 each	Baked Potato w/skin - medium	0.06	13.42	0.68	12.20	0.37	1.66
1 oz-wt	Cheddar Cheese-Shredded	0.10	5.16	0.12	204.40	0.01	0.19
4 oz-wt	Broccoli Pieces-Steamed	0.54	68.27	0.58	54.32	0.05	1.00
1/2 cup	Rich Vanilla Ice Cream	0	3.70	0.27	86.58	0.02	0.04
1/2 cup	Fresh Strawberries-Slices-Cup	0.12	14.69	0.28	11.62	0.04	0.32
2 tbs	Frozen Dessert Topping-Semi Solid	0.02	0	0	0.59	0.00	0.01
1 cup	Brewed Coffee	0	0.24	0.00	4.74	0.02	0.12
1 tsp	White Granulated Sugar	0	0	0	0.04	0.00	0.00
	Totals	3.79	440.36	4.87	665.59	1.24	12.83

From Vivian H. Heyward, 2002, *Advanced Fitness Assessment and Exercise Prescription,* 4th ed. (Champaign, IL: Human Kinetics).

Spreadsheet

Amount	Food Item	Magn (mg)	Mang (mg)	Phos (mg)	Potas (mg)	Sel (mcg)	Sod (mg)
1/2 cup	Orange Juice prepared from frozen	12.45	0.02	19.92	236.55	0.25	1.25
2 oz-wt	Kelloggs Corn Flakes Cereal	6.80	0.05	35.72	52.16	2.89	580.04
1 each	Banana--Medium size	34.22	0.18	23.60	467.28	1.18	1.18
1/2 cup	Skim Milk-Vitamin A Added	13.97	0.00	123.73	203.35	1.23	63.09
1 piece	Whole Wheat Bread-Toasted	24.25	0.65	64.50	70.75	10.25	148.00
2 tsp	Jelly	0.76	0.02	0.63	8.11	0.25	4.56
1 each	White Pita Pocket Bread 6 1/2"diameter	15.60	0.29	58.20	72.00	18.00	321.60
1/2 cup	Tuna Salad	19.47	0.04	182.45	182.45	70.01	412.05
1/4 cup	Alfalfa Sprouts-Raw	2.23	0.02	5.78	6.52	--	0.50
2 piece	Fresh Tomato Wedge(1/4 of Medium Tomato)	6.82	0.07	14.88	137.64	0.25	5.58
8 oz-wt	Diet soda pop - average assorted	0	0	90.72	34.02	0	113.40
1 each	Medium Apple w/Peel	6.90	0.06	9.66	158.70	0.41	0
4 oz-wt	Chicken light meat - roasted	26.08	0.02	246.08	267.62	28.92	57.83
1 each	Baked Potato w/skin - medium	32.94	0.28	69.54	509.96	1.95	9.76
1 oz-wt	Cheddar Cheese-Shredded	7.88	0.00	145.15	27.90	4.03	176.05
4 oz-wt	Broccoli Pieces-Steamed	28.35	0.25	74.73	367.42	--	30.62
1/2 cup	Rich Vanilla Ice Cream	8.14	0.01	70.30	117.66	4.00	41.44
1/2 cup	Fresh Strawberries-Slices-Cup	8.30	0.24	15.77	137.78	0.75	0.83
2 tbs	Frozen Dessert Topping-Semi Solid	0.17	0.01	0.72	1.71	--	2.37
1 cup	Brewed Coffee	11.85	0.06	2.37	127.98	0.11	4.74
1 tsp	White Granulated Sugar	0	0.00	0.08	0.08	0.01	0.04
	Totals	267.18	2.25	1254.53	3187.63	144.48	1974.93

Amount	Food Item	Zinc (mg)
1/2 cup	Orange Juice prepared from frozen	0.06
2 oz-wt	Kelloggs Corn Flakes Cereal	0.16
1 each	Banana--Medium size	0.19
1/2 cup	Skim Milk-Vitamin A Added	0.49
1 piece	Whole Wheat Bread-Toasted	0.55
2 tsp	Jelly	0.01
1 each	White Pita Pocket Bread 6 1/2"diameter	0.50
1/2 cup	Tuna Salad	0.57
1/4 cup	Alfalfa Sprouts-Raw	0.08
2 piece	Fresh Tomato Wedge(1/4 of Medium Tomato)	0.06
8 oz-wt	Diet soda pop - average assorted	0
1 each	Medium Apple w/Peel	0.06
4 oz-wt	Chicken light meat - roasted	0.88
1 each	Baked Potato w/skin - medium	0.39
1 oz-wt	Cheddar Cheese-Shredded	0.88
4 oz-wt	Broccoli Pieces-Steamed	0.45
1/2 cup	Rich Vanilla Ice Cream	0.30
1/2 cup	Fresh Strawberries-Slices-Cup	0.11
2 tbs	Frozen Dessert Topping-Semi Solid	0.00
1 cup	Brewed Coffee	0.05
1 tsp	White Granulated Sugar	0.00
	Totals	5.78

The Food Processor® Nutrition Analysis program from ESHA Research, Salem, Oregon.

From Vivian H. Heyward, 2002, *Advanced Fitness Assessment and Exercise Prescription*, 4th ed. (Champaign, IL: Human Kinetics).

Physical Activity Log

Name: _____ Date: _____

Day and date	Activity	Duration (min)	X	kcal/min	= Total (kcal)

From Vivian H. Heyward, 2002, *Advanced Fitness Assessment and Exercise Prescription,* 4th ed. (Champaign, IL: Human Kinetics).

Gross Energy Expenditure for Conditioning Exercises, Sports, and Recreational Activities

METs	Description
Conditioning exercises	
5.0	Aerobic dancing, low impact
7.0	Aerobic dancing, high impact
8.5	Aerobics, step, with 6-8 in. step
10.0	Aerobics, step, with 10-12 in. step
3.0	Bicycling, stationary, 50 W, very light effort
5.5	Bicycling, stationary, 100 W, light effort
7.0	Bicycling, stationary, 150 W, moderate effort
10.5	Bicycling, stationary, 200 W, vigorous effort
12.5	Bicycling, stationary, 250 W, very vigorous effort
8.0	Calisthenics (e.g., push-ups, pull-ups, jumping jacks, sit-ups), vigorous
3.5	Calisthenics, light or moderate effort
8.0	Circuit resistance training, including some aerobic activity and minimal rest (e.g., super circuit resistance training)
8.0	Elliptical training, machine, 125 strides/min with resistance
3.5	Rowing (machine), 50 W, light effort
7.0	Rowing (machine), 100 W, moderate effort
8.5	Rowing (machine), 150 W, vigorous effort
12.0	Rowing (machine), 200 W, very vigorous effort
8.0	Running, 5 mph (12 min/mile)
9.0	Running, 5.2 mph (11.5 min/mile)
10.0	Running, 6.0 mph (10 min/mile)
11.0	Running, 6.7 mph (9 min/mile)
11.5	Running, 7.0 mph (8.5 min/mile)
12.5	Running, 7.5 mph (8 min/mile)
13.5	Running, 8 mph (7.5 min/mile)
14.0	Running, 8.6 mph (7 min/mile)
15.0	Running, 9 mph (6.5 min/mile)
16.0	Running, 10 mph (6 min/mile)
18.0	Running, 10.9 mph (5.5 min/mile)
9.0	Running, cross country
7.0	Jogging, general
6.0	Jogging/walking combination (jogging component less than 10 min)

From Vivian H. Heyward, 2002, *Advanced Fitness Assessment and Exercise Prescription,* 4th ed. (Champaign, IL: Human Kinetics).

4.5	Jogging on a mini-trampoline
12.5	Rollerblading, in-line skating, vigorous effort
8.0	Rope skipping, slow
10.0	Rope skipping, moderate
12.0	Rope skipping, fast
9.5	Skiing, Nordic (machine)
6.0	Slimnastics, jazzercize
9.0	Stair climbing (machine), step ergometer
2.5	Stretching, hatha yoga
10.0	Swimming, laps, freestyle, fast, vigorous effort
7.0	Swimming, laps, freestyle, slow, moderate or light effort
7.0	Swimming, backstroke
10.0	Swimming, breaststroke
11.0	Swimming, butterfly
11.0	Swimming, crawl, fast, vigorous effort
8.0	Swimming, crawl, slow, moderate or light effort
8.0	Swimming, sidestroke
4.0	Swimming, treading water, moderate effort
4.0	Tai chi
5.0	Treading™, walking, variable speed 2.5-4.0 mph and grade 0-10%
11.0	Treading™, running, variable speed 5.8-7.5 mph and grade 0-10%
2.5	Walking, 2.0 mph
3.0	Walking, 2.5 mph
3.3	Walking, 3.0 mph
3.8	Walking, 3.5 mph
5.0	Walking, 4.0 mph
6.3	Walking, 4.5 mph
4.0	Water aerobics, water calisthenics
8.0	Water jogging
3.0	Weightlifting (free weights/machines), light to moderate effort
6.0	Weightlifting (free weights/machines), power lifting, bodybuilding, vigorous effort
Sports and recreational activities	
3.5	Archery (non-hunting)
7.0	Badminton, competitive
4.5	Badminton, social singles or doubles
5.0	Baseball, general
8.0	Basketball, game
4.5	Basketball, shooting baskets
6.5	Basketball, wheelchair
8.5	Bicycling, BMX or mountain
4.0	Bicycling, <10 mph, leisure, pleasure

(continued)

From Vivian H. Heyward, 2002, *Advanced Fitness Assessment and Exercise Prescription,* 4th ed. (Champaign, IL: Human Kinetics).

6.0	Bicycling, 10-11.9 mph
8.0	Bicycling, 12-13.9 mph
10.0	Bicycling, 14-15.9 mph
12.0	Bicycling, 16-19 mph
16.0	Bicycling, ≥20 mph
5.0	Bicycling, unicycle
2.5	Billiards, pool
2.5	Bird watching
3.0	Bowling
3.0	Bowling, lawn
12.0	Boxing, in ring
6.0	Boxing, punching bag
9.0	Boxing, sparring
7.0	Broomball
3.0	Canoeing, 2.0-3.9 mph, light effort
7.0	Canoeing, 4.0-5.9 mph, moderate effort
12.0	Canoeing, ≥6.0 mph, vigorous effort
5.0	Children's games, hopscotch, dodgeball, T-ball, tetherball, playground
5.0	Cricket (batting and bowling)
2.5	Croquet
4.0	Curling
4.8	Dancing, ballet or modern, twist, jazz, tap, jitterbug
4.5	Dancing, Greek, Middle Eastern, belly, hula, flamenco, swing
4.5	Dancing, ballroom, fast, disco, folk, square, line dancing, Irish step dancing, polka, contra, country
3.0	Dancing, slow, waltz, foxtrot, samba, tango, mambo, cha-cha
5.5	Dancing, traditional American Indian dancing
2.5	Darts, wall or lawn
3.0	Diving, springboard or platform
6.0	Fencing
4.0	Fishing and hunting from river bank and walking
2.5	Fishing and hunting from boat, sitting
6.0	Fishing in stream, in waders
2.0	Fishing, ice, sitting
2.5	Fishing and hunting, bow and arrow, crossbow
2.5	Fishing and hunting, pistol shooting, trap shooting, standing
9.0	Football, competitive
2.5	Football or baseball, playing catch
8.0	Football, touch, flag
3.0	Frisbee, playing, general
8.0	Frisbee, ultimate
3.0	Gardening, lawn work, general

From Vivian H. Heyward, 2002, *Advanced Fitness Assessment and Exercise Prescription*, 4th ed. (Champaign, IL: Human Kinetics).

4.5	Golfing, walking and carrying clubs
3.0	Golfing, miniature, driving range
4.3	Golfing, walking and pulling clubs
3.5	Golfing, power cart
4.0	Gymnastics, general
4.0	Hacky sack
12.0	Handball, general
8.0	Handball, team
3.5	Hang gliding
6.0	Hiking, cross country
8.0	Hockey, field
8.0	Hockey, ice
4.0	Horseback riding, general
3.0	Horseshoe pitching, quoits
12.0	Jai alai
10.0	Judo, jujitsu, kick boxing, tae kwon do
4.0	Juggling
5.0	Kayaking and whitewater rafting
7.0	Kickball
8.0	Lacrosse
4.0	Motor-cross
9.0	Orienteering
10.0	Paddleball, competitive
6.0	Paddleball, casual, general
4.0	Paddle boating
8.0	Polo
6.5	Race walking
10.0	Racquetball, competitive
7.0	Racquetball, casual, general
11.0	Rock climbing, ascending
8.0	Rock climbing, rappelling
10.0	Rugby
3.0	Sailing, boat and board sailing, wind surfing, ice surfing
7.0	Scuba diving, skin diving
3.0	Shuffleboard
5.0	Skateboarding
7.0	Skating, roller or ice
15.0	Skating, speed skating
7.0	Skiing, cross-country, 2.5 mph, light effort
8.0	Skiing, cross-country, 4.0-4.9 mph, moderate effort
9.0	Skiing, cross-country, 5.0-7.9 mph, vigorous effort

(continued)

From Vivian H. Heyward, 2002, *Advanced Fitness Assessment and Exercise Prescription,* 4th ed. (Champaign, IL: Human Kinetics).

(continued)

14.0	Skiing, cross-country, >8.0 mph, racing
5.0	Skiing, downhill, light effort
6.0	Skiing, downhill, moderate effort
8.0	Skiing, downhill, vigorous effort, racing
6.0	Skiing, water
7.0	Skimobiling
3.5	Skydiving
7.0	Sledding, tobogganing, bobsledding, luge
5.0	Snorkeling
8.0	Snow shoeing
10.0	Soccer, competitive
7.0	Soccer, casual, general
5.0	Softball, fast or slow pitch
6.0	Softball, pitching
12.0	Squash
3.0	Surfing, body or board
6.0	Swimming, leisurely, not laps
8.0	Swimming, synchronized
4.0	Table tennis, ping-pong
7.0	Tennis, general
5.0	Tennis, doubles
8.0	Tennis, singles
4.0	Track and field, shot, discus, hammer throw
6.0	Track and field, high jump, long jump, triple jump, javelin, pole vault
10.0	Track and field, steeplechase, hurdles
3.5	Trampoline
8.0	Volleyball, competitive
8.0	Volleyball, beach
3.0	Volleyball, noncompetitive
10.0	Water polo
3.0	Water volleyball
7.0	Wallyball
6.0	Wrestling

From Vivian H. Heyward, 2002, *Advanced Fitness Assessment and Exercise Prescription,* 4th ed. (Champaign, IL: Human Kinetics). Data from Ainsworth, B.E., et al. (2000). Compendium of physical activities: An update of activity codes and MET intensities. *Medicine & Science in Sports & Exercise* 32(supplement): S498-S516.

Flexibility Exercises, Low Back Care Exercises, and Stress Assessment

Appendix F.1 describes and illustrates selected static stretching exercises for flexibility. This information is organized by body region and muscle groups. Appendix F.2 summarizes Exercise Do's and Don'ts. For each contraindicated exercise, a safe alternative exercise is presented.

Recomended exercises for low back care programs are illustrated in appendix F.3. This appendix provides a description and identifies muscle groups involved for each exercise. Appendix F.4 outlines testing and scoring procedures for the Rathbone Manual Tension Test. This test may be used to assess the relative amont of neuromuscular tension in your client's wrist, elbow, shoulder, knee, hip, and neck joints at rest.

Selected Flexibility Exercises

ANTERIOR THIGH REGION

Muscle Groups: Quadriceps and Hip Flexors

Exercise 1
Description: From a standing position, raise one foot toward hips and grasp ankle. Pull leg upward toward buttocks.

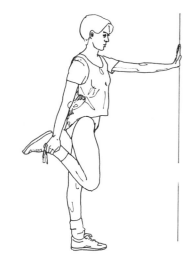

Exercise 2
Description: Lying on your side, flex the knee and grasp the ankle. Press the foot into the hand and squeeze the pelvis forward. Do not pull the foot.

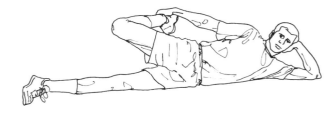

Exercise 3
Description: In a prone position, flex the knee and grasp ankle or foot with both hands. Do not pull on the foot. Keep knees on the floor and do not arch the back.

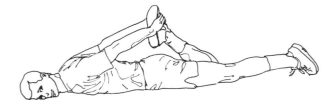

From Vivian H. Heyward, 2002, *Advanced Fitness Assessment and Exercise Prescription,* 4th ed. (Champaign, IL: Human Kinetics).

APPENDIX F.1

POSTERIOR THIGH REGION

Muscle Groups: Hamstrings and Hip Extensors

Exercise 1

Description: In a supine position, grasp knee and pull knee toward chest, then flex head to knee.

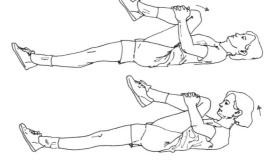
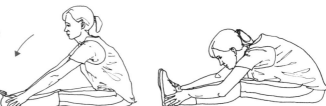

Exercise 2

Description: From a long-sitting position, grasp ankles and flex trunk to legs.

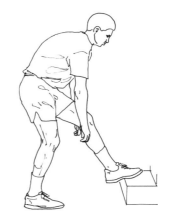

Exercise 3

Description: From a standing position, place your foot on a low step, keep the knee flexed slightly, and bend from the hips until you feel the stretch.

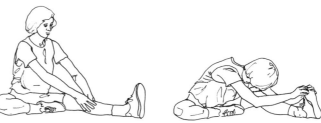

Exercise 4

Description: From a sitting position, with one knee flexed, flex the trunk keeping the spine extended until you feel tension.

Exercise 5

Description: From a lying position, with one leg extended and the other leg flexed, grasp leg with both hands and flex thigh to trunk.

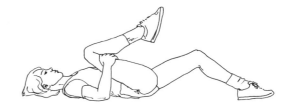

From Vivian H. Heyward, 2002, *Advanced Fitness Assessment and Exercise Prescription,* 4th ed. (Champaign, IL: Human Kinetics).

GROIN REGION (MEDIAL THIGH REGION)

Muscle Groups: Hip Adductors

Exercise 1
Description: From a tailor-sitting position, with soles of feet together, place hands on inside of knees and push downward slowly.

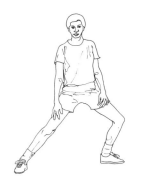

Exercise 2
Description: From a straddle-standing position, flex one knee and hip, lowering body closer to floor.

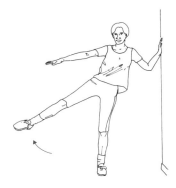

Exercise 3
Description: Standing on one leg while supporting yourself against wall or chair abduct hip, keeping leg straight. Have partner grasp ankle and passively stretch the muscle further.

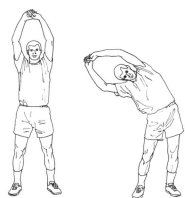

LATERAL THIGH-TRUNK REGION

Muscle Groups: Hip Abductors and Trunk Lateral Flexors

Exercise 1
Description: From standing position, with arms overhead, clasp hands together and laterally flex trunk to side no more than 20°.

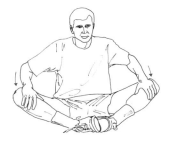

From Vivian H. Heyward, 2002, *Advanced Fitness Assessment and Exercise Prescription,* 4th ed. (Champaign, IL: Human Kinetics).

APPENDIX F.1

Exercise 2

Description: From a crossed-leg sitting position, rotate trunk to the right. Place hands on right side of thigh and pull. Repeat to opposite side.

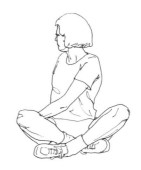

POSTERIOR LEG REGION

Muscle Group: Plantar Flexors

Exercise 1
Description: Assume front-leaning position against wall with one foot ahead of the other. Flex hip, knee, and ankle to lower your body closer to ground, keeping feet flat on floor.

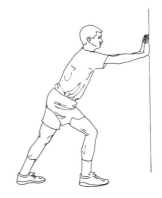

Exercise 2
Description: Standing with balls of feet on stairs, curb, or wood block, lower heels to floor.

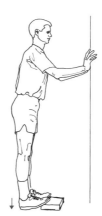

ANTERIOR LEG REGION

Muscle Group: Dorsiflexors

Exercise 1
Description: Standing with ankle of the non-supporting leg fully extended, stretch the dorsiflexors by slowly flexing the knee of the supporting leg.

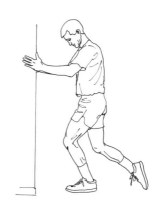

From Vivian H. Heyward, 2002, *Advanced Fitness Assessment and Exercise Prescription,* 4th ed. (Champaign, IL: Human Kinetics).

UPPER AND LOWER BACK REGIONS

Muscle Group: Trunk Extensors

Exercise 1

Description: Sit with legs crossed and arms relaxed. Tuck chin and curl forward attempting to touch forehead to knees.

Exercise 2

Description: In a supine position, with knees flexed, grasp thighs below the knee caps and bring knees to chest. Flatten lower back to floor.

Exercise 3

Description: From a kneeling position, bring chin to chest. Contract abdomen and buttocks muscles while rounding lower back.

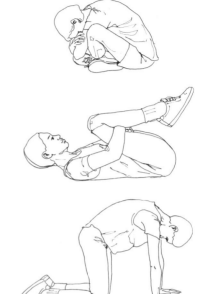

ANTERIOR CHEST, SHOULDER, AND ABDOMINAL REGIONS

Muscle Groups: Shoulder Flexors and Adductors, Trunk Flexors

Exercise 1

Description: In a prone position, push up until elbows are fully extended. Keep pelvis and hips on floor.

Exercise 2

Description: Grasp towel or rope with both hands. Rotate arms overhead behind trunk.

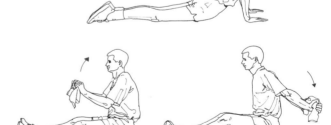

Exercise 3

Description: Clasp hands together behind trunk with elbows extended. Slowly raise arms upward.

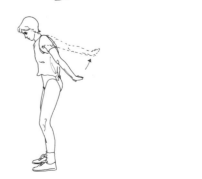

From Vivian H. Heyward, 2002, *Advanced Fitness Assessment and Exercise Prescription,* 4th ed. (Champaign, IL: Human Kinetics).

APPENDIX F.1

Exercise Do's and Don'ts

DON'T: Neck Hyperextension

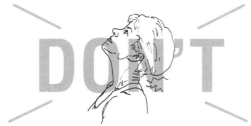

DO: Neck Lateral Flexion

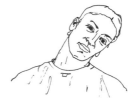

DON'T: Head Throws in a Crunch

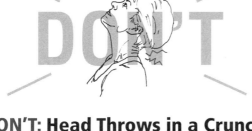

DO: Partial Sit-Up (see Appendix F.3, p. 344)

DON'T: Unsupported Hip/Trunk Flexion

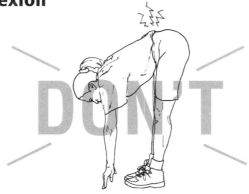

DO: Seated Hip/Trunk Flexion (see Appendix F.1, Exercise 4, p. 337)

DON'T: The Plow

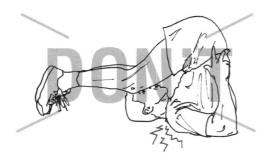

DO: Camel (see Appendix F.3, p. 344)

From Vivian H. Heyward, 2002, *Advanced Fitness Assessment and Exercise Prescription,* 4th ed. (Champaign, IL: Human Kinetics).

DON'T: Swan Lifts

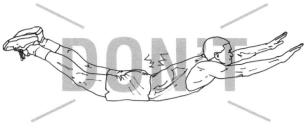

DO: Trunk Extensions

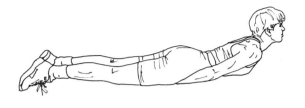

DON'T: V-Sits

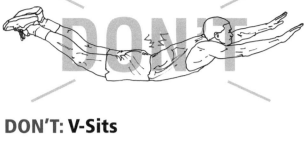

DO: Partial Sit-Up (see Appendix F.3, p. 344)

DON'T: Leg Lifts With Trunk Hyperextended

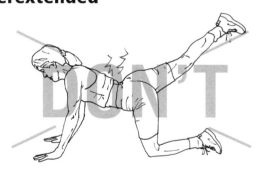

DO: Leg Lifts With Trunk and Leg in Straight Line

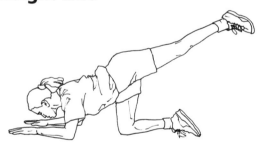

DON'T: Hamstring Stretch—Leg on Bar

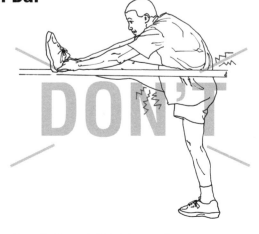

DO: Hamstring Stretch—Knee to Chest (see Appendix F.1, Exercise 5, p. 337)

From Vivian H. Heyward, 2002, *Advanced Fitness Assessment and Exercise Prescription,* 4th ed. (Champaign, IL: Human Kinetics).

APPENDIX F.2

DON'T: Hurdler's Stretch

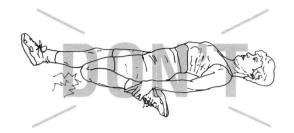

DON'T: Squats & Deep Knee Bends

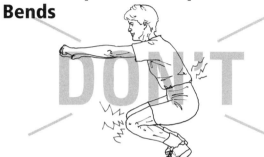

DON'T: Lunges (with knee forward of supporting foot)

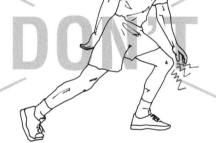

DON'T: Fast Twists & Jump Twists

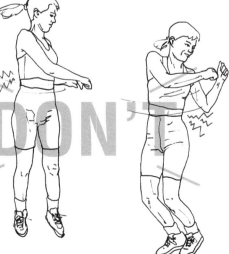

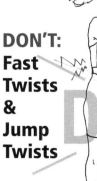

DO: Quad Stretch (see Appendix F.1, Exercise 2, p. 336)

DO: Half-Squats

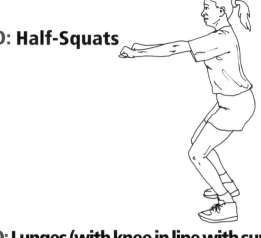

DO: Lunges (with knee in line with supporting heel)

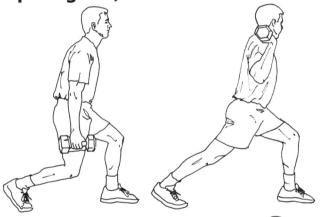

DO: Jump Without Twist

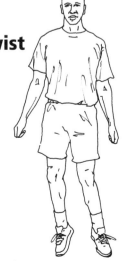

From Vivian H. Heyward, 2002, *Advanced Fitness Assessment and Exercise Prescription,* 4th ed. (Champaign, IL: Human Kinetics).

Exercises for Low Back Care

Pelvic Tilt (stretches abdominal muscles)
Lie on your back with knees bent, feet flat on the floor, and arms at your sides. Flatten the small of your back against the floor. (Your hips will tilt upward.) Hold.

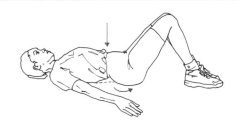

Double Knee to Chest (stretches hip, buttock, and lower back muscles)
Lie on your back with knees bent, feet flat on the floor, and arms at your sides. Raise both knees, one at a time, to your chest and hold with your hands. Lower your legs, one at a time, to the floor and rest briefly.

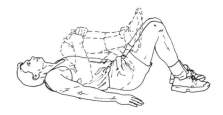

Trunk Flex (stretches back, abdominal, and leg muscles)
On your hands and knees, tuck in your chin and arch your back. Slowly sit back on your heels, letting your shoulders drop toward the floor. Hold.

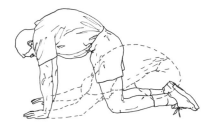

Cat and Camel (strengthens back and abdominal muscles)
On your hands and knees with your head parallel to the floor, arch your back and then let it slowly sag toward the floor. Try to keep your arms straight.

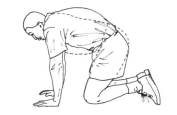

Partial Sit-Up (strengthens abdominal muscles)
Lie on your back with knees bent, feet flat on the floor, and arms crossed over your chest. Keeping your middle and lower back flat on the floor, raise your head and shoulders off the floor, and hold. Gradually increase your holding time.

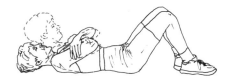

Single Leg Extension (strengthens hip and buttock muscles, and stretches abdominal and leg muscles)
Lie on your stomach with your arms folded under your chin. Slowly lift one leg—not too high—without bending it, while keeping your pelvis flat on the floor. Slowly lower your leg and repeat with the other leg.

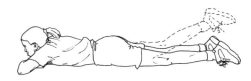

From Vivian H. Heyward, 2002, *Advanced Fitness Assessment and Exercise Prescription*, 4th ed. (Champaign, IL: Human Kinetics).

APPENDIX F.3

Single-Leg Extension Hold (strengthens the trunk extensors)

On your hands and knees with your head parallel to the floor, extend your thigh and leg and hold this position. Raising the contralateral arm simultaneously is more difficult and increases the extensor muscle activity and spinal compression.

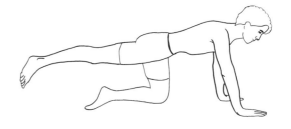

Curl-Up with Leg Extended (strengthens abdominal muscles)

Lie on your back with one knee flexed (foot flat on floor) and the other knee extended. Place your hands under the lumbar spine to preserve the neutral spine position. Slowly raise your head and shoulders off the floor.

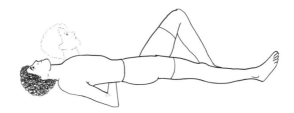

Isometric Side Support or Side Bridge (strengthens the lateral muscles of trunk and abdomen)

Assume a side support position with body supported by the knee, thigh, and forearm (flexed to 90°), and hold this position. Supporting the body with the feet, instead of the knee and thigh, increases the muscle activity and spinal load.

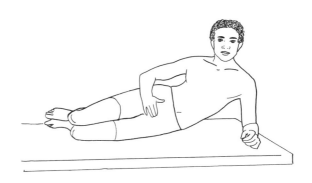

Notes

From Vivian H. Heyward, 2002, *Advanced Fitness Assessment and Exercise Prescription,* 4th ed. (Champaign, IL: Human Kinetics).

Rathbone Manual Tension Test

Purpose. This test was developed to assess neuromuscular tension in the wrist, elbow, shoulder, knee, hip, and neck joints at rest. Neuromuscular tension is measured during passive movement of the joints throughout the range of motion using a 4-point scale. 0 = no tension, 1 = slight tension, 2 = moderate tension, 3 = marked tension.

Tension Factors. Four tension factors are evaluated and scored:

1. *Assistance*—the client anticipated the movement and aids the tester in moving the body segment.
2. *Resistance*—the client resists the passive movement of the joint, limiting the range of motion or making the limb seem heavier than usual.
3. *Posturing*—the client maintains a static position against the pull of gravity when support of the limb by the tester is removed.
4. *Perseveration*—the client repeats the movement of the body segment after it is released by the tester.

Procedure

1. Tell the client to assume a relaxed, back-lying position on a padded table or mat and to be passive, allowing the tester to move the body segments.
2. To test each joint, support the client's body segment and passively rotate the body segment through the range of motion (e.g., flexion, extension, abduction, adduction, and circumduction of the shoulder joint) in a flowing, rhythmical manner.
3. Move the wrist, elbow, and shoulder joints while supporting the client's forearm and hand.
4. Move knee and hip joints while supporting the client's thigh and lower leg.
5. Move the neck by holding the client's head posterolaterally with both hands.
6. Use the 4-point scale to evaluate each tension factor for both right and left body segments. Record scores on the data sheet.

Data Sheet

Joint	Assistance R/L	Resistance R/L	Posturing R/L	Perseveration R/L
Wrist	_____	_____	_____	_____
Elbow	_____	_____	_____	_____
Shoulder	_____	_____	_____	_____
Knee	_____	_____	_____	_____
Hip	_____	_____	_____	_____
Neck	_____	_____	_____	_____
Total	_____	_____	_____	_____

Scoring

Score each joint movement for assistance, resistance, posturing, and perseveration on a 0 to 3 scale. Use the following hints for scoring:

Assistance—the client aids in lifting the limb.
Resistance—the client does not "let go," but offers opposition.

Posturing—when the limb is lifted and then released, it does not fall, but floats down or stays in the new position.
Perseveration—the client independently continues a motion.

_____

Adapted from Rathbone and Hunt (1965).

From Vivian H. Heyward, 2002, *Advanced Fitness Assessment and Exercise Prescription,* 4th ed. (Champaign, IL: Human Kinetics).

APPENDIX F.4

List of Abbreviations

Terms	
%BF	Relative body fat
AAHPERD	American Alliance for Health, Physical Education, Recreation and Dance
ACSM	American College of Sports Medicine
AI	Adequate intake
ATP	Adenosine triphosphate
AV	Atrioventricular
BIA	Bioelectrical impedance analysis
BM	Body mass
BMI	Body mass index
BMR	Basal metabolic rate
BP	Blood pressure
BSA	Body surface area
BV	Body volume
BW	Body weight
C	Circumference
CDC	Centers for Disease Control
CHD	Coronary heart disease
CP	Creatine phosphate
CRAC	Contract-relax with agonist contraction
CSA	Cross-sectional area
CSEP	Canadian Society for Exercise Physiology
CV	Cardiovascular
CVD	Cardiovascular disease
D	Distance
Db	Body density
DOMS	Delayed-onset muscle soreness
DXA	Dual-energy X-ray absorptiometry
ECG	Electrocardiogram
EMG	Electromyography
F	Force

Terms	
FFB	Fat-free body
FFM	Fat-free mass
FM	Fat mass
FRC	Functional residual lung capacity
GH	Growth hormone
GI	Glycemic index
GV	Volume of air in gastrointestinal tract
GXT	Graded exercise test
HDL-C	High-density lipoprotein cholesterol
HR	Heart rate
HRmax	Maximal heart rate
HRrest	Resting heart rate
HRA	Health risk appraisal
HRR	Heart rate reserve
HT	Standing height
HT^2/R	Resistance index
HW	Hydrostatic weighing
LDL-C	Low-density lipoprotein cholesterol
MET	Metabolic equivalent
MRI	Magnetic resonance imaging
MVC	Maximal voluntary contraction
N	Sample size
NCEP	National Cholesterol Education Program
NIDDM	Non-insulin-dependent diabetes mellitus
NIH	National Institutes of Health
NIR	Near-infrared interactance
P	Power output
p	Specific resistivity
PAR-Q	Physical Activity Readiness Questionnaire

Terms

PARmed-X	Physical Activity Readiness Medical Examination Questionnaire
PEI	Physical efficiency index
$\dot{Q}$	Cardiac output
R	Resistance for bioimpedance analysis
r	Pearson product-moment correlation
RDA	Recommended dietary allowance
rep	Repetition
RER	Respiratory exchange ratio
RM	Repetition maximum
R_{mc}	Multiple correlation coefficient
RMR	Resting metabolic rate
ROM	Range of motion
RPE	Rating of perceived exertion
RV	Residual lung volume
SEE	Standard error of estimate
SKF	Skinfold
SV	Stroke volume
TBW	Total body water
TC	Total cholesterol
TC/HDL-C	Ratio of total cholesterol to HDL-cholesterol
TLC	Total lung capacity
TLCNS	Total lung capacity, head not submerged
UWW	Underwater weighing
VC	Vital capacity
$\dot{V}O_2$	Volume of oxygen consumed per minute
$\dot{V}O_2max$	Maximal oxygen uptake
$\dot{V}O_2R$	Oxygen uptake reserve
WHR	Waist-to-hip ratio
X_c	Reactance
YMCA	Young Men's Christian Association
Z	Impedance
ΣSKF	Sum of skinfolds

Units of Measure

bpm	beats per minute
C	Celsius
cc	cubic centimeter
cm	centimeter
dl	deciliter
F	Fahrenheit
ft-lb	foot-pound
g	gram
hr	hour
in.	inch
kcal	kilocalorie
kg	kilogram
kgm	kilogram-meter
km	kilometer
L	liter
lb	pound
m	meter
meq	milli-equivalent
mg	milligram
min	minute
ml	milliliter
mm	millimeter
mm Hg	millimeters of mercury
mph	miles per hour
Nm	newton-meter
rpm	revolutions per minute
sec	second
W	watt
wk	week
yr	year
μg	microgram
μg RE	retinol equivalent
Ω	ohm

Glossary

absolute $\dot{V}O_2$—Measure of rate of oxygen consumption and energy cost of non-weight-bearing activities; measured in L/min or ml/min.

accommodating-resistance exercise—Type of exercise in which fluctuations in muscle force throughout the range of motion are matched by an equal counterforce as the speed of limb movement is kept at a constant velocity; isokinetic exercise.

acquired immune deficiency syndrome (AIDS)—Disease characterized as a deficiency in the body's immune system, caused by human immunodeficiency virus (HIV).

acute-onset muscle soreness—Soreness or pain occurring during or immediately after exercise; caused by ischemia and accumulation of metabolic waste products in the muscle.

air displacement plethysmography—Densitometric method to estimate body volume using air displacement and pressure-volume relationships.

alarm reaction stage—First stage of stress reaction in which the body perceives the stress and activates the fight-or-flight response.

android obesity—Type of obesity in which excess body fat is localized in the upper body; upper-body obesity; apple-shaped body.

aneurysm—Dilation of a blood vessel wall causing a weakness in the vessel's wall; usually caused by atherosclerosis and hypertension.

angina pectoris—Chest pain.

ankylosis—Limited range of motion at a joint.

anorexia nervosa—Eating disorder characterized by excessive weight loss.

anthropometry—Measurement of body size and proportions including skinfold thicknesses, circumferences, bony widths and lengths, stature, and body weight.

aortic stenosis—Narrowing of the aortic valve that obstructs blood flow from the left ventricle into the aorta.

Archimedes' principle—Principle stating that weight loss underwater is directly proportional to the volume of water displaced by the body's volume.

arrhythmia—Abnormal heart rhythm.

arteriosclerosis—Hardening of the arteries, or thickening and loss of elasticity in the artery walls, that obstruct blood flow; caused by deposits of fat, cholesterol, and other substances.

assistance—In manual tension testing, a measure of how much the client aids the tester in moving the body segment.

asthma—Respiratory disorder characterized by difficulty in breathing and wheezing due to constricted bronchi.

ataxia—Impaired ability to coordinate movement characterized by staggering gait or postural imbalance.

atherosclerosis—Buildup and deposition of fat and fibrous plaque in the inner walls of the coronary arteries.

atrial fibrillation—Cardiac dysrhythmia in which the atria quiver instead of pumping in an organized fashion.

atrial flutter—Type of atrial tachycardia in which the atria contract at rates of 230 to 380 bpm.

atrophy—A wasting or decrease in size of a body part.

augmented unipolar leads—Three ECG leads (aVF, aVL, aVR) that compare voltage across each limb lead to the average voltage across the two opposite electrodes.

auscultation—Method used to measure heart rate or blood pressure by listening to heart and blood sounds.

autogenic relaxation—Series of mental exercises used to elicit a relaxation response.

ballistic stretching—Type of stretching exercise that uses a fast bouncing motion to produce stretch and increase range of motion.

basal metabolic rate (BMR)—Measure of minimal amount of energy needed to maintain basic and essential physiological functions.

behavior modification theory—Psychological theory of change; clients become actively involved with the change process by setting short- and long-term goals.

biaxial joint—Joint allowing movement in two planes; condyloid and saddle joints.

bioelectrical impedance analysis (BIA)—Field method for estimating the total body water or fat-free mass using measures of impedance to current flowing through the body.

biofeedback—Use of visual and auditory signals to control unconscious bodily functions.

body composition—A component of physical fitness; absolute and relative amounts of muscle, bone, and fat tissues composing body mass.

body density (Db)—Overall density of fat, water, mineral, and protein components of the human body; total body mass expressed relative to total body volume.

body mass (BM)—Measure of the size of the body; body weight.

body mass index (BMI)—Crude index of obesity; body mass (kg) divided by height squared (m^2).

body volume (BV)—Measure of body size estimated by water or air displacement.

body weight (BW)—Mass or size of the body; body mass.

bone strength—Function of mineral content and density of bone tissue; related to risk of bone fracture.

bradycardia—Resting heart rate <60 bpm.

bronchitis—Acute or chronic inflammation of the bronchi of lungs.

caloric threshold—Method to estimate duration of exercise based on the caloric cost of the exercise and to estimate the total amount of exercise needed per week for health benefits.

cardiac arrest—Sudden loss of heart function usually caused by ventricular fibrillation.

cardiomyopathy—Any disease that affects the structure and function of the heart.

cardiorespiratory endurance—Ability of heart, lungs, and circulatory system to supply oxygen to working muscles efficiently.

cardiovascular disease—Disease of the heart and/ or blood vessels; types of cardiovascular disease include atherosclerosis, hypertension, coronary heart disease, congestive heart failure, and stroke.

chest leads—Six ECG leads (V_1 to V_6) used to measure voltage across specific areas of the chest.

cirrhosis—Chronic, degenerative disease of the liver in which the lobes are covered with fibrous tissue; associated with chronic alcohol abuse.

claudication—Cramp-like pain in the calves due to poor circulation to leg muscle.

compound sets—Advanced resistance training system in which two sets of exercises for the same muscle group are performed consecutively, with little or no rest between sets.

concentric contraction—Type of dynamic muscle contraction in which muscle shortens as it exerts tension.

congestive heart failure—Impaired cardiac pumping caused by myocardial infarction, ischemic heart disease, or cardiomyopathy.

constant-resistance exercise—Type of exercise in which the external resistance remains the same throughout the range of motion (e.g., lifting free weights or dumbbells).

continuous training—One continuous, aerobic exercise bout performed at low-to-moderate intensity.

contract-relax agonist contract (CRAC) technique—Type of proprioceptive neuromuscular facilitation technique in which the target muscle is isometrically contracted and then stretched; stretching is assisted by a submaximal contraction of the agonistic muscle group.

contract-relax (CR) technique—Type of proprioceptive neuromuscular facilitation technique in which the target muscle is isometrically contracted and then stretched.

contracture—Shortening of resting muscle length caused by disuse or immobilization.

coronary heart disease—Disease of the heart caused by a lack of blood flow to heart muscle, resulting from atherosclerosis.

criterion method—Gold standard or reference method; typically a direct measure of a component used to validate other tests.

cross training—Type of training in which the client participates in a variety of exercise modes to develop one or more components of physical fitness.

cyanosis—Bluish discoloration of skin caused by lack of oxygenated hemoglobin in the blood.

delayed-onset muscle soreness (DOMS)—Soreness in the muscle occurring 24 to 48 hr after exercise.

densitometry—Measurement of total body density; hydrodensitometry and air displacement plethysmography are densitometry methods.

diabetes—Complex disorder of carbohydrate, fat, and protein metabolism resulting from a lack of insulin secretion (type 1) or defective insulin receptors (type 2).

diastolic blood pressure (DBP)—Lowest pressure in the artery during the cardiac cycle.

diminishing return principle—Training principle; as genetic ceiling is approached, rate of improvement slows or evens off.

discontinuous training—Several intermittent, low- to high-intensity aerobic exercise bouts interspersed with rest or relief intervals.

dual-energy X-ray absorptiometry (DXA)—Method used to measure total body bone mineral density, bone mineral content, fat, and lean soft-tissue mass.

dynamic contraction—Type of muscle contraction producing visible joint movement; concentric, eccentric, or isokinetic contraction.

dynamic flexibility—Measure of the rate of torque or resistance developed during stretching throughout the range of joint motion.

dyslipidemia—Abnormal blood lipid profile.

dyspnea—Shortness of breath or difficulty breathing caused by certain heart conditions, anxiety, or strenuous exercise.

eccentric contraction—Type of muscle contraction in which the muscle lengthens as it produces tension to resist gravity or decelerate a moving body segment.

edema—Accumulation of interstitial fluid in tissues such as pericardial sac and joint capsules.

elastic deformation—Deformation of the muscle-tendon unit that is proportional to the load or force applied during stretching.

electrocardiogram (ECG)—A composite record of the electrical events in the heart during the cardiac cycle.

electromyography (EMG)—Method used to measure muscle activity during rest and exercise.

embolism—Piece of tissue or thrombus that circulates in the blood until it lodges in a vessel.

emphysema—Pulmonary disease causing damage in alveoli and loss of lung elasticity.

exercise-induced hypertrophy—Increase in size of muscle as a result of resistance training.

exhaustive stage—Final stage of stress response in which the body loses its ability to combat stressors; characterized by illness or death.

fat-free body (FFB)—All residual, lipid-free chemicals and tissues in the body, including muscle, water, bone, connective tissue, and internal organs.

fat-free mass (FFM)—See fat-free body; weight or mass of the fat-free body.

fat mass (FM)—All extractable lipids from adipose and other tissues in the body.

flexibility—Ability to move joints fluidly through complete range of motion without injury.

flexometer—Device for measuring range of joint motion using a weighted 360° dial and pointer.

generalized prediction equations—Prediction equations that are applicable to a diverse, heterogeneous group of individuals.

glucose intolerance—Inability of body to metabolize glucose.

glycemic index (GI)—Rating of the body's glycemic response to a food compared to the reference value (GI = 100 for white bread or glucose).

goniometer—Protractor-like device used to measure joint angle at the extremes of the range of motion.

graded exercise test (GXT)—A multistage submaximal or maximal exercise test requiring the client to exercise at gradually increasing workloads; may be continuous or discontinuous; used to estimate $\dot{V}O_2max$.

Graves disease—Disease associated with an overactive thyroid gland that secretes greater-than-normal amounts of thyroid hormones; also known as hyperthyroidism or thyrotoxicosis.

gross $\dot{V}O_2$—Total rate of oxygen consumption, reflecting the caloric cost of both rest and exercise.

group I aerobic activities—Aerobic exercise modalities that provide constant intensity and are not skill dependent.

group II aerobic activities—Aerobic exercise modalities that provide constant or variable intensity, depending on skill.

group III aerobic activities—Aerobic exercise modalities that provide variable intensity and are highly skill dependent.

gynoid obesity—Type of obesity in which excess fat is localized in the lower body; lower-body obesity; pear-shaped body.

HDL-cholesterol (HDL-C)—Cholesterol transported in the blood by high-density lipoproteins.

healthy body weight—Body mass index from 18.5 to 25 kg/m^2.

heart block—Interference in the normal conduction of electrical impulses that control normal contraction of the heart muscle; may occur at sinoatrial node, atrioventricular node, bundle of HIS, or at combination of these sites.

heart rate reserve (HRR)—Maximal heart rate minus the resting heart rate.

hepatitis—Inflammation of the liver characterized by jaundice and gastrointestinal discomfort.

high CHD risk—One or more signs/symptoms of cardiovascular and pulmonary disease; or characterizing individuals with known cardiovascular, pulmonary, or metabolic disease.

high intensity-low repetitions—Optimal training stimulus for strength development; 85% to 100% 1-RM or 1- to 6-RM.

hydrodensitometry—Method used to estimate body volume by measuring weight loss when the body is fully submerged; underwater weighing.

hydrostatic weighing (HW)—See hydrodensitometry.

hypercholesterolemia—Excess of total cholesterol and/or LDL-cholesterol in blood.

hyperlipidemia—Excess lipids in blood.

hypermobility—Excessive range of motion at a joint.

hyperplasia—Increase in number of cells.

hypertension—High blood pressure; chronic elevation of blood pressure.

hyperthyroidism—Overactive thyroid gland that secretes greater-than-normal amounts of thyroid hormones; also known as thyrotoxicosis or Graves disease.

hypertrophy—Increase in size of cells.

hypoglycemia—Low blood glucose level.

hypokalemia—Inadequate amount of potassium in the blood characterized by an abnormal ECG, weakness, and flaccid paralysis.

hypomagnesemia—Inadequate amount of magnesium in the blood resulting in nausea, vomiting, muscle weakness, and tremors.

hypothyroidism—Underactive thyroid gland that secretes lower-than-normal amounts of thyroid hormones; also known as myxedema.

hypoxia—Inadequate oxygen at the cellular level.

imagery—Form of autosuggestion or self-hypnosis that uses visual images to produce a relaxed state.

impedance (Z)—Measure of total amount of opposition to electrical current flowing through the body; function of resistance and reactance.

improvement stage—Stage of exercise program in which client improves most rapidly; frequency, intensity, duration are systematically increased; usually lasting 16 to 20 weeks.

inclinometer—Gravity-dependent goniometer used to measure the angle between the long axis of the moving segment and the line of gravity.

initial conditioning stage—Stage of exercise program used as primer to familiarize client with exercise training; usually lasting four weeks.

initial values principle—Training principle; the lower the initial value of a component, the greater the relative gain and the faster the rate of improvement in that component; the higher the initial value, the slower the improvement rate.

interindividual variability principle—Training principle; individual responses to training stimulus are variable and depend on age, initial fitness level, and health status.

interval training—A repeated series of exercise work bouts interspersed with rest or relief periods.

ischemia—Decreased supply of oxygenated blood to body part or organ.

ischemic heart disease—Pathologic condition of the myocardium caused by lack of oxygen to the heart muscle.

isokinetic contraction—Maximal contraction of a muscle group at a constant velocity throughout entire range of motion.

isometric contraction—Type of muscle contraction in which there is no visible joint movement; static contraction.

isotonic contraction—Type of muscle contraction producing visible joint movement; dynamic contraction.

joint laxity—Looseness or instability of a joint, increasing risk of musculoskeletal injury.

Karvonen method—Method to prescribe exercise intensity as a percentage of the heart rate reserve added to the resting heart rate; percent heart rate reserve method.

kilocalorie (kcal)—Amount of heat needed to raise the temperature of 1 kg of water 1 °C; measure of energy need and expenditure.

LDL-cholesterol (LDL-C)—Cholesterol transported in the blood by low-density lipoproteins.

limb leads—Three ECG leads (I, II, III) measuring the voltage differential between left and right arms (I) and between the left leg and right (II) and left (III) arms.

line of best fit—Regression line depicting relationship between reference measure and predictor variables in an equation.

low back pain—Pain produced by muscular weakness or imbalance resulting from lack of physical activity.

low CHD risk—Characterizing younger individuals (men <45 years and women <55 years) who are asymptomatic and have no more than one risk factor.

lower-body obesity—Type of obesity in which excess body fat is localized in the lower body; gynoid obesity; pear-shaped body.

low intensity-high repetitions—Optimal training stimulus for development of muscular endurance; ≤60% 1-RM or 15- to 20-RM.

lumbar stabilization—Maintaining a static position of the lumbar spine by isometrically co-contracting the abdominal wall and low back muscles during exercise.

macrocycle—Phase of periodized resistance training program usually lasting one year.

maintenance stage—Stage of exercise program designed to maintain level of fitness achieved by end of improvement stage; should be continued on a regular, long-term basis.

manual tension test—Test used to assess degree of muscular tension during passive movement of the limbs.

maximal exercise test—Graded exercise test in which exercise intensity increases gradually until the $\dot{V}O_2$ plateaus or fails to rise with a further increase in workload.

maximum oxygen uptake ($\dot{V}O_2$max)—Maximum rate of oxygen utilization of muscles during aerobic exercise.

McArdle's syndrome—Inherited metabolic disease characterized by inability to metabolize muscle glycogen, resulting in excessive amounts of glycogen stored in skeletal muscles.

mesocycles—Parts of a macrocycle of a periodized resistance training program in which training volume progressively decreases as training intensity increases throughout the program.

moderate CHD risk—Characterizing older individuals (men ≥45 years and women ≥55 years), or individuals of any age having two or more risk factors.

multicomponent model—Body composition model that takes into account interindividual variations in water, protein, and mineral content of the fat-free body.

multimodal exercise program—Type of exercise program that uses a variety of aerobic exercise modalities.

multiple correlation coefficient (R_{mc})—Correlation between reference measure and predictor variables in a prediction equation.

murmur—Low-pitched fluttering or humming sound.

muscle balance—Ratio of strength between opposing muscle groups, contralateral muscle groups, and upper- and lower-body muscle groups.

muscular endurance—Ability of muscle to maintain submaximal force levels for extended periods.

muscular strength—Maximal force or tension level produced by a muscle or muscle group.

musculoskeletal fitness—Ability of skeletal and muscular systems to perform work.

myocardial infarction—Heart attack.

myocardial ischemia—Lack of blood flow to the coronary arteries.

myocarditis—Inflammation of the heart muscle caused by viral, bacterial, or fungal infection.

myxedema—Disease associated with an underactive thyroid gland that secretes lower-than-normal amounts of thyroid hormones; also known as hypothyroidism.

near-infrared interactance (NIR)—Field method that estimates %BF based on optical density of tissues at the measurement site; presently, validity of this method is questionable.

negative energy balance—Excess of energy expenditure in relation to energy intake.

net $\dot{V}O_2$—Rate of oxygen consumption in excess of the resting $\dot{V}O_2$; used to describe the caloric cost of exercise.

neuromuscular relaxation—Ability to reduce or eliminate unnecessary tension or contraction in a muscle group.

nonaxial joint—Type of joint allowing only gliding, sliding, or twisting rather than movement about an axis of rotation; gliding joint.

obesity—Excessive amount of body fat relative to body mass; BMI of 30 kg/m² or more.

objectivity—Intertester reliability; ability of test to yield similar scores for given individual when same test is administered by different technicians.

objectivity coefficient—Correlation between pairs of test scores measured on same individuals by two different technicians.

occlusion—Blockage of blood flow to body part or organ.

omnikinetic exercise—Type of accommodating-resistance exercise that adjusts for fluctuations in both muscle force and speed of joint rotation throughout range of motion.

one-repetition maximum (1-RM)—Maximal weight that can be lifted for one complete repetition of a movement.

osteoarthritis—Degenerative disease of the joints characterized by excessive amounts of bone and cartilage in the joint.

osteoporosis—Disorder characterized by low bone mineral and bone density; occurring most frequently in postmenopausal women and sedentary individuals.

overload principle—Training principle; physiological systems must be taxed beyond normal to stimulate improvement.

overweight—BMI between 25 to 29.9 kg/m².

pallor—Unnatural paleness or absence of skin color.

palpation—Method used to measure heart rate by feeling the pulse at specific anatomical sites.

palpitations—Racing or pounding of the heart.

peak $\dot{V}O_2$—Measure of highest rate of oxygen consumption when GXT is terminated before a plateau in $\dot{V}O_2$ is reached.

pelvic stabilization—Maintaining a static position of the pelvis while performing exercises for the low back extensor muscles.

percent body fat (%BF)—Fat mass expressed relative to body mass; relative body fat.

percent heart rate maximum (%HRmax)—Method used to prescribe exercise intensity as a percentage of the measured or age-predicted maximum heart rate.

percent heart rate reserve (%HRR)—Method used to prescribe exercise intensity as a percentage of the heart rate reserve (HRR = HRmax – HRrest) added to the resting heart rate; Karvonen method.

percent $\dot{V}O_2$reserve (%$\dot{V}O_2$R)—Method used to prescribe exercise intensity as a percentage of $\dot{V}O_2$reserve ($\dot{V}O_2$R = $\dot{V}O_2$max – $\dot{V}O_2$rest) added to the resting $\dot{V}O_2$.

pericarditis—Inflammation of the pericardium caused by trauma, infection, uremia, or heart attack.

periodization—Advanced form of training that systematically varies the volume and intensity of the training exercises.

perseveration—In manual tension testing, a measure of how much the client continues to move or repeats the movement of the body segment after it is released by the tester.

physical fitness—Ability to perform occupational, recreational, and daily activities without undue fatigue.

population-specific equations—Prediction equations intended only for use with individuals from a specific homogenous group.

positive energy balance—Excess of energy intake in relation to energy expenditure.

posturing—In manual tension testing, a measure of whether the client maintains the position of the limb after it is released by the tester.

PR interval—Part of ECG tracing that indicates delay in the impulse at the atrioventricular node.

progression principle—Training principle; training volume must be progressively increased to overload and stimulate further improvements.

progressive relaxation—Technique used to reduce muscular tension through conscious contraction and relaxation of muscle groups.

proprioceptive neuromuscular facilitation (PNF)—Mode of stretching designed to increase range of joint motion through spinal reflex mechanisms such as reciprocal inhibition.

prosthesis—An artificial replacement of a missing body part, such as an artificial limb or joint.

pulse pressure—Difference between the systolic and diastolic blood pressures.

P wave—Part of ECG tracing that reflects depolarization of the atria.

pyramiding—Advanced resistance training system in which a relatively light weight is lifted in the first set and progressively heavier weights are lifted in subsequent sets; light-to-heavy system.

QRS complex—Part of ECG tracing reflecting ventricular depolarization and contraction.

range of motion—Degree of movement at a joint; measure of static flexibility.

rating of perceived exertion (RPE)—A scale used to measure a client's subjective rating of exercise intensity.

reactance (X_c)—Measure of opposition to electrical current flowing through body due to the capacitance of cell membranes; a vector of impedance.

readiness for change theory—Psychological theory of behavior change; ability to make long-term behavioral change is based on client's emotional and intellectual readiness; stages of readiness are precontemplation, contemplation, preparation, action, and maintenance.

reference method—Gold standard or criterion method; typically a direct measure of a component used to validate other tests.

regression line—Line of best fit depicting relationship between reference measure and predictor variables.

relative body fat (%BF)—Fat mass expressed as a percentage of total body mass; percent body fat.

relative strength—Muscular strength expressed relative to the body mass or lean body mass; 1-RM/BM.

relative $\dot{V}O_2$—Rate of oxygen consumption expressed relative to the body mass or lean body mass; measured in $ml \cdot kg^{-1} \cdot min^{-1}$.

reliability—Ability of test to yield consistent and stable scores across trials and over time.

reliability coefficient—Correlation depicting relationship between trial 1 and trial 2 scores or day 1 and day 2 scores of a test.

repetition maximum (RM)—Measure of intensity for resistance exercise expressed as maximum weight that can be lifted for a given number of repetitions.

repetitions—Number of times a specific exercise movement is performed in a set.

residual volume (RV)—Volume of air remaining in lungs following a maximal expiration.

resistance—In manual muscle testing, a measure of how much the client resists the passive movement of a body segment.

resistance (R)—Measure of pure opposition to electrical current flowing through body; a vector of impedance.

resistance and adaptation stage—Second stage of stress reaction in which body continues to counteract and adapt to the stressor.

resistance index (ht^2/R)—Predictor variable in some BIA regression equations that is calculated by dividing standing height squared by resistance.

respiratory exchange ratio (RER)—Ratio of expired CO_2 to inspired O_2.

resting metabolic rate (RMR)—Energy required to maintain essential physiological processes in a relaxed, awake, and reclined state.

reversibility principle—Training principle; physiological gains from training are lost when individual stops training (detraining).

rheumatic heart disease—Condition in which the heart valves are damaged by rheumatic fever, contracted from a streptococcal infection (strep throat).

rheumatoid arthritis—Chronic, destructive disease of the joints characterized by inflammation and thickening of the synovial membranes and swelling of the joints.

self-efficacy—Individuals' perception of their ability to perform a task and their confidence in making a specific behavioral change.

set—Defines the number of times a specific number of repetitions of a given exercise is repeated; single or multiple sets.

skinfold—Measure of the thickness of two layers of skin and the underlying subcutaneous fat.

social cognitive theory—Psychological theory of behavior change; based on concepts of self-efficacy and outcome expectation.

specificity principle—Training principle; physiological and metabolic responses and adaptations to exercise training are specific to type of exercise and muscle groups involved.

sphygmomanometer—Device used to measure blood pressure manually, consisting of a blood pressure cuff and a manometer.

split routine—Advanced resistance training system in which different muscle groups are targeted on consecutive days to avoid overtraining.

standard error of estimate *(SEE)*—Measure of error for prediction equation; quantifies the average deviation of individual data points around the line of best fit.

static contraction—Type of muscle contraction in which there is no visible joint movement; isometric contraction.

static flexibility—Measure of the total range of motion at a joint.

static stretching—Mode of exercise used to increase range of motion by placing the joint at the end of its range of motion and slowly applying torque to the muscle to stretch it further.

stress relaxation—Decreased tension within musculotendinous unit when it is held at a fixed length during static stretching.

stress response—Generalized physiological response of the body to physical, psychological, or environmental demands.

stroke—Rupture or blockage of blood flow to the brain caused by a blood clot or some other particle.

ST segment—Part of ECG tracing reflecting ventricular repolarization; used to detect coronary occlusion and myocardial infarct.

submaximal exercise test—Graded exercise test in which exercise is terminated at some predetermined submaximal heart rate or workload; used to estimate $\dot{V}O_2max$.

super circuit resistance training—Type of circuit resistance training that intersperses a short, aerobic exercise bout between each resistance training exercise station.

supersetting—Advanced resistance training system in which exercises for agonistic and antagonistic muscle groups are done consecutively without rest.

syncope—Brief lapse in consciousness caused by lack of oxygen to the brain.

systolic blood pressure (SBP)—Highest pressure in the arteries during systole of the heart.

tachycardia—Resting heart rate >100 bpm.

thrombophlebitis—Inflammation of a vein often accompanied by formation of a blood clot.

thrombus—Lump of cellular elements of the blood attached to inner walls of an artery or vein, sometimes blocking blood flow through the vessel.

thyrotoxicosis—Overactive thyroid gland that secretes greater-than-normal amounts of thyroid hormones; also known as Graves disease or hyperthyroidism.

total cholesterol (TC)—Absolute amount of cholesterol in the blood.

training volume—Total amount of training as determined by the number of sets and exercises for a muscle group, intensity, and frequency of training.

Treading™—Type of group-led interval training that involves walking, jogging, and running at various speeds and grades on a treadmill with relief intervals interspersed.

triaxial joint—Type of joint allowing movement in three planes; ball-and-socket joint.

tri-sets—Advanced resistance training system in which three different exercises for the same muscle group are performed consecutively with little or no rest between the exercises.

T wave—Part of ECG tracing corresponding to ventricular repolarization.

two-component model—Body composition model that divides the body into fat and fat-free body components.

type 1 diabetes—Insulin-dependent diabetes caused by lack of insulin production by the pancreas.

type 2 diabetes—Non-insulin-dependent diabetes caused by decreased insulin receptor sensitivity.

type A behavior—Personality type characterized by speed, impatience, competitiveness, hard-driving behavior, and aggressiveness.

type B behavior—Personality type characterized by a relaxed and easygoing nature.

underwater weighing—Method used to estimate body volume by measuring weight loss when the body is fully submerged; hydrostatic weighing.

underweight—BMI <18.5 kg/m².

uniaxial joint—Type of joint allowing movement in one plane; hinge or pivot joint.

upper-body obesity—Type of obesity in which excess fat is localized to the upper body; android obesity; apple-shaped body.

uremia—Excessive amounts of urea and other nitrogen waste products in the blood associated with kidney failure.

validity—Ability of a test to accurately measure, with minimal error, a specific component.

validity coefficient—Correlation between reference measure and predicted scores.

valvular heart disease—Congenital disorder of a heart valve characterized by obstructed blood flow, valvular degeneration, and regurgitation of blood.

variable-resistance exercise—Type of exercise in which resistance changes during the range of motion due to levers, pulleys, and cams.

ventricular ectopy—Premature (out of sequence) contraction of the ventricles.

ventricular fibrillation—Cardiac dysrhythmia marked by rapid, uncoordinated, and unsynchronized contractions of the ventricles, so that no blood is pumped by the heart.

vertigo—Dizziness or inability to maintain normal balance in a standing or seated position.

viscoelastic properties—Tension within the muscle-tendon unit caused by the elastic and viscous deformation of the unit when force is applied during stretching.

viscous deformation—Deformation of the muscle-tendon unit that is proportional to the speed at which tension is applied during stretching.

$\dot{V}O_2max$—Maximum rate of oxygen utilization of muscles during exercise.

$\dot{V}O_2reserve$—The $\dot{V}O_2max$ minus the $\dot{V}O_2rest$.

waist-to-hip ratio (WHR)—Waist circumference divided by hip circumference; used as a measure of upper-body or abdominal obesity.

Index

Note: Tables are indicated by an italicized t following the page number; figures by an italicized f.

About the Author

Vivian H. Heyward, PhD, is a Regents professor emerita at the University of New Mexico, where she has taught physical fitness assessment and exercise prescription courses for more than 25 years. Extensively published, Dr. Heyward is the author of three previous editions of *Advanced Fitness Assessment and Exercise Prescription* as well as *Applied Body Composition Assessment*. She also has written more than 60 articles in research and professional journals dealing with various aspects of physical fitness assessment and exercise prescription. Dr. Heyward has given numerous presentations at international, national, and regional meetings of professional organizations in the field. The American College of Sports Medicine named her a fellow in 1997. Her hobbies include weightlifting, rock hounding, and woodcarving.

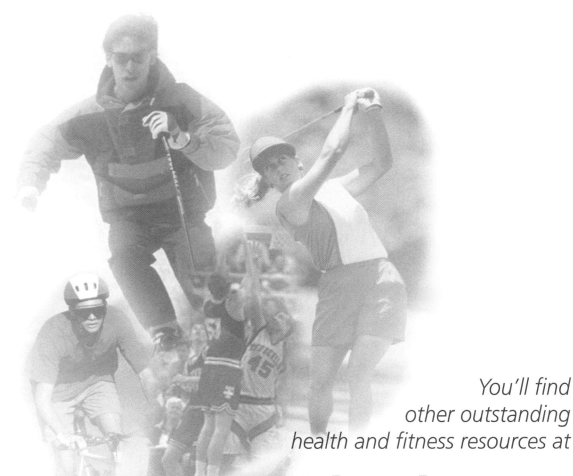